Days of our Lives
BETTER LIVING

CAST SECRETS FOR A HEALTHIER, BALANCED LIFE

GREG MENG & EDDIE CAMPBELL

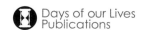
Days of our Lives
Publications

Published by Sourcebooks, Inc.
P.O. Box 4410, Naperville, Illinois 60567-4410
(630) 961-3900
Fax: (630) 961-2168
www.sourcebooks.com

Library of Congress Cataloging-in-Publication Data

Meng, Greg.
  Days of our lives better living / Greg Meng and Eddie Campbell.
      pages cm
  Includes index.
  1. Days of our lives (Television program) 2. Reducing diets—Recipes. 3. Motion picture actors and actresses—Health and hygiene. I. Campbell, Eddie II. Title. III. Title: Better living.

RM222.2.M4573 2013
641.5'63—dc23

2012038439
Printed and bound in China.

LEO 10 9 8 7 6 5 4 3 2 1

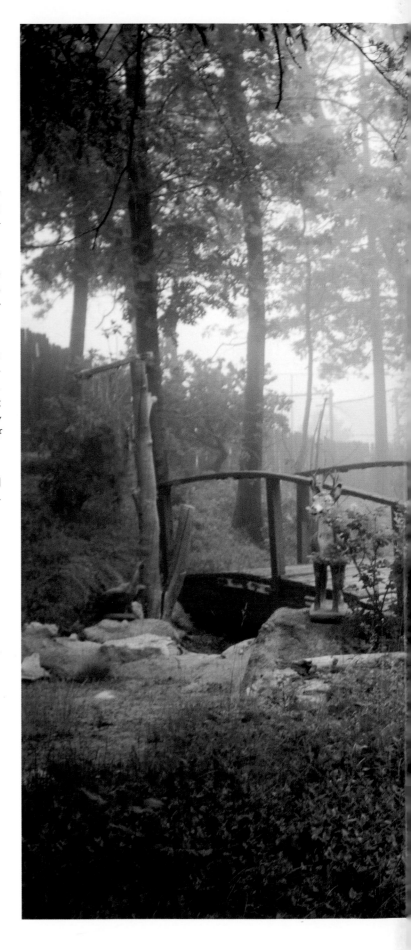

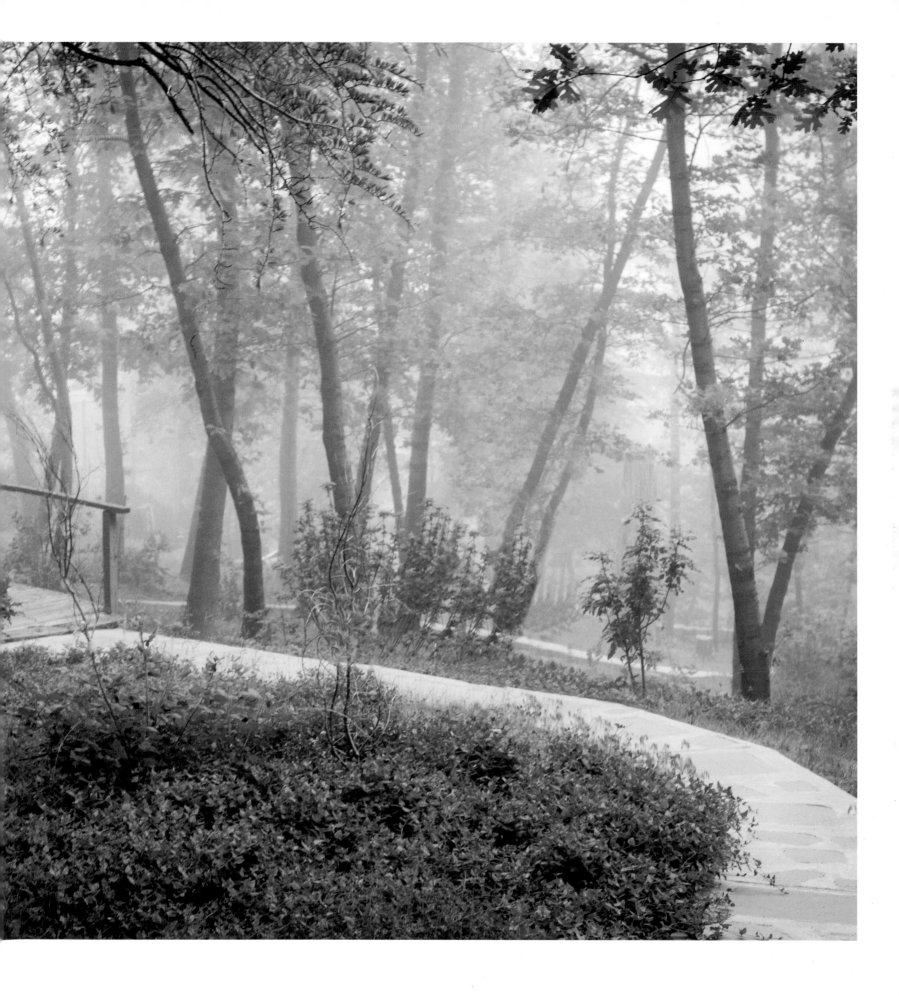

To Ken Corday,
who keeps the sands flowing
through the hourglass.

Days of our Lives
BETTER LIVING

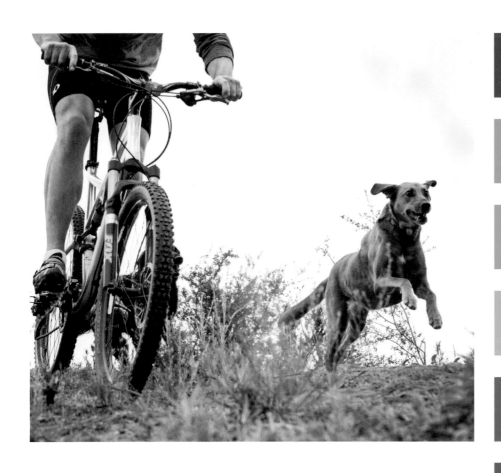

GREG MENG
& EDDIE CAMPBELL

INTRODUCTION

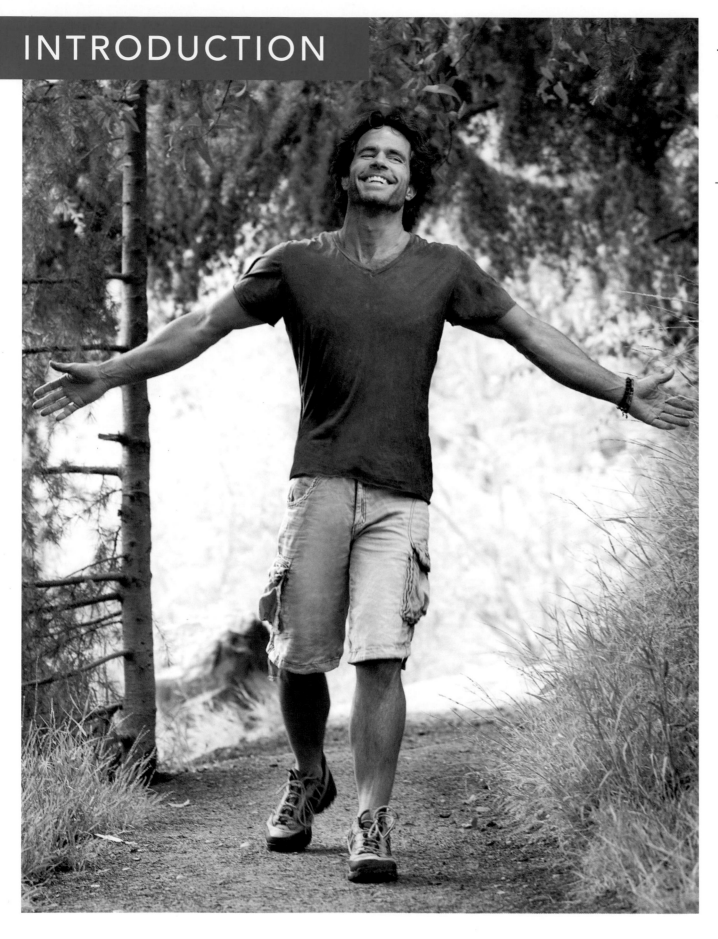

The way you live your life is reflected in the way you portray your character.
—*Betty Corday*

MILLIONS OF FANS IN MORE THAN 20 COUNTRIES have come to love and admire the characters on *Days of our Lives*, which has been airing on NBC since November 8, 1965. In fact, many fans have grown so close to these characters, as they are portrayed by the talented cast, that they view them as if they were members of their own family! It wasn't until several of us spent time with our cast members, traveling around the country promoting the *Days of our Lives 45 Years: A Celebration in Photos* book, that we grew to know some of them on a personal level. We began to discover that they are multidimensional individuals, each involved in some other fascinating endeavor. They not only have lives beyond acting on *Days*, but they have a wide variety of interests, worthy goals and important causes that inspire them. These actors continue to face the same hurdles and challenges we all meet as we strive to attain our own goals. However, we found that they are genuinely happy, fulfilled individuals. We became intrigued as to how they achieve that. What are their secrets to being not only physically attractive, but well-rounded and happy, too? And wouldn't this be valuable information to share with others?

After an interview with magazine editor Michael Maloney, it occurred to me that we could use his help in uncovering these "secrets" from the cast. He had interviewed most of them before, so I knew they would be comfortable talking with him. Michael loved the idea, so we created a list of categories for him to use as he formulated questions for each cast member. He went home and started making phone calls. These interviews and meetings continued for months.

As coauthor Eddie Campbell and I started compiling the information, it became clear that many cast members share quite a few of the same traits. We noticed that a pattern was developing. None of the cast members are on extreme diets or attempting impossible exercise routines. Their approach to style is wearing clothes that are comfortable, affordable and practical. None of them are living a crazy, glamorous, "Hollywood" lifestyle. And as they strive to attain their goals, each one of them is either involved in some type of charitable organization or somehow finding a way to help others.

Each of the actors in this book has succeeded in creating his or her own unique lifestyle, yet they share many of the same qualities. They have learned how to nurture and maintain their bodies and minds as they search for their inner values. So, here is their secret: it's about balance. They have found a realistic approach to balancing the way they live in the following five categories, each of which we have created as a chapter for this book:

NUTRITION, EXERCISE, STYLE, INSPIRATION and BALANCE.

Come build a better, happier and balanced life for yourself with *Days of our Lives*.

Greg Meng
Executive in Charge of Production
Days of our Lives

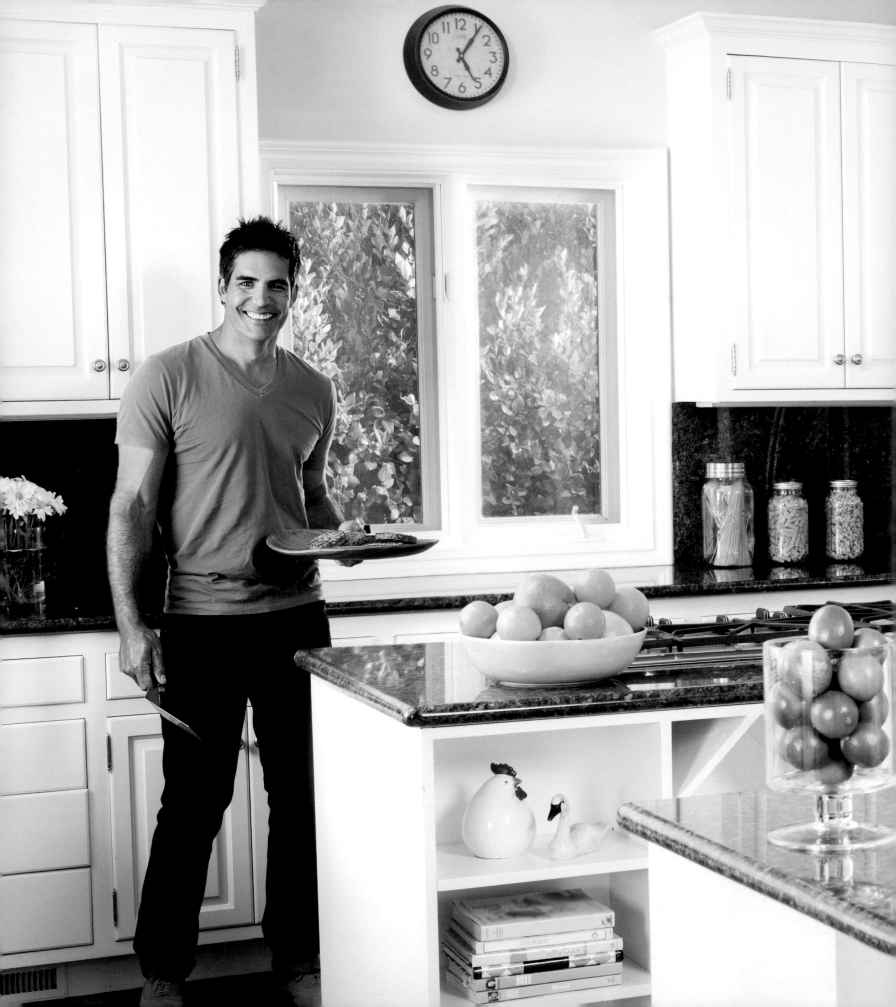

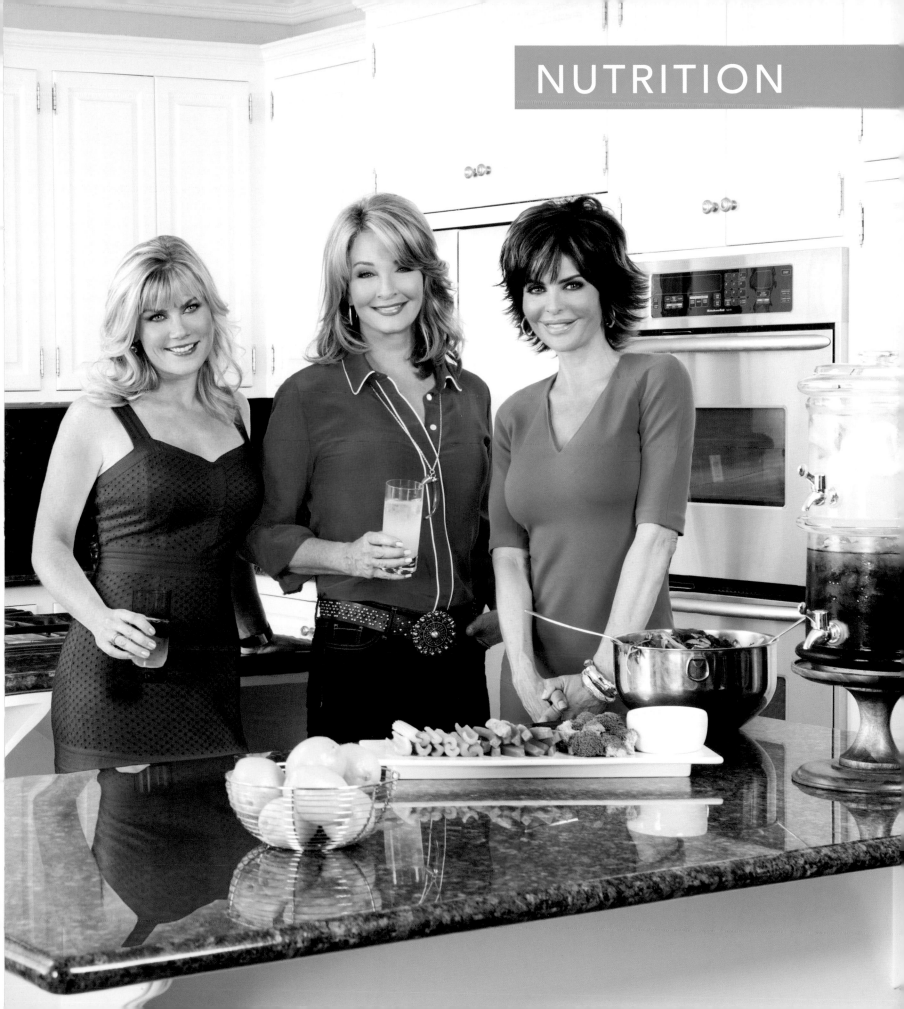

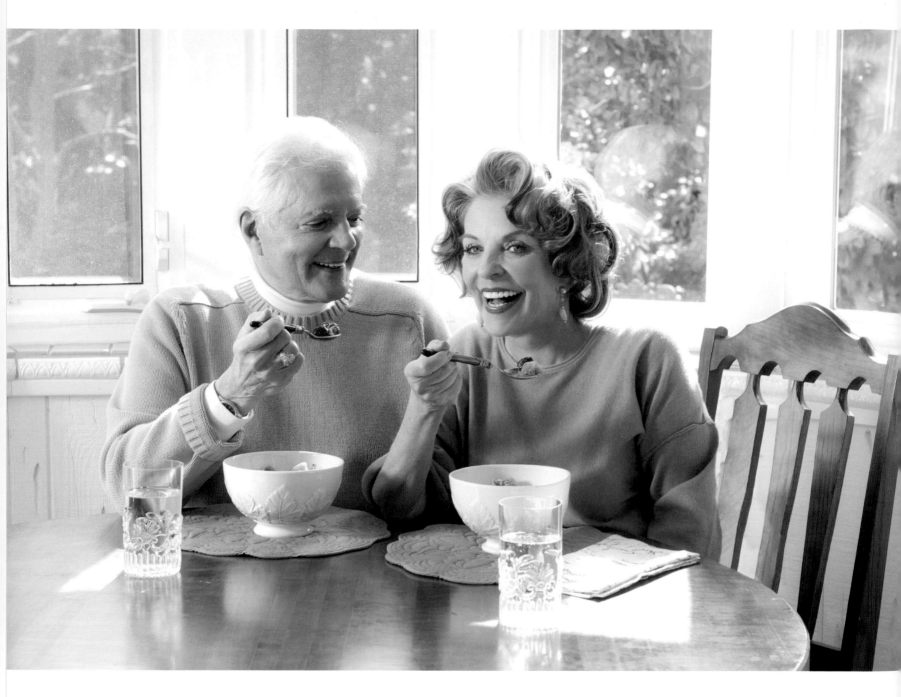

"Breakfast is the meal that Bill enjoys the most—he can eat heartily and right away," says Susan. "I have a hard time doing that but the first thing I do when I'm out of bed in the morning is to make sure he gets his breakfast.

"I spend a lot of time thinking about the meals (like yogurt for breakfast) and

preparing them. I'm proud of the fact that we're still pretty active and I think a lot of it has to do with good nutrition."

"Susan doesn't go for yogurt as much as I do," Bill notes. "But we enjoy a good bowl of yogurt about twice a week. We both love fresh fruit."

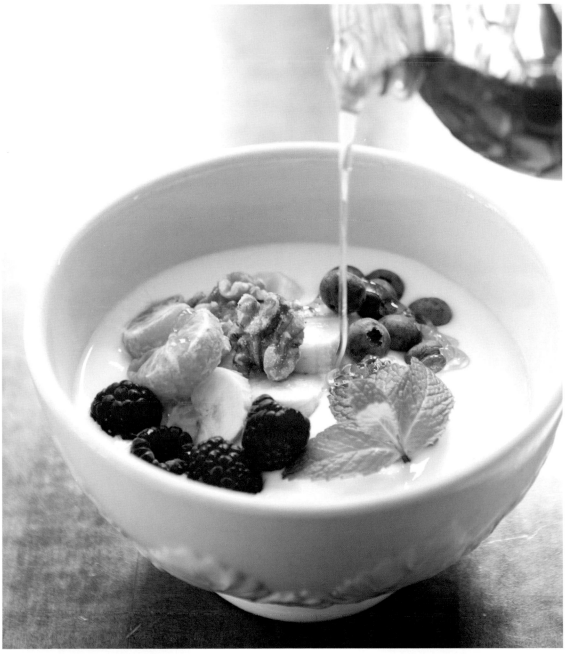

MORNING BOOST

By Bill and Susan Hayes

Start your day off on the fast track with a mixture of yogurt and super foods like walnuts and berries.

INGREDIENTS:

12 ounces 0% fat Greek yogurt
1 cup raspberries
1 cup blueberries
¾ cup walnuts
½ sliced banana
Mint leaf (not just for decoration but good for digestion)

*You do not have to use the same fruits and nuts each morning. Mix it up. Or top with a touch of organic, sugar-free honey.

METHOD:

Combine ingredients in a bowl and enjoy!

SERVES: 2

Approximate nutritional analysis per serving: 487.3 calories, 26.29 grams of protein, 38.3 grams of carbohydrates, 29.34 grams of fat, 9.55 grams of fiber and 67.25 milligrams of sodium.

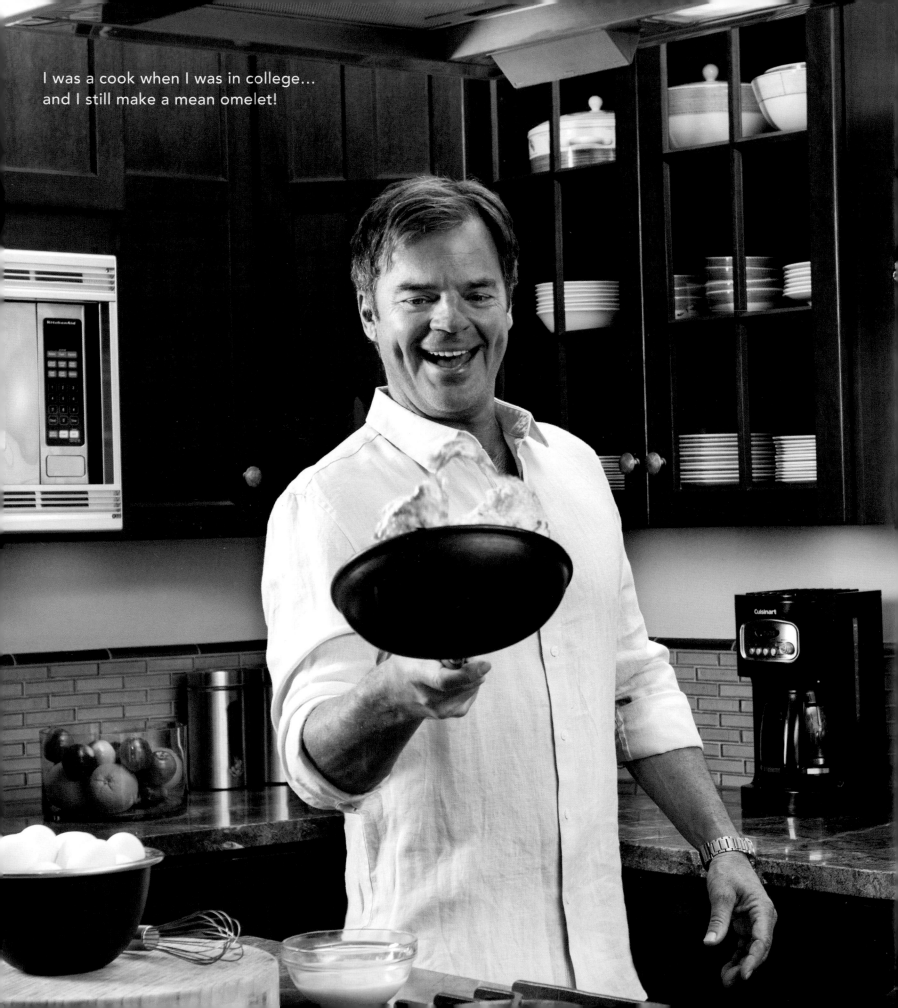

I was a cook when I was in college...
and I still make a mean omelet!

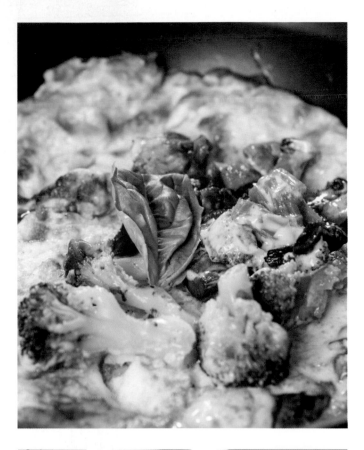

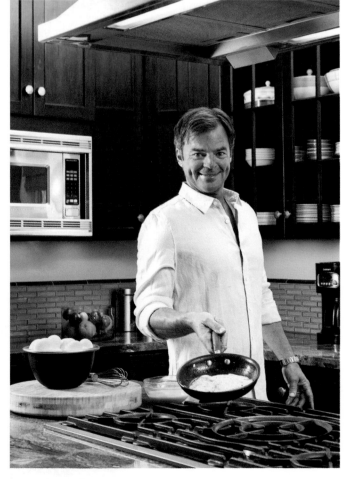

VEGETABLE OMELET

By Wally Kurth

Ready…set…veggie omelet. Let's go!

INGREDIENTS:

2 tablespoons extra-virgin olive oil
½ small onion, chopped (optional)
1 green bell pepper, chopped
2 large eggs
2 large egg whites
Freshly ground black pepper to taste
½ ounce shredded Swiss cheese (or cheese of your choosing)

METHOD:

1. Heat 1 tablespoon oil in a medium skillet over medium heat. Place onion and bell pepper in skillet. Cook for 4 to 5 minutes, stirring occasionally until vegetables are just tender. While the vegetables are cooking, blend and beat the whole eggs and egg whites, and add pepper. Shred the cheese into a small bowl and set it aside. Remove the vegetables from heat, transfer them to another bowl and sprinkle additional pepper as desired.

2. Over medium heat add 1 tablespoon oil (in the skillet just used to cook the vegetables). When skillet is ready, add egg mixture and cook the eggs for 2 minutes or until the eggs begin to set on the bottom of the pan. Gently lift the edges of the omelet with a spatula to let the uncooked part of the eggs flow toward the edges and cook. Continue cooking for 2 to 3 minutes or until the center of the omelet starts to look dry.

3. Sprinkle the cheese over the omelet and spoon the vegetable mixture into the center of the omelet. Using a spatula gently fold one edge of the omelet over the vegetables. Let the omelet cook for another 2 minutes or until the cheese melts to your desired consistency. Slide the omelet out of the skillet and onto a plate.

SERVES: 1

Approximate nutritional analysis per serving: 548 calories, 25.9 grams of protein, 17.44 grams of carbohydrates, 41 grams of fat, 4.2 grams of fiber and 270 milligrams of sodium.

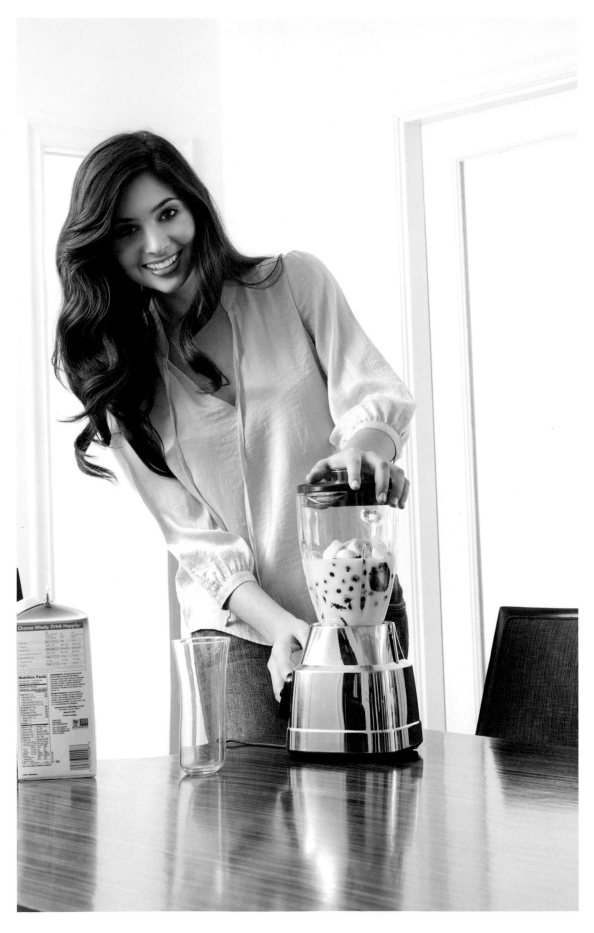

I try to make smoothies at home so I know exactly what's going into them. I'll have a smoothie maybe once or twice a week. I enjoy drinking juices. I'd rather have a glass of juice than a full plate of food. I try to vary it. I add protein to my juices. There are just so many things. I add goji berries to my drinks. Chi seeds are good, too. I don't usually have milk shakes. I really like sour smoothies more than sweet ones so I'll have citrus in them.

I'll go to Jamba Juice and have a Caribbean Passion. That has passion fruit sorbet, orange juice and peaches. It's kind of tart. Check out the calorie count—that's why I go to the gym. I come out dripping. But I'd rather have a smoothie than a burger any day.

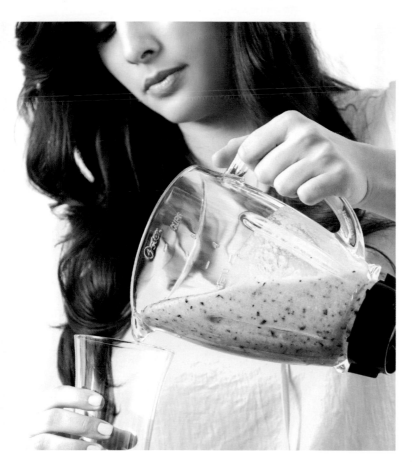

BERRY BANANA SHAKE
By Camila Banus

With 5 ingredients and easy blending you are enjoying a smoothie—delicious!

INGREDIENTS:
1 cup blueberries (fresh or frozen)
1 cup strawberries (fresh or frozen)
½ medium banana
1 cup soy milk (skim, hemp or other
 alternatives)
1 scoop vanilla whey protein powder*
1 cup crushed ice (optional)

METHOD:
Blend all ingredients together until the desired consistency is reached. Add water as needed.

*Choose a protein powder that has no more than 7 grams of total carbohydrates and 15 to 30 grams of protein per serving.

SERVES: 1

Approximate nutritional analysis per serving: 384.5 calories, 33.25 grams of protein, 59.1 grams of carbohydrates, 9.7 grams of fat, 10 grams of fiber and 204 milligrams of sodium.

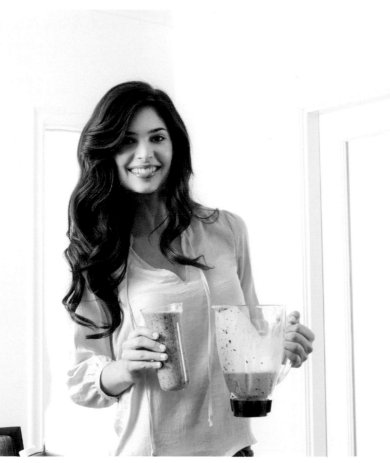

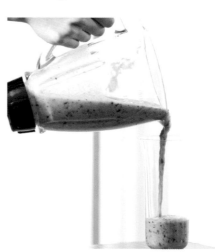

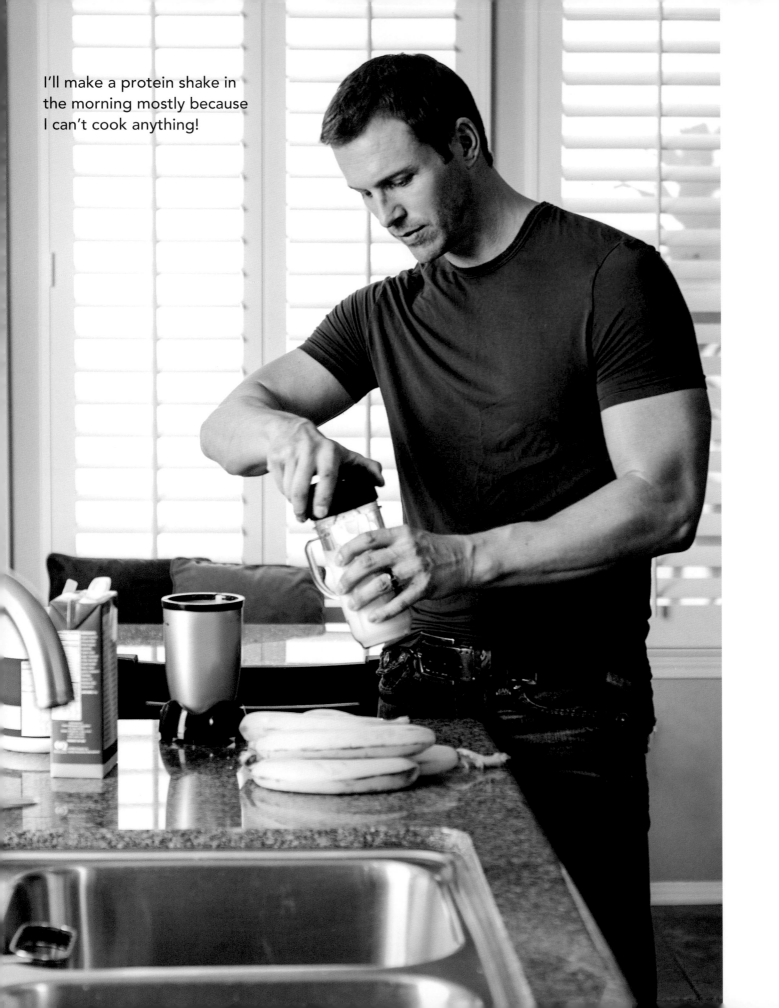

I'll make a protein shake in the morning mostly because I can't cook anything!

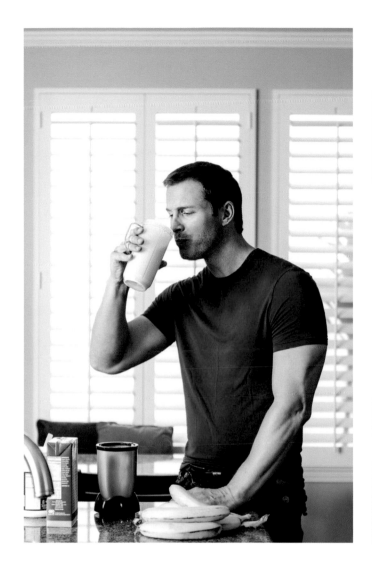
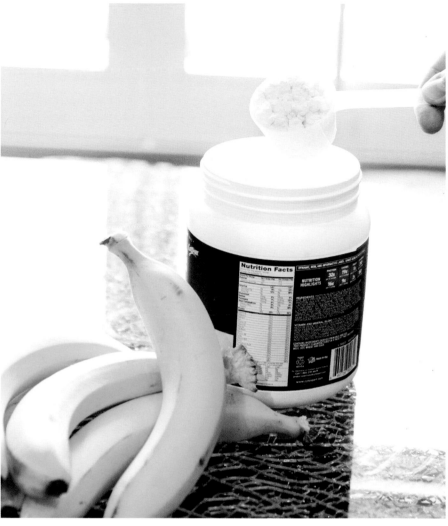

PROTEIN ON-THE-GO SHAKE

By Eric Martsolf

Get satiated and energized with a boost of protein, milk of your choice and ripe banana!

INGREDIENTS:

*1 cup of soy milk (skim, hemp or other
   alternatives)*
1 scoop vanilla whey protein powder*
1 banana (ripe)
½ cup crushed ice (optional)

METHOD:

Blend all ingredients together until the
desired consistency is reached. Add water
as needed.

*Choose a protein powder that has no more
than 7 grams of total carbohydrates and 15 to
30 grams of protein per serving.

SERVES: 1

Approximate nutritional analysis per serving: 405
calories, 44.29 grams of protein, 46.94 grams of
carbohydrates, 8.39 grams of fat, 4.1 grams of fiber
and 279 milligrams of sodium.

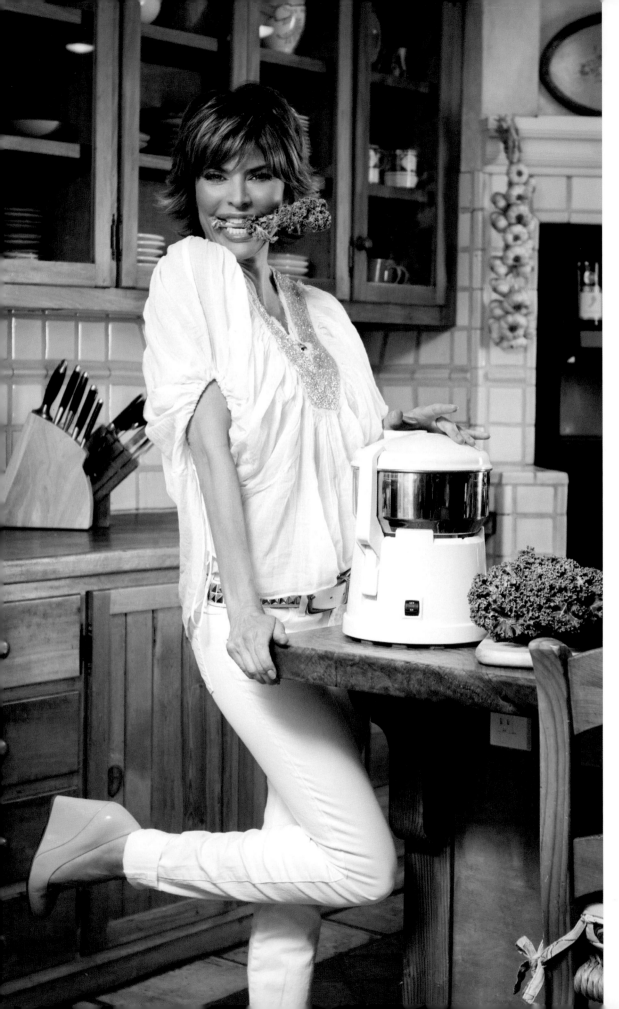

I am doing a gluten-free diet. We found out my daughter, Delilah, has a gluten intolerance. She and I were having the same kind of stomach problems. I decided to do the gluten-free diet with her and it has made us both feel so much better. I've always eaten healthy. It's all about moderation. I certainly eat a cookie if I want a cookie. But now that I'm eating gluten-free, all my stomach issues are gone. And so are Delilah's. I think that's pretty fantastic. I feel so good and I have much more energy.

We're going to continue the gluten-free diet.

There's an app about gluten-free foods for your iPhone. There's so much gluten-free food now that it's so easy to be gluten-free. It forces you to eat more organically and to eat less processed food.

When time is of the essence and you want to keep your metabolism on the fast track, give this smoothie a try. Packed with veggie protein, fiber and healthy fat—in minutes you can enjoy a delicious and nutritious smoothie!

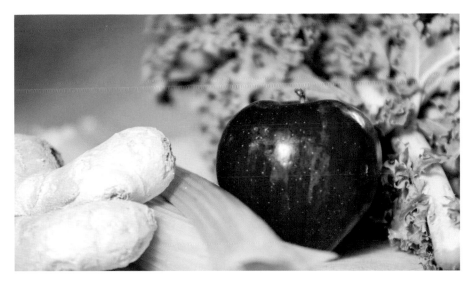

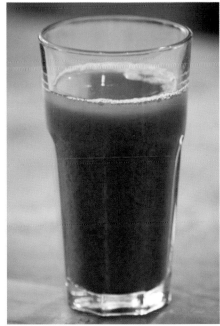

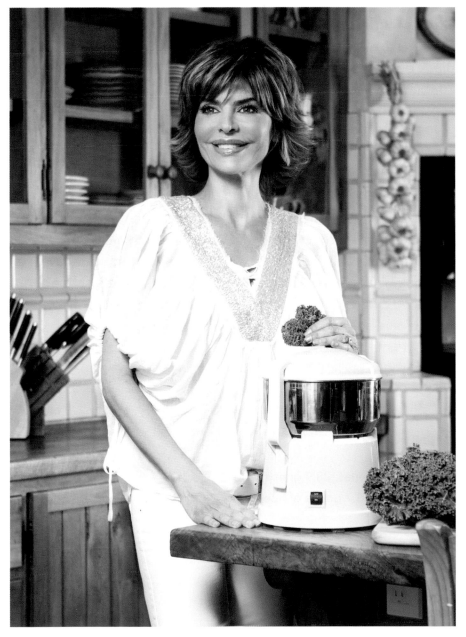

THE BRAZILIAN BOMBSHELL SMOOTHIE

By Lisa Rinna

INGREDIENTS:

½ cup organic apple juice
½ cup green tea
3 stalks organic kale leaves
1 handful fresh organic spinach leaves
1 sprig parsley
½ medium-size avocado
¼ teaspoon cinnamon
Chunk ginger
Ice

METHOD:

Blend all ingredients together until the desired consistency is reached. Add water as needed.

SERVES: 1

Approximate nutritional analysis per serving: 323 calories, 9.1 grams of protein, 44.4 grams of carbohydrates, 18.1 grams of fat, 11.4 grams of fiber and 107 milligrams of sodium.

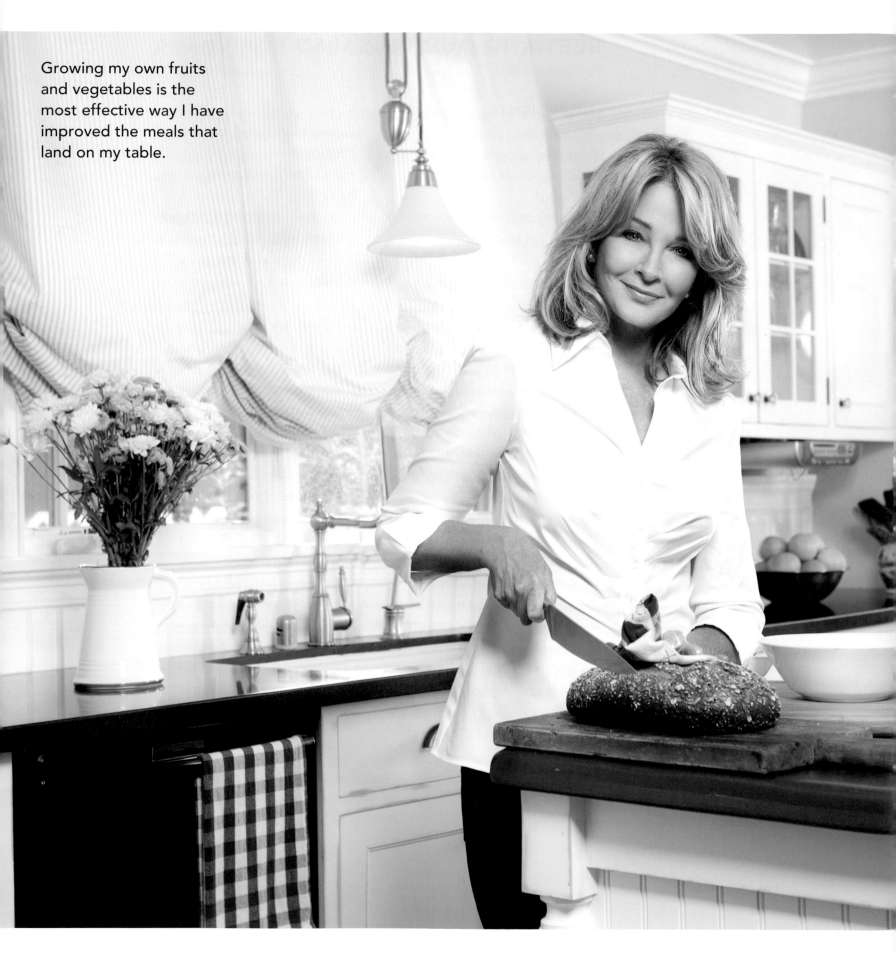

Growing my own fruits and vegetables is the most effective way I have improved the meals that land on my table.

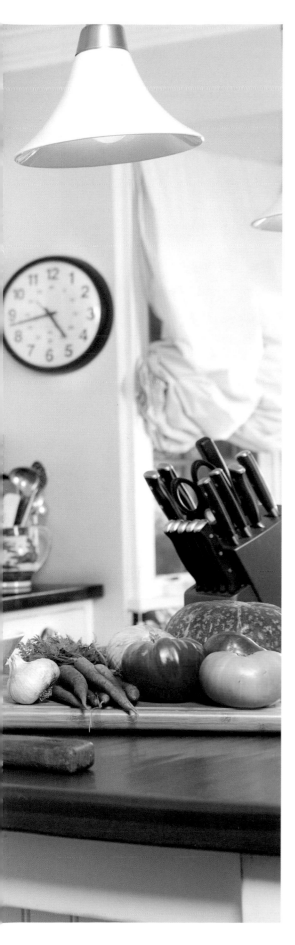

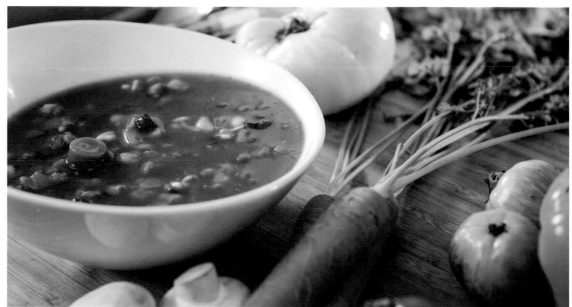

RED PEPPER SOUP

By Deidre Hall

INGREDIENTS:

1 medium onion, chopped
1 tablespoon butter
2 red peppers, cubed
1 garlic clove
1 large carrot or zucchini, chopped
1 cup chicken or vegetable broth, low sodium
Fresh black pepper to taste
¼ cup feta cheese
Yogurt for garnish (optional)

METHOD:

1. Sauté the onion in butter.
2. Add the red pepper, garlic, carrot and broth to the pan. Cook until the vegetables are tender.
3. Combine all ingredients in the blender with pepper and a bit of feta until it's creamy (about 30 seconds).
4. Dish up in pretty bowls and garnish with a dab of yogurt.

SERVES: 1

Approximate nutritional analysis per serving: 300 calories, 13.2 grams of protein, 34 grams of carbohydrates, 13.8 grams of fat, 9.1 grams of fiber and 1107 milligrams of sodium.

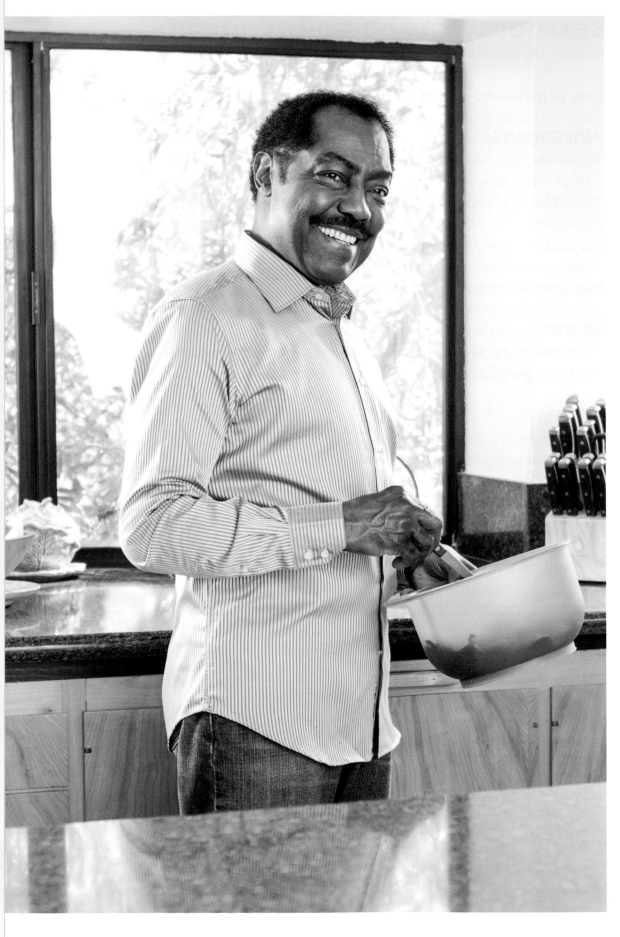

I enjoy cooking. One of my favorite recipes is crab cakes.

That's one of the meals I make. I love crab cakes. I've learned about good crab cakes over time. Crab cakes are great. They're wonderful. I don't usually bread them although most people do. I make enough to last a few days.

I find different foods from different countries to be interesting. Whatever area I'm in or visiting I try to take part in the food there—when I'm in Kansas, I'll go to barbeque places, for example.

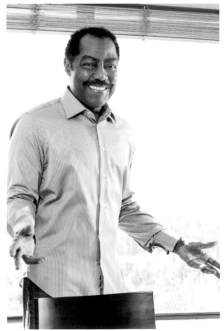

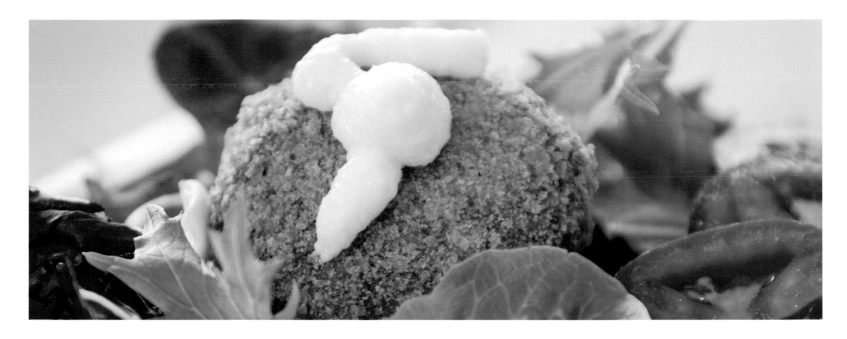

REYNOLDS'S CRAB CAKES

By James Reynolds

Engaging and talk-about-able crab cakes with lots of flavor!

INGREDIENTS:

4 large eggs
⅓ cup chopped celery
⅓ cup chopped carrots
8 ounces shredded lump crab
2 tablespoons minced garlic
2 tablespoons mustard

2 tablespoons reduced-fat
  mayonnaise
Seasoned black pepper
  to taste
4 tablespoons extra-virgin
  olive oil

METHOD:

1. Beat eggs in mixing bowl. Add celery, carrots and crab. Mix in garlic, mustard, mayonnaise and pepper to taste. Set aside.
2. Heat oil in a large skillet over medium heat.
3. Spoon crab mixture, about 5 tablespoons, on the skillet until it forms one cake. You may have to push egg run-off back onto the cake while they cook. Avoid this by using a spoon with holes to let the excess egg drip back into mixing bowl. Keep heat at medium. Sauté crab cakes, turning once, until golden brown, about 3 minutes per side. Transfer to a paper towel–lined plate. Serve immediately.

BREADING TIP: To bread your crab cakes there are two additional steps. First, whisk 3 large eggs in a small bowl in which you will dip each crab cake. Second, in another bowl, place 2 cups bread crumbs and dip the egg-covered crab cake before placing in skillet.

SERVES: 8

Approximate nutritional analysis per serving: 126.8 calories, 8.3 grams of protein, 2.4 grams of carbohydrates, 9.5 grams of fat, .5 grams of fiber and 347.5 milligrams of sodium.

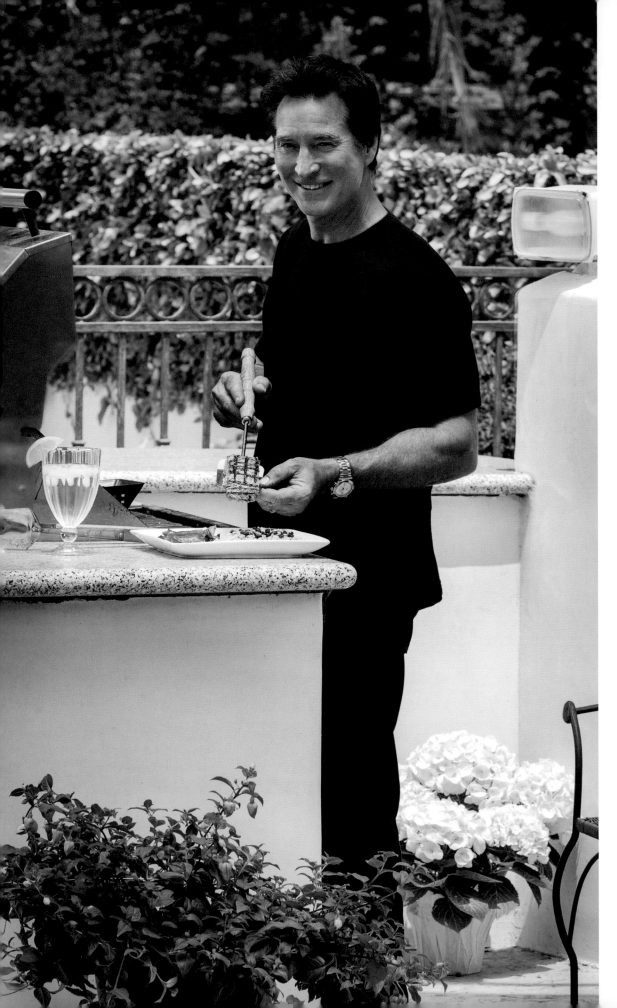

For dinner, I will have a salmon steak, grilled red and yellow peppers and black beans and brown rice. You have to have colorful fruits and vegetables. I get my protein and essential fats from the salmon, fibrous carbohydrates from the peppers and starch from the rice and beans.

I try to avoid pasta. I retain water from pasta and I become puffy. It is important to eat clean, healthy foods.

I try not to eat anything that is processed. The more you process food the more you break down all the natural elements.

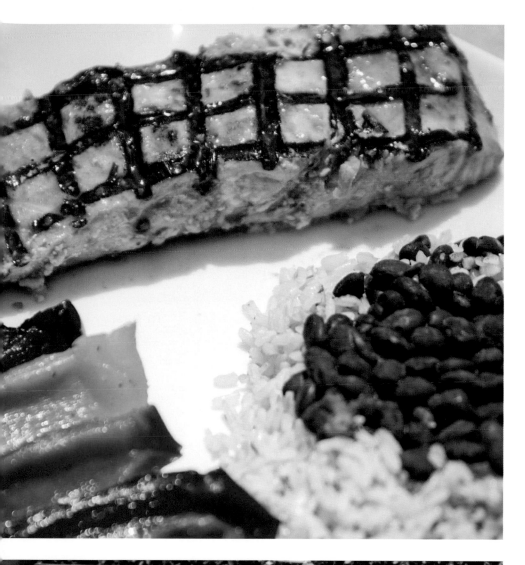

GRILLED SIZZLING SALMON
By Drake Hogestyn

Here's a simple marinade with hints of lemon and garlic to complement rich salmon fillets.

INGREDIENTS:
4 (5-ounce) wild salmon fillets
Lemon pepper as desired
Garlic powder as desired
¼ cup soy sauce
¼ cup natural brown sugar
¼ cup extra-virgin olive oil
Freshly squeezed lemon juice as desired

METHOD:
1. Season salmon fillets with lemon pepper and garlic powder.
2. In a small bowl, stir together soy sauce, brown sugar and olive oil until sugar is dissolved.
3. Place fish in a large re-sealable plastic bag with the mixture from the bowl, seal and turn to coat. Refrigerate for at least 2 hours.
4. Preheat grill to medium heat.
5. Lightly oil grill grate. Place salmon on the preheated grill, and discard marinade. Sprinkle lemon pepper and garlic powder as desired. Cook salmon for 6 to 8 minutes per side, or until the fish flakes easily with a fork. Sprinkle lemon juice over fillets when done and serve!

RECOMMENDATION: Serve with grilled asparagus and some colorful peppers. Also goes well with a side of black beans and brown rice and topped with feta cheese.

SERVES: 4

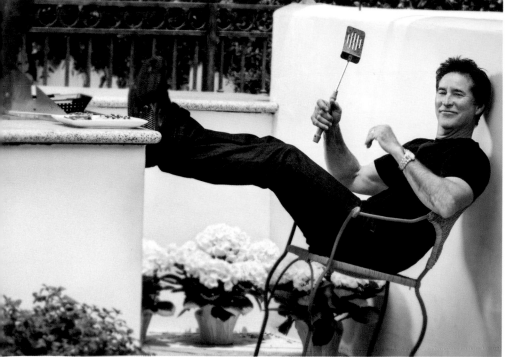

Approximate nutritional analysis per serving: 422 calories, 32 grams of protein, 19 grams of carbohydrates, 30 grams of fat, .2 grams of fiber and 1026 milligrams of sodium.

SPICY TUNA ROLL

By Chandler Massey

Take the flavors of your favorite sushi bar home with these homemade spicy tuna rolls.

INGREDIENTS:

½ pound sushi/sashimi grade tuna (maguro)
1 tablespoon mayonnaise
½ teaspoon ichimi-togarashi* (ground dried red chili pepper)
4 sheets nori (dried seaweed)
6 cups prepared sushi rice (brown optional)
1 tablespoon white sesame seeds

*adjust the amount to your preference.

METHOD:

1. Chop sashimi/sushi grade tuna and mix with mayonnaise and ichimi-togarashi. Put a nori sheet on top of a bamboo mat. Spread a quarter portion of sushi rice on top of the nori sheet. Sprinkle sesame seed on top of the sushi rice.
2. Place a quarter portion of tuna mixture lengthwise on the rice. Roll up the bamboo mat, pressing forward to shape the sushi into a cylinder. Press the bamboo mat firmly and remove it from the sushi. Make more rolls. Wipe a knife with a wet cloth before slicing sushi. Cut the rolled sushi into bite-size pieces.

SERVES: 20

Approximate nutritional analysis per serving: 229.5 calories, 10.1 grams of protein, 46.7 grams of carbohydrates, 1.8 grams of fat, 2.1 grams of fiber and 10.6 milligrams of sodium.

TURKEY LOAF

By Josh Taylor

The ease of meatloaf without the calories is what you get with this recipe!

INGREDIENTS:

2 one-pound packages lean ground turkey
1 green bell pepper, chopped
2 large whole eggs
2 pieces whole grain wheat nugget bread (cut in small pieces)
1 package dried onion soup mix
¾ cup water
⅓ cup ketchup

METHOD:

Preheat oven to 400°F. Mix all ingredients together in bowl and put in a loaf pan. After it browns (about 30 minutes) turn down heat to 300°F for 30 minutes. Total cook time is about 1 hour.

SERVES: 10

Approximate nutritional analysis per serving: 199.2 calories, 24.3 grams of protein, 7.6 grams of carbohydrates, 8.4 grams of fat, .9 grams of fiber and 261 milligrams of sodium.

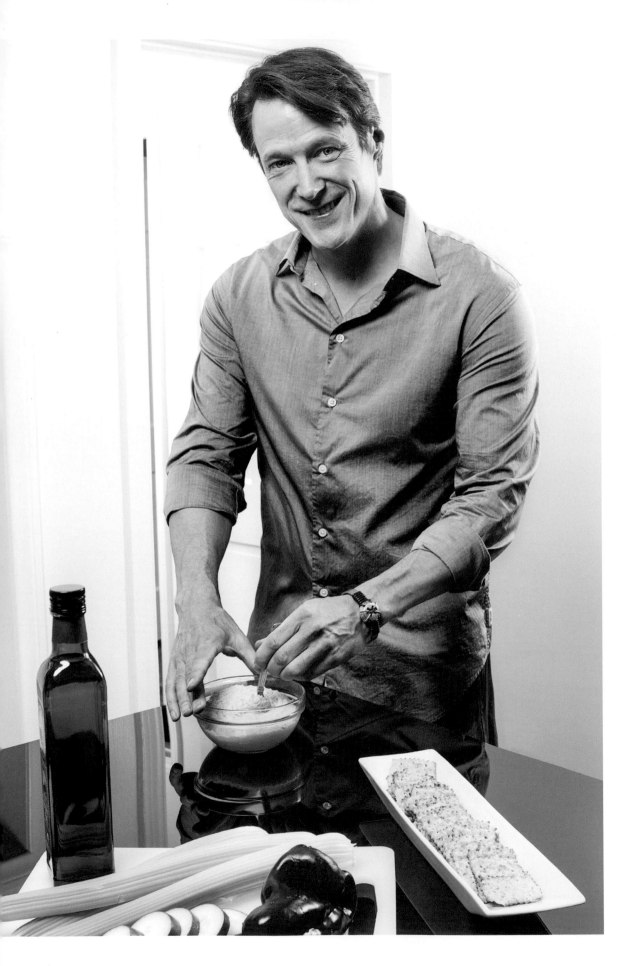

I'll have hummus with raw vegetables as a meal several times a week. It's wonderful!

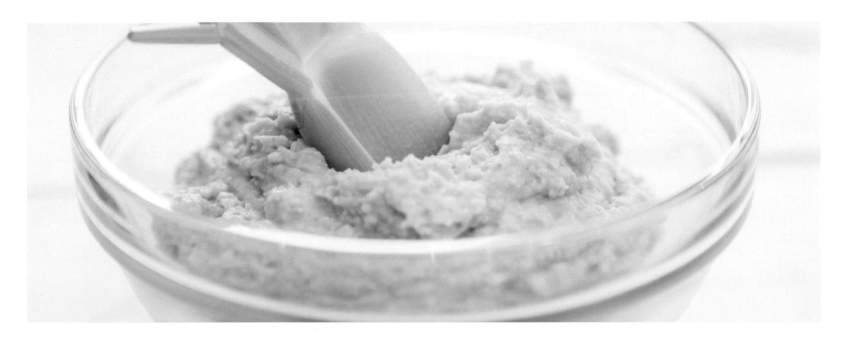

SPICY HUMMUS

by Matthew Ashford

INGREDIENTS:

1½ cups raw chickpeas
3 medium cloves garlic, minced
Juice from 2 medium lemons
¾ cup Tahini
¼ cup (packed) finely minced parsley
Fresh black pepper to taste
Dash of cayenne
Dash of Tamari sauce
¼ cup minced scallion

METHOD:

1. Soak raw chickpeas for 90 minutes and boil until very soft (about 90 minutes).
2. Mash chickpeas into a thick paste using a food mill, grinder or masher.
3. Combine all ingredients and chill thoroughly.
4. To achieve desired taste, add additional garlic, Tamari or Tahini.

SERVES: 6

Approximate nutritional analysis per serving: 110.3 calories, 4.5 grams of protein, 11.7 grams of carbohydrates, 13.8 grams of fat, .3 grams of fiber and 7.1 milligrams of sodium.

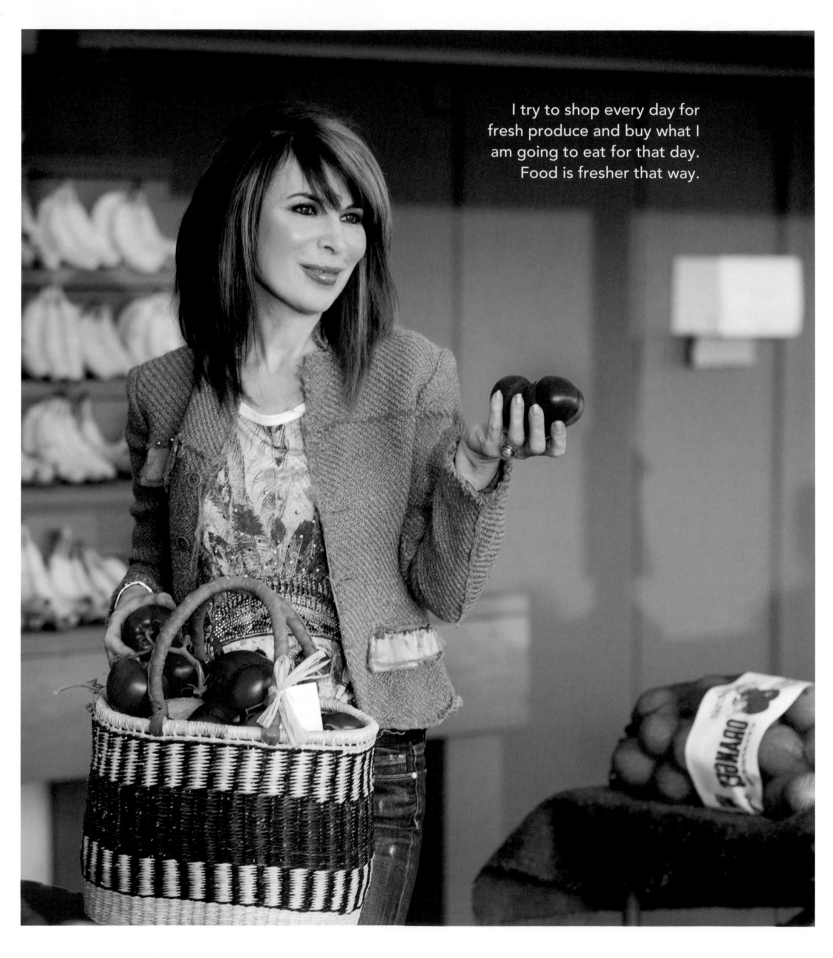

I try to shop every day for fresh produce and buy what I am going to eat for that day. Food is fresher that way.

EGGPLANT WITH BUTTERMILK SAUCE

By Lauren Koslow

If eggplant sounds foreign, it won't after you put this recipe to the test. Topped with a soulful buttermilk sauce, eggplant is sure to become a staple in your diet.

INGREDIENTS:

2 large and long eggplants
⅓ cup extra-virgin olive oil
1½ teaspoons lemon thyme
Fresh black pepper to taste
1 medium pomegranate
1 teaspoon za'atar

SAUCE
9 tablespoons buttermilk, low-fat
½ cup 0% fat Greek yogurt
1½ tablespoons extra-virgin olive oil
1 small garlic clove, crushed

METHOD:

1. Preheat oven to 350°F. Cut the eggplants in half lengthways—cutting straight through the green stalk. Use a small sharp knife to make three or four parallel incisions in the cut side of each eggplant half, without cutting through to the skin. Repeat at a 45-degree angle to get a diamond-shaped pattern.

2. Place the eggplant halves, cut-side up, on a baking sheet lined with parchment paper. Brush them with olive oil and continue brushing until all of the oil has been absorbed by the flesh. Sprinkle with the lemon thyme leaves and some pepper. Roast for 35 to 40 minutes, at which point the flesh should be soft, flavorful and nicely browned. Remove from the oven and let cool completely.

3. While eggplants are in the oven, cut the pomegranate into two horizontally. Hold 1 half over a bowl, with the cut side against your palm, and use the back of a wooden spoon or a rolling pin to gently knock on the pomegranate skin. Continue beating with increasing power until the seeds start coming out naturally and falling through your fingers into the bowl. Once all are there, sift through the seeds and remove any bits of white skin or membrane.

4. To make the sauce, whisk together all of the ingredients. Taste for seasoning, then keep cold until needed.

5. To serve, spoon plenty of buttermilk sauce over the eggplant halves without covering the stalks. Sprinkle za'atar and plenty of pomegranate seeds on top and garnish with lemon thyme. Finish with a drizzle of olive oil.

SERVES: 6

Approximate nutritional analysis per serving:
223 calories, 5 grams of protein, 19.7 grams of carbohydrates, 15.7 grams of fat, 7.1 grams of fiber and 37.2 milligrams of sodium.

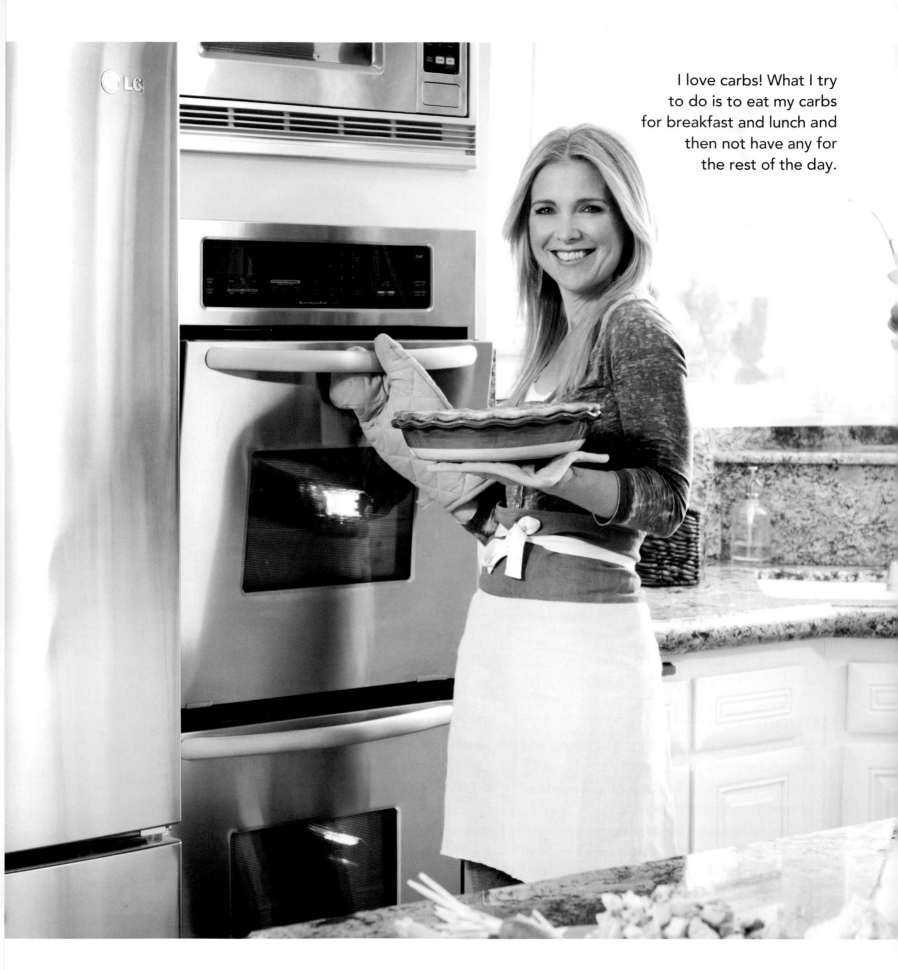

I love carbs! What I try to do is to eat my carbs for breakfast and lunch and then not have any for the rest of the day.

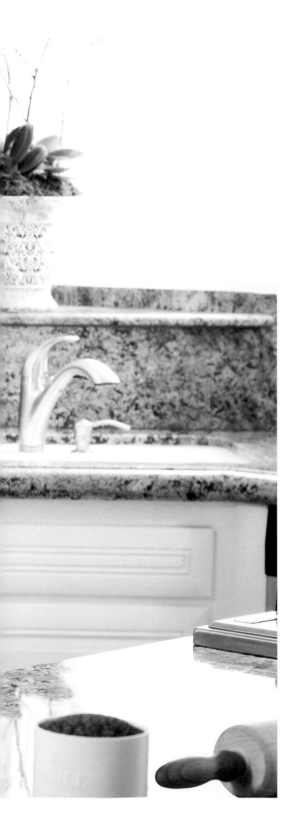

CHICKEN POT PIE

By Melissa Reeves

Made from scratch, this recipe is not only delicious to taste but also heartwarming and packed with comfort.

INGREDIENTS:

1 pound skinless, boneless chicken breast halves, cubed
1 cup sliced carrots
1 cup frozen green peas
½ cup sliced celery
⅓ cup chopped onion
⅓ cup margarine

⅓ cup unbleached all-purpose flour
Pinch salt
¼ teaspoon black pepper
¼ teaspoon celery seed
1¾ cups chicken broth, low sodium
⅔ cup skim milk (or soy milk)
2 (9-inch) unbaked pie crusts

METHOD:

1. Preheat oven to 425°F.
2. In a saucepan, combine chicken, carrots, peas and celery. Add water to cover and boil for 15 minutes. Remove from heat, drain and set aside.
3. In the saucepan over medium heat, cook onions in margarine until soft and translucent. Stir in flour, salt, pepper and celery seed. Slowly stir in chicken broth and milk. Simmer over medium-low heat until thick. Remove from heat and set aside.
4. Place the chicken mixture in bottom pie crust. Pour hot liquid mixture over. Cover with top crust, seal edges and cut away excess dough. Make several small slits in the top to allow steam to escape.
5. Bake in the preheated oven for 30 to 35 minutes, or until pastry is golden brown and filling is bubbly. Cool for 10 minutes before serving.

SERVES: 8

Approximate nutritional analysis per serving: 337.4 calories, 22.1 grams of protein, 25.3 grams of carbohydrates, 15.5 grams of fat, 2.1 grams of fiber and 449 milligrams of sodium.

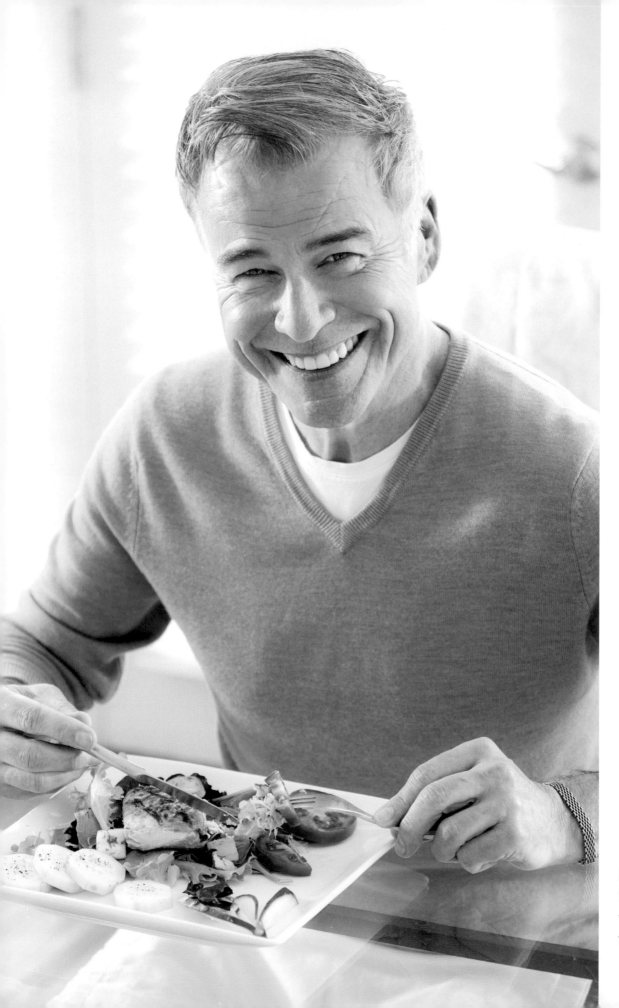

I love salmon. I'll either grill it or steam it and have it with vegetables. Salmon is my favorite fish.

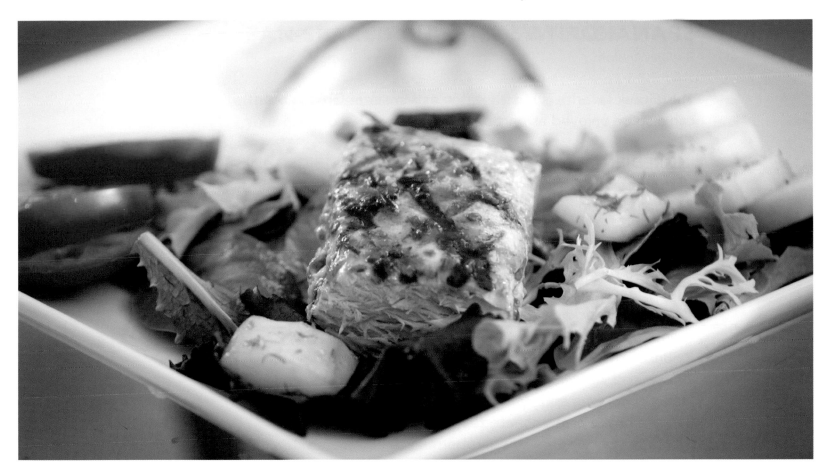

LEMON PEPPER SALMON

By Ian Buchanan

Top your choice of greens with a healthy fillet filled with flavor!

INGREDIENTS:
4 (5-ounce) salmon fillet (wild when possible)
2 tablespoons margarine, melted
2 tablespoons soy sauce
Lemon pepper to taste

METHOD:
1. Preheat the oven broiler. Lightly grease a baking sheet.
2. Once salmon is cleaned, place on baking sheet. Mix melted margarine with soy sauce in a small bowl, and brush over the salmon. Sprinkle salmon with lemon pepper.
3. Broil salmon for 5 to 8 minutes, until easily flaked or at desired doneness.

SERVES: 4

Approximate nutritional analysis per serving: 223.5 calories, 29.21 grams of protein, .5 grams of carbohydrates, 10.73 grams of fat, 0 grams of fiber and 663 milligrams of sodium.

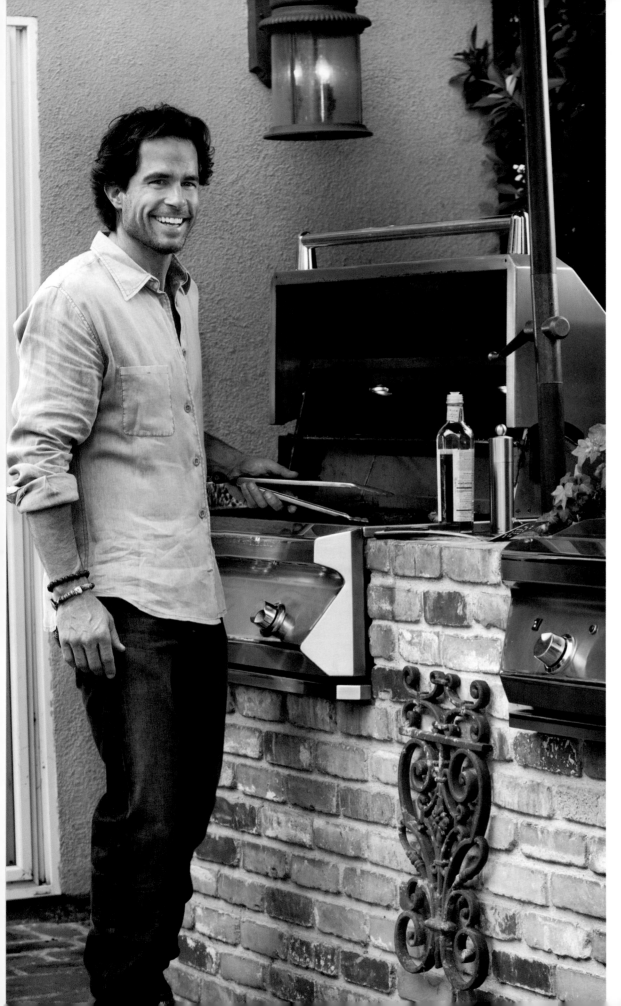

I'm not a nutritionist, but you want to put out more than you take in. Every body, and I mean every "body," is different. The way that people metabolize foods is different. The greatest nutritional and exercise advice is to do what works for you, what makes you feel good on the inside. The rest can and should take care of itself. You have to mix it up, too. If something's not working for you, then why do it?

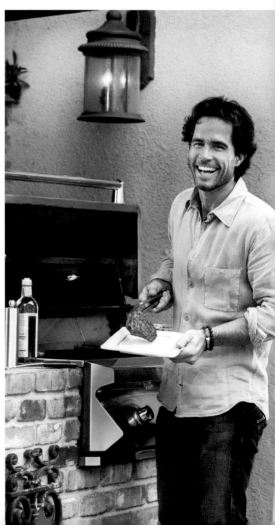

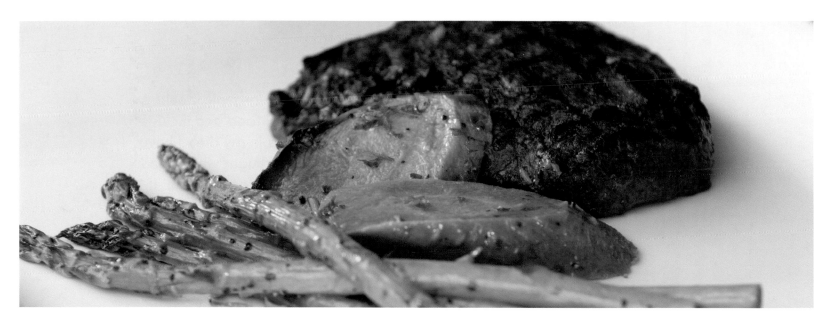

GRILLED RIB-EYE STEAK

By Shawn Christian

This recipe uses the natural fat marbling contained in the rib-eye to make a very flavorful and juicy steak without a lot of effort.

INGREDIENTS:

4 (4-ounce) rib-eye steaks (at least an inch thick), boneless

4 tablespoons extra-virgin olive oil
Fresh ground pepper to taste

METHOD:

1. Preheat your grill to high.
2. Remove the rib-eye steaks from their packaging and rub each with a tablespoon of olive oil and then coat with a generous amount of freshly ground black pepper. The olive oil provides just enough fat to help the pepper create a great, caramelized crust.
3. Clean and lubricate your grill grates with some cooking oil on a rolled-up piece of paper towel (using tongs, of course).
4. Place the rib-eye steaks on the hottest part of the grill and keep the tongs near. If you experience a flare-up, use your tongs to slide the steaks away from the open flame. Once the flame dies, however, move back to original position.
5. Continue to grill each side of the rib-eye with the lid open for about 4 to 6 minutes.

6. Once steaks are done to your preference, place to the side for about 5 minutes before serving.

COOKING TIP: Consider grilling a jalapeño right along with the steak. Keep it pure and simple.

RECOMMENDATION: Serve rib-eye with wild rice and greens sautéed with freshly chopped garlic and olive oil.

SERVES: 4

Approximate nutritional analysis per serving: 227 calories, 26.6 grams of protein, 1.8 grams of carbohydrates, 26.4 grams of fat, 0 grams of fiber and 428 milligrams of sodium.

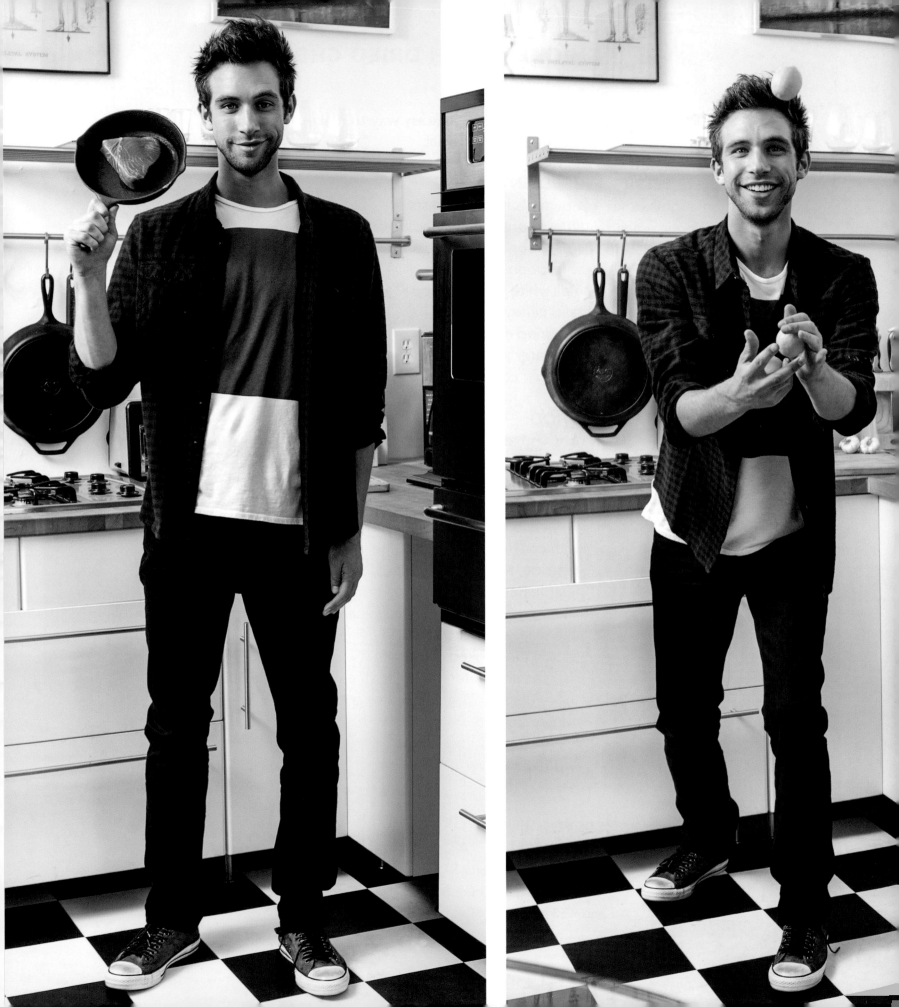

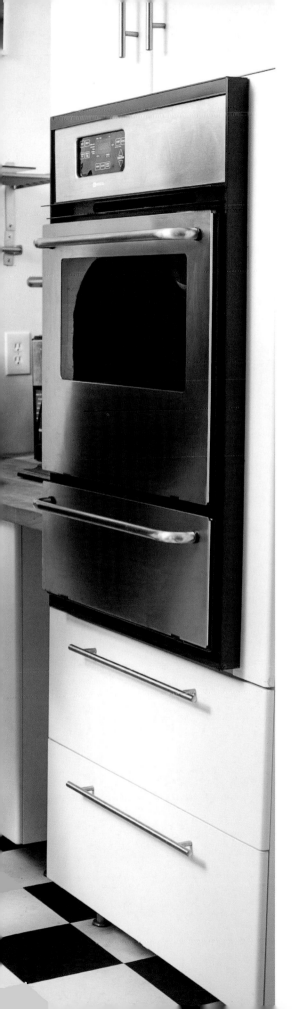

CHIMICHURRI SAUCE
by Blake Berris

INGREDIENTS:
¼ cup fresh lemon juice
2 cloves garlic
1 seeded jalapeno pepper (to taste—some peppers are hotter than others)
⅓–½ cup flat-leaf parsley (regular curly-leaf parsley has a very strong flavor, but can be used if necessary)
⅓–½ cup cilantro (can use all parsley if you prefer)
⅔ cup extra-virgin olive oil

METHOD:
1. Add first 5 ingredients to food processor and blend.
2. Then, slowly through the top of the machine, add olive oil in a steady stream until thickened.
3. Adjust flavors—add more lemon, chives, red pepper flakes—make it your own.

RECOMMENDATION: Use on top of steak, grilled fish or veggie burgers

SERVES: 10

Approximate nutritional analysis per serving: 126.1 calories, .2 grams of protein, 1.4 grams of carbohydrates, 14 grams of fat, .2 grams of fiber and 25.5 milligrams of sodium.

I keep it simple when I cook.
To make preparing food less
of a chore, I try to have fun in the
kitchen while I am cooking.

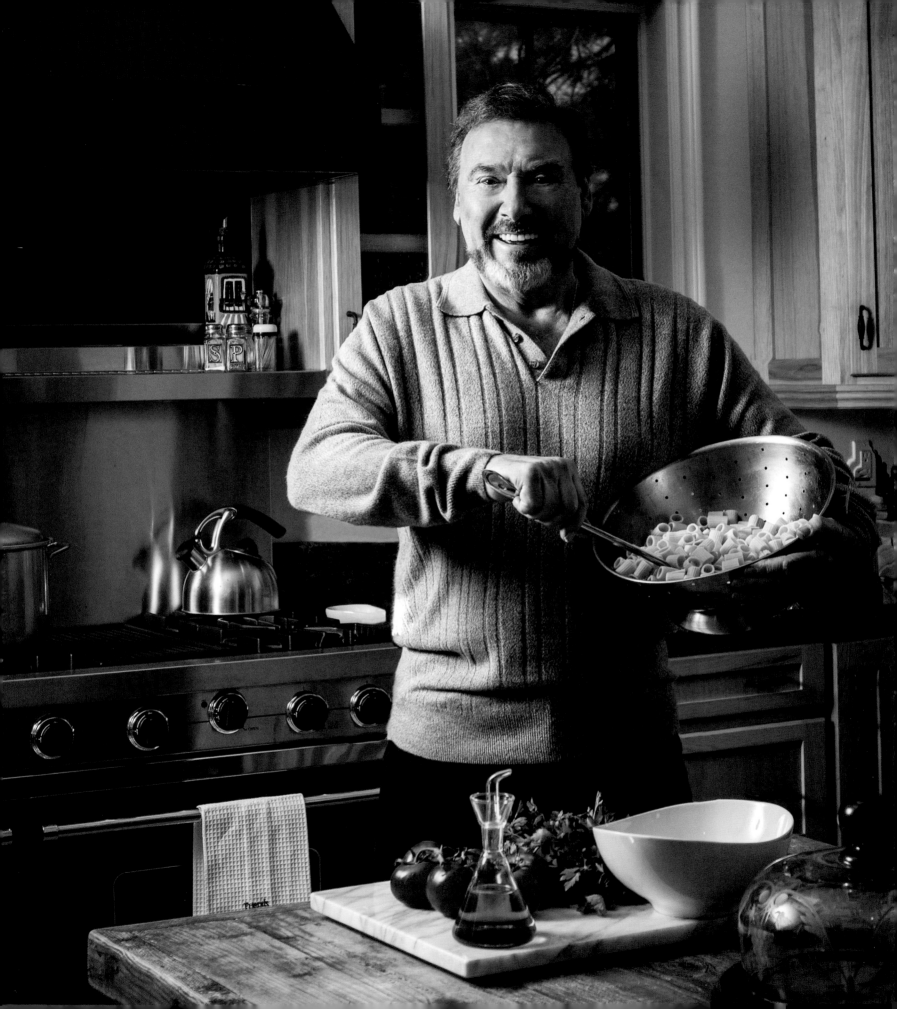

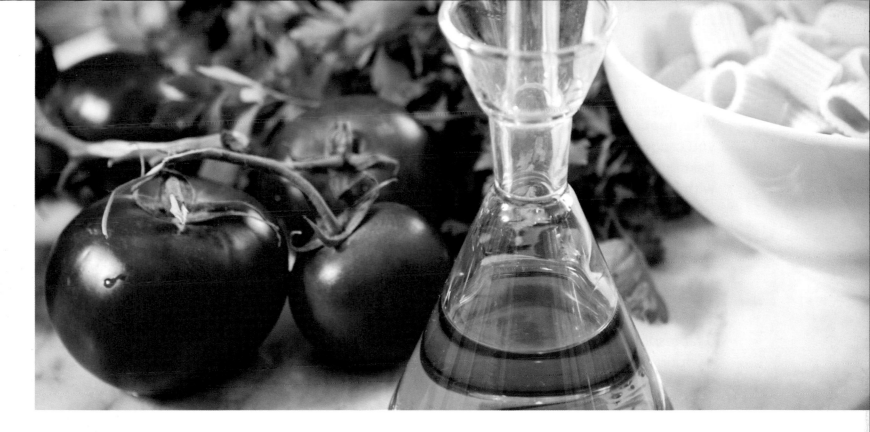

PASTA MISTO MARE

By Joe Mascolo

Did someone say pasta, pasta, PASTA? This is delicious and nutritious!

INGREDIENTS:
2 tablespoons extra-virgin olive oil
1 clove garlic, chopped
1 teaspoon parsley
1 teaspoon oregano

2 teaspoons black pepper
1 cup marinara sauce
8 ounces penne pasta (or pasta of choice)
1 pound fresh shrimp, calamari and scallops

METHOD:
Heat olive oil in pan. Add garlic, parsley, oregano and pepper. Add marinara sauce and heat together. In the meantime, prepare pasta according to package directions. In a separate pan, grill shrimp in small amount of olive oil, add calamari and scallops and grill just a few minutes on each side. Add seafood to sauce just to warm. Pour sauce and seafood combination over penne pasta, or pasta of your choice.

RECOMMENDATION: Serve with a lovely glass of red wine!

SERVES: 4

Approximate nutritional analysis per serving: 290.8 calories, 28.1 grams of protein, 22.6 grams of carbohydrates, 10.1 grams of fat, 2 grams of fiber and 557 milligrams of sodium.

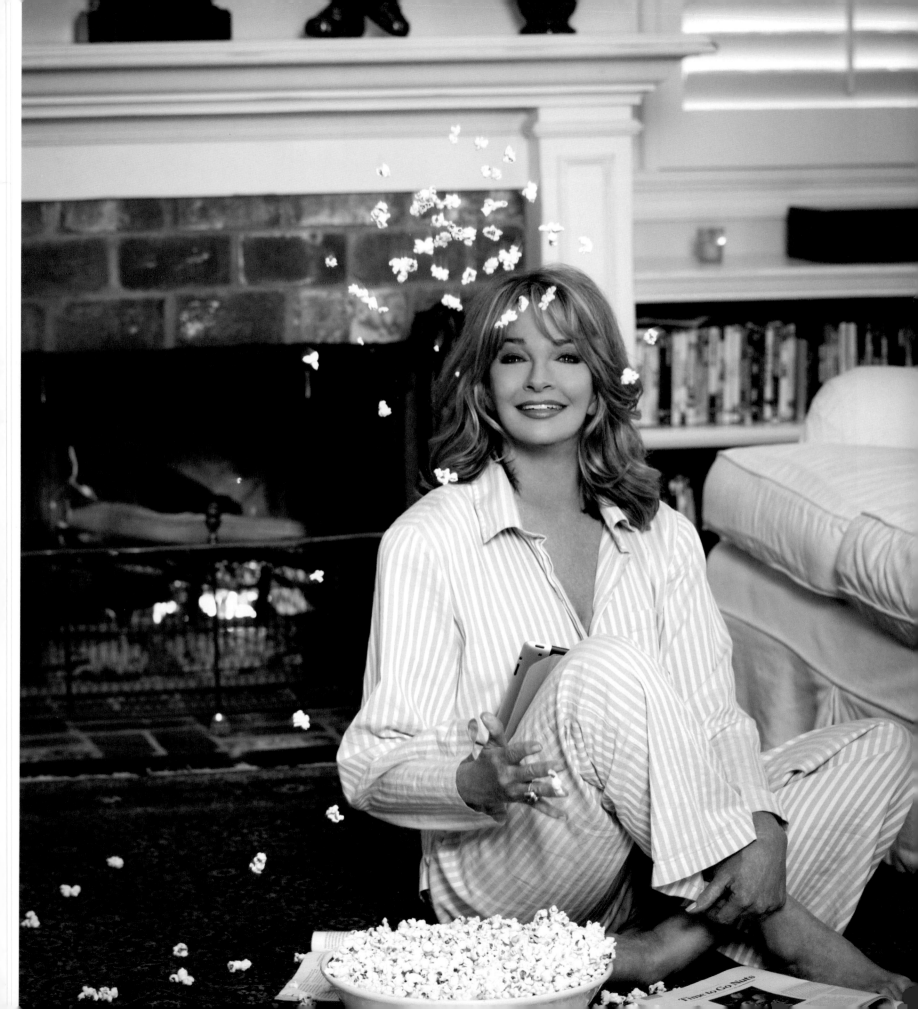

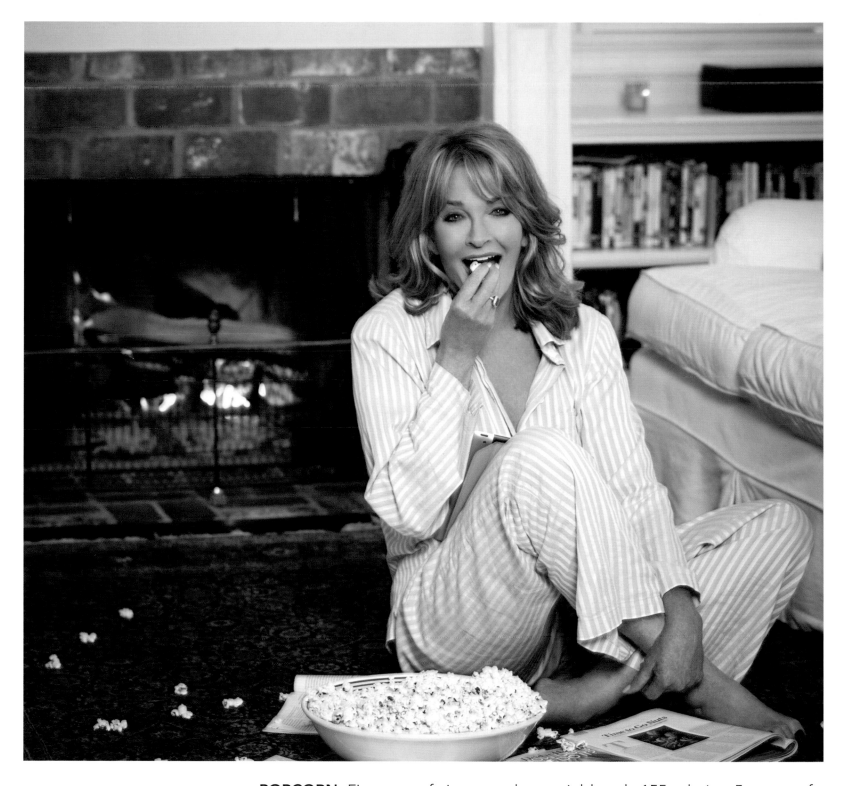

I love popcorn! However, I don't add salt and butter like I used to.
—*Deidre Hall*

POPCORN: Five cups of air-popped corn yields only 155 calories, 5 grams of protein, 6 grams of fiber and only 2 milligrams of sodium. Keep the butter in balance or consider topping it with brewer's yeast and you have a super food that tastes fabulous! Popcorn is a whole grain, which is great for fighting a number of chronic diseases. It's also packed with polyphenols, which is also one of the primary reasons fruits and vegetables rank high on the healthy list.

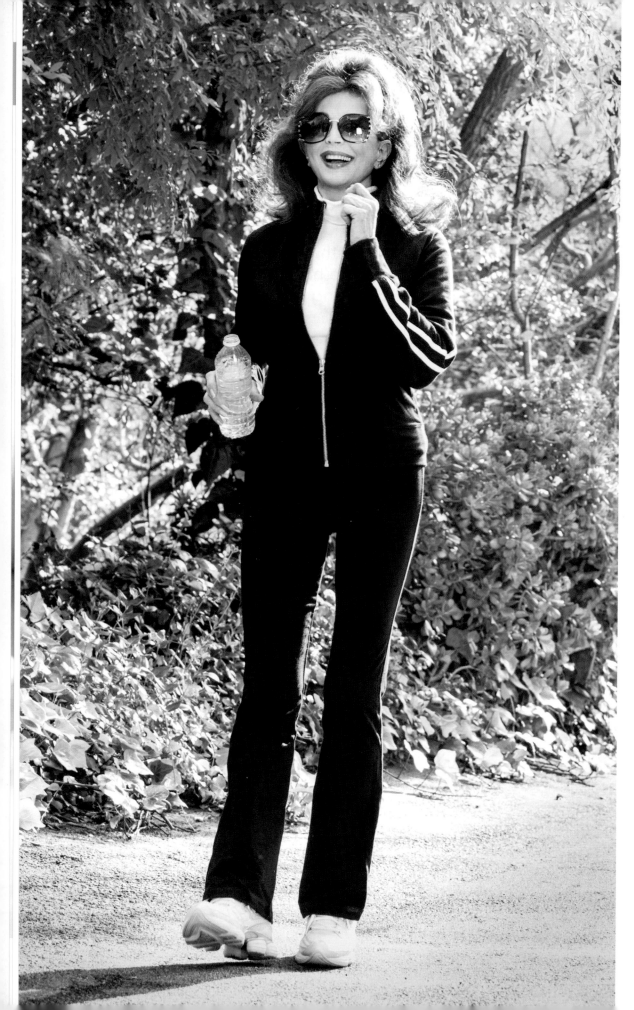

I walk every day to keep my legs in shape. The importance of physical fitness stems from my days as a professional dancer performing as one of the Rockettes (at Radio City Music Hall in New York City) and in several Broadway musicals including *Coco*, *Hallelujah Boys* and *Follies*.

I bring a bottle of water with me everywhere I go even as I walk up and down the streets of my neighborhood. I get a nice cardio workout this way. To change my walking routine, occasionally I will play a round of golf not only for the golf itself but also to enjoy the beautifully manicured greens. This is a great workout for me as well. One of these days I'm going to get back out there and play 18 holes! One piece of advice: try not to use golf carts when you play—you'll get a better cardio workout if you walk the course.

Because I'm fair-skinned I know the importance of protecting myself from the sun, so I always cover myself with sunscreen.
—*Suzanne Rogers*

My best girlfriend and her husband are avid golfers. They invited me along to a course one time in Oxnard. That's how I got started playing golf! An interesting thing about the sport is that you can do it alone. There's a wonderful social element to golf as well when you join people you meet on the course for a round.

Playing golf allows you to focus and forget everything else…because if you don't you're not going to play as well as you can. You may have an occasional lucky day where you'll go out and hit great, but you need to practice on a regular basis if you want to continue to play well. That's the game of golf…and if nothing else, it gets you outdoors!!

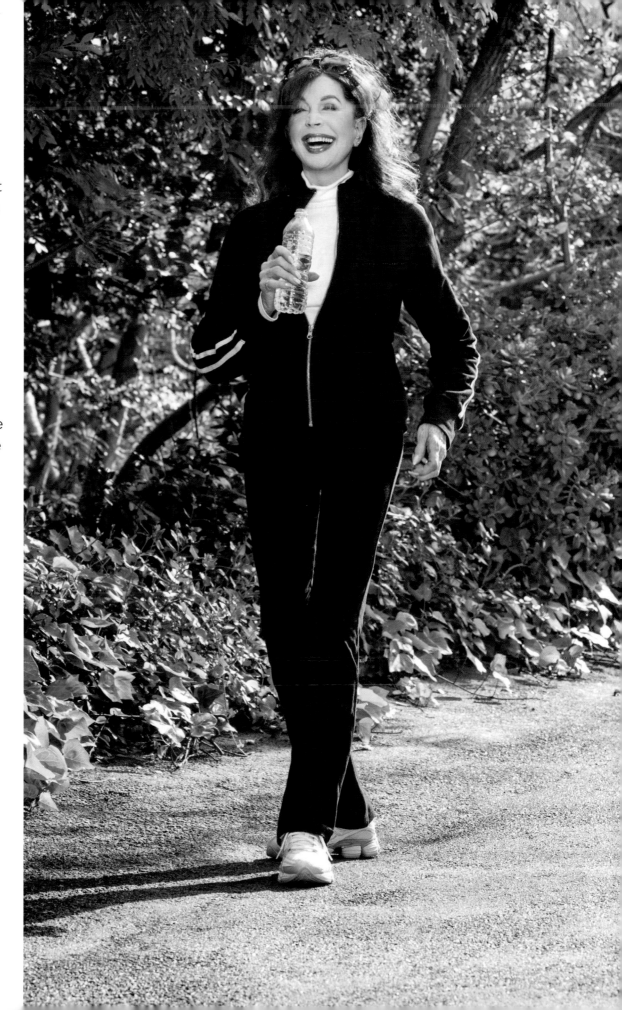

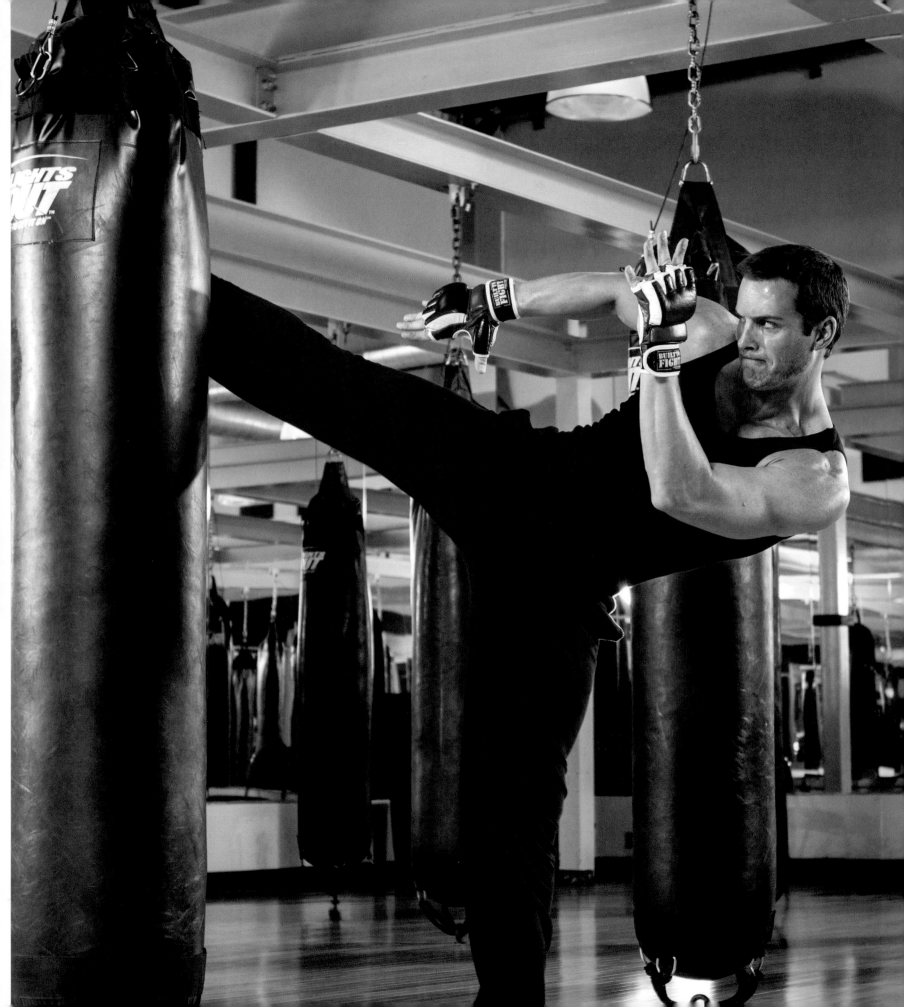

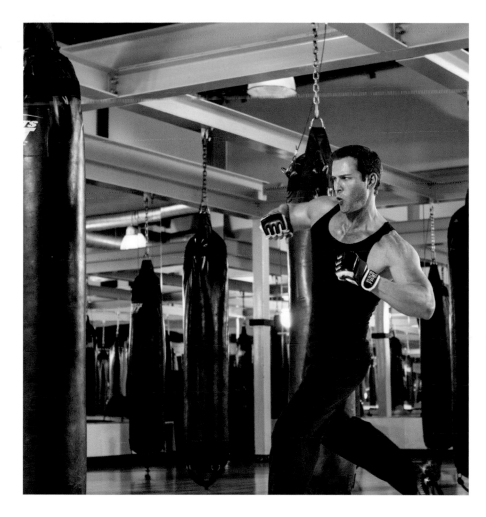

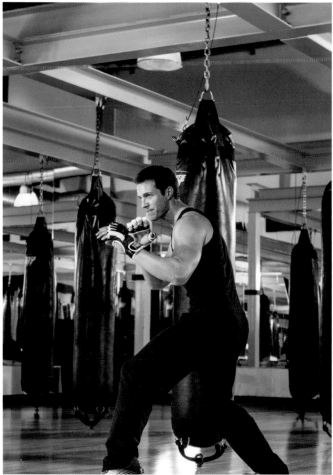

I found it increasingly difficult to get motivated at the gym. I realized that I needed someone to kick my butt, so classes and training sessions work very well for me. I've always hated cardiovascular activity. I'd rather lift 600 pounds over my head than run a mile. It's important to be a fan of what you do to work out so you'll do it more.

Right now, kickboxing is my "go to" regime. I kickbox not because of its defensive tactics. I take it because it's constant movement for 60 minutes. I sweat more when I do kickboxing than anything else. Your muscles can become accustomed to doing the same workout. I truly try to change the furniture, for lack of a better phrase, in my routine to avoid that.

There's monotony in everything we do. I've never met a person who's excited to get on that treadmill.
—Eric Martsolf

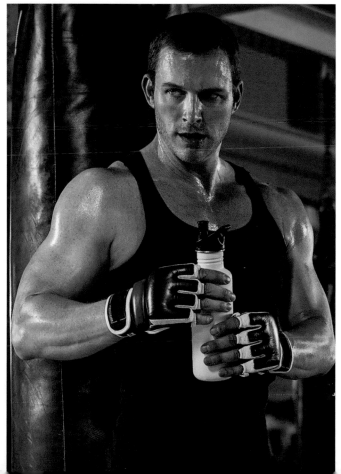

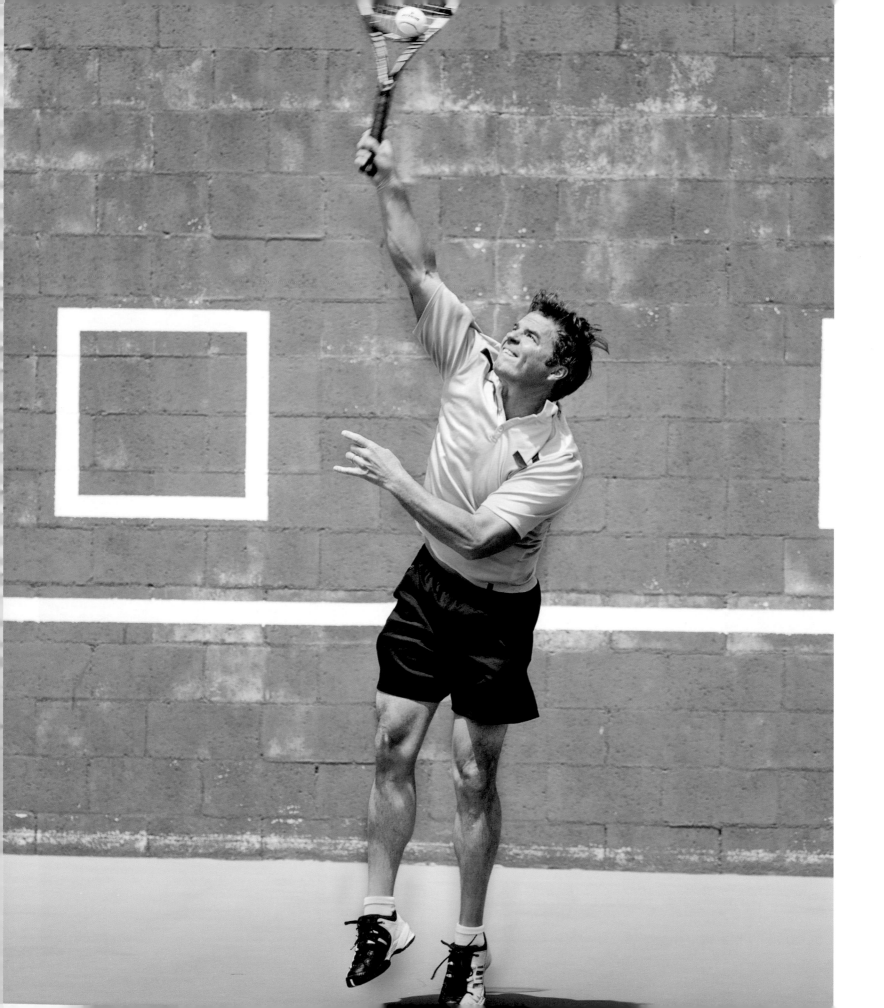

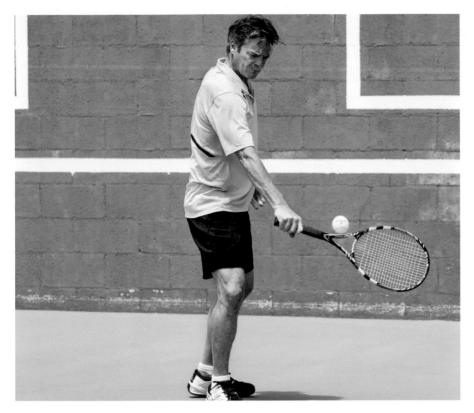

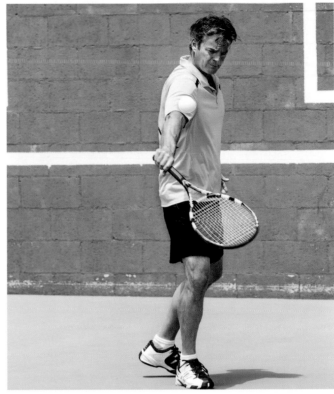

I played baseball up until I was 15 years old and then I took up tennis in high school. My first summer job was stringing tennis rackets at the club. I took one summer of tennis classes. It's actually the only sport that I've ever played competitively. I recently picked up playing tennis after about a 20-year gap. I started taking lessons again and I had to laugh when my instructor said to me, "Wally, you hit forehand like they taught two decades ago!" There's a whole different grip now. The techniques changed over the years, but I didn't let that stop me from getting back into the game. It didn't take me long to learn the new methods. I've learned the new forehand grip and I use it now. It's absolutely better. I'll watch tennis on television and I see the players use the new grips. Your wrist and arm move forward in a slightly different way than how I was taught.

Now, I play for an hour each weekend with a buddy. We're equally matched so our sets can go either way. We'll go down to the wire with scores of 6-4 or 7-5. Sometimes I'll win and other times he will. We've been doing this for about a year and a half, off and on. I have other forms of exercise that I do, too. I'll do a hot (Bikram) yoga class after I drop my son off at school during the week. Other days, I'll do a swim class with a group. We swim well over 2,000 yards. It's a hard workout.

I find that a good combination for me is yoga, swimming and playing tennis.
—*Wally Kurth*

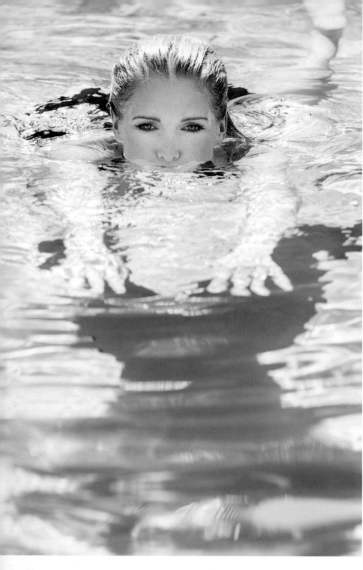

Swimming has always been a part of my life. I grew up on the East Coast and went to camp a lot as a kid where I learned freestyle, butterfly and backstroke. I find that I remember all those lessons now as I swim for exercise in my pool in Los Angeles.

We do have a little chlorine in our saltwater pool, but I don't have to worry about it affecting my hair because I wet my hair before I go in. I get a total low-impact cardio workout that works a lot of my muscle groups at the same time through swimming.

Living in California is great because you can swim all year round.
—*Melissa Reeves*

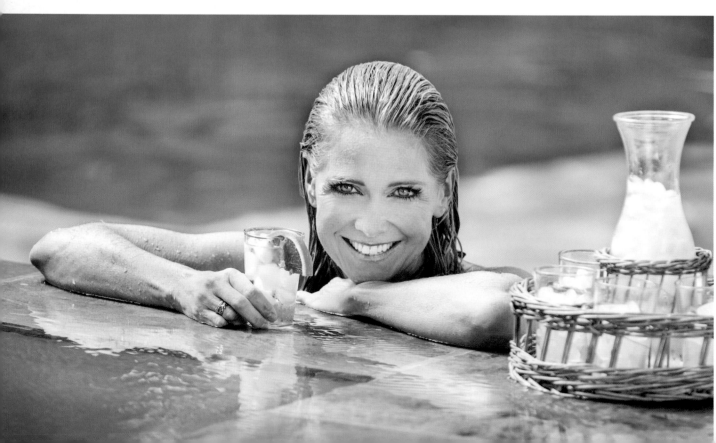

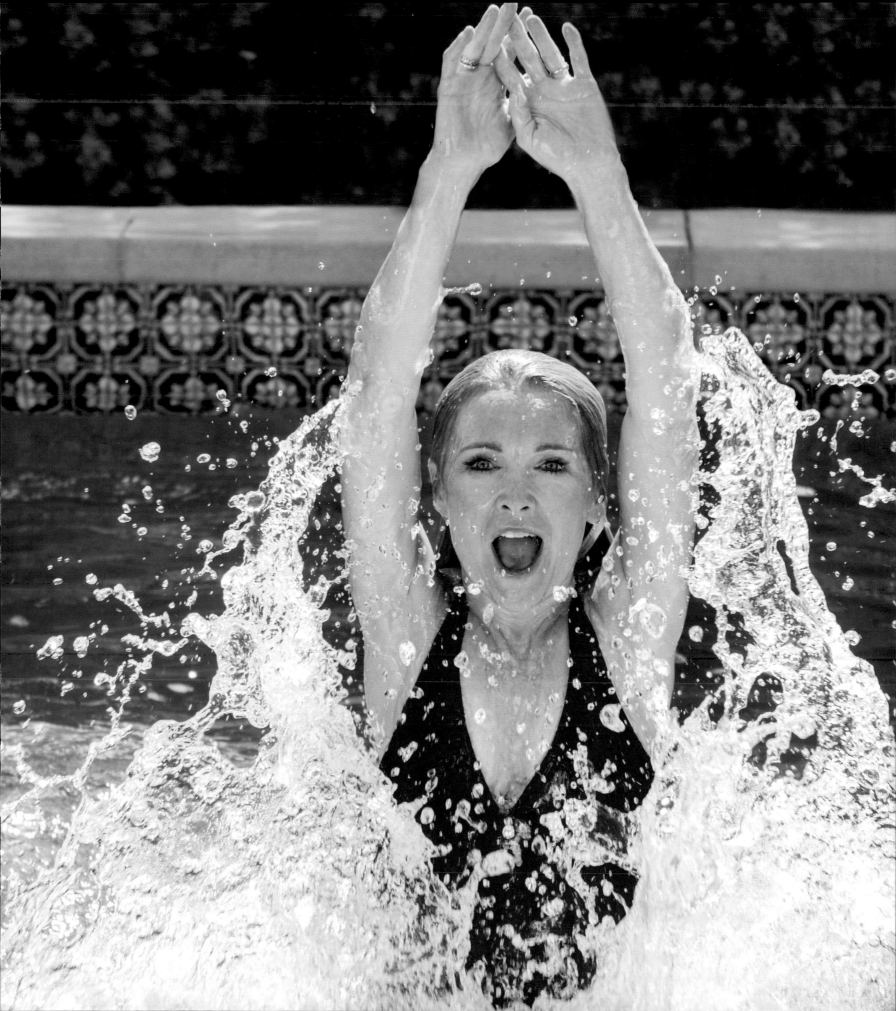

I've always loved dancing. I was a dancer on Broadway in *Bye Bye Birdie* and *Me and Juliet*. When my wife Susan and I were hired to do a production of *42nd Street*, I began taking tap classes. I was 65 years old when I started. Susan's character in the musical had been a tap dancer, so I suggested that we take a tap dance class together. I prefer to dance and exercise my blues away rather than go through the push and pull of a gym routine. I still enjoy tap classes now and then.

I get up every day and stretch immediately upon waking. Susan and I also go on long walks together to stay active.

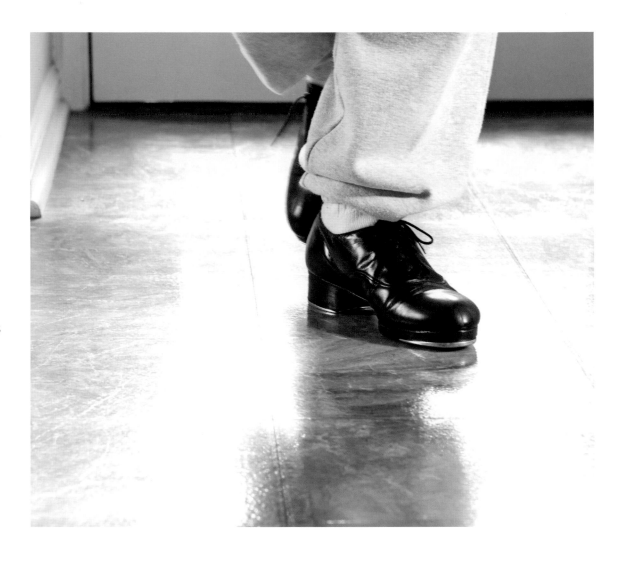

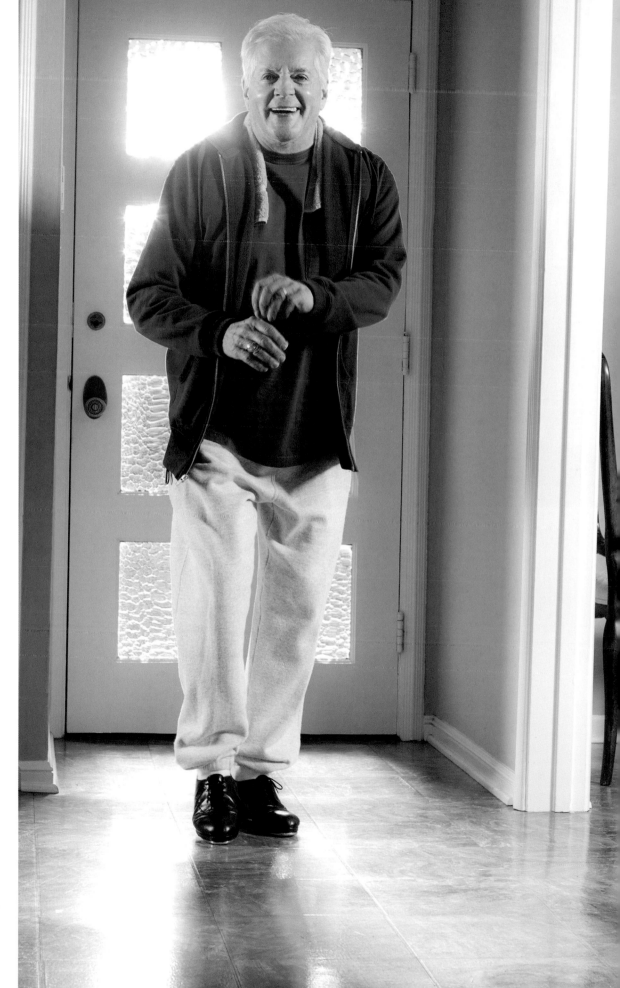

When I was a kid, I could not force myself to go to tap class, which was filled with girls. Now, if my class has a dozen women and me in it, I'm extremely happy.

—*Bill Hayes*

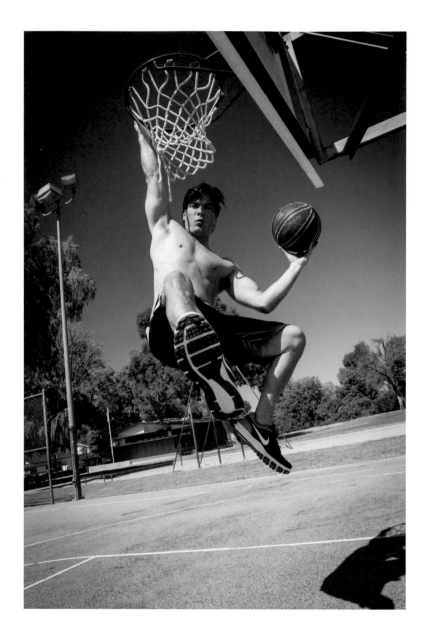

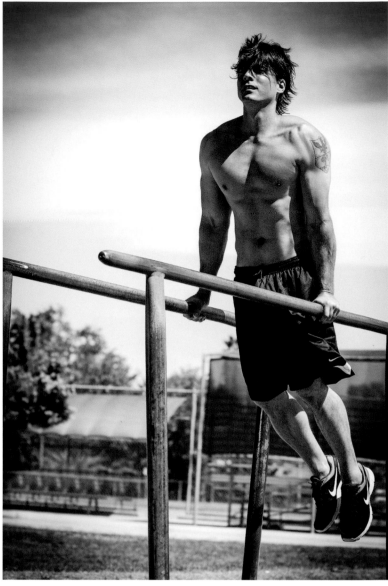

I regularly play basketball with my son, Gabe. We have a court in the backyard and we'll go one on one for hours. I've taught him how to shoot and I make sure his form is good. Now, he beats me! He'll shoot 250 times a day from different spots on the court to hone his skill.

I have a makeshift gym in my garage. It's not glamorous at all, but it gets the job done. If I have a big dinner at night I don't have far to go to work it off.

—Bryan Dattilo

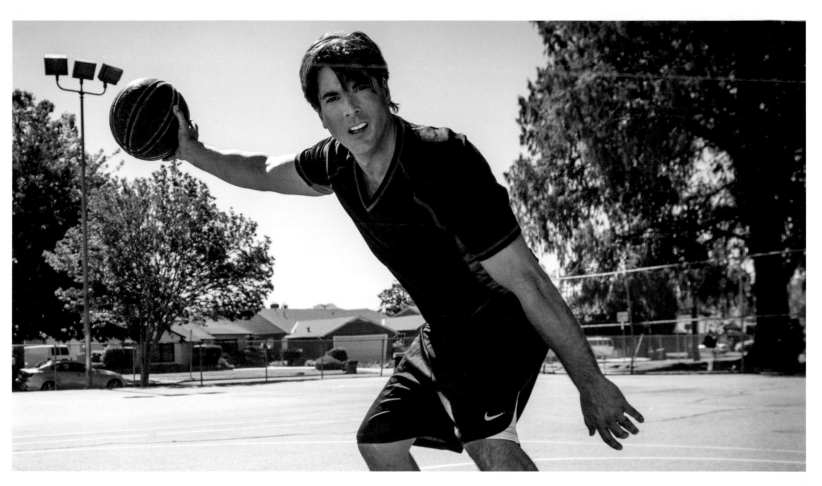

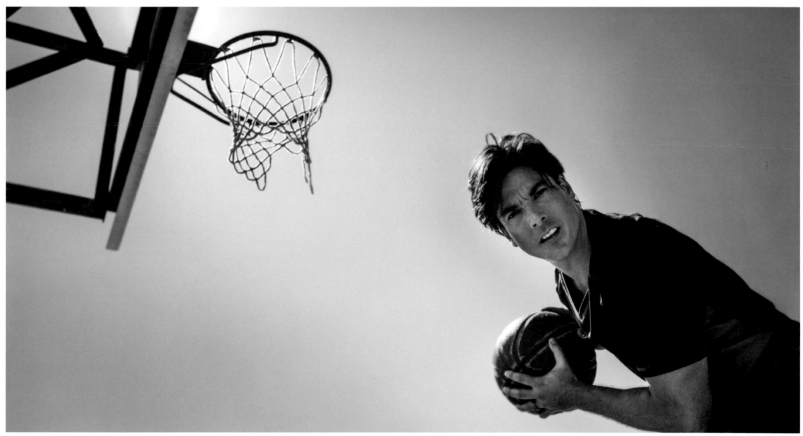

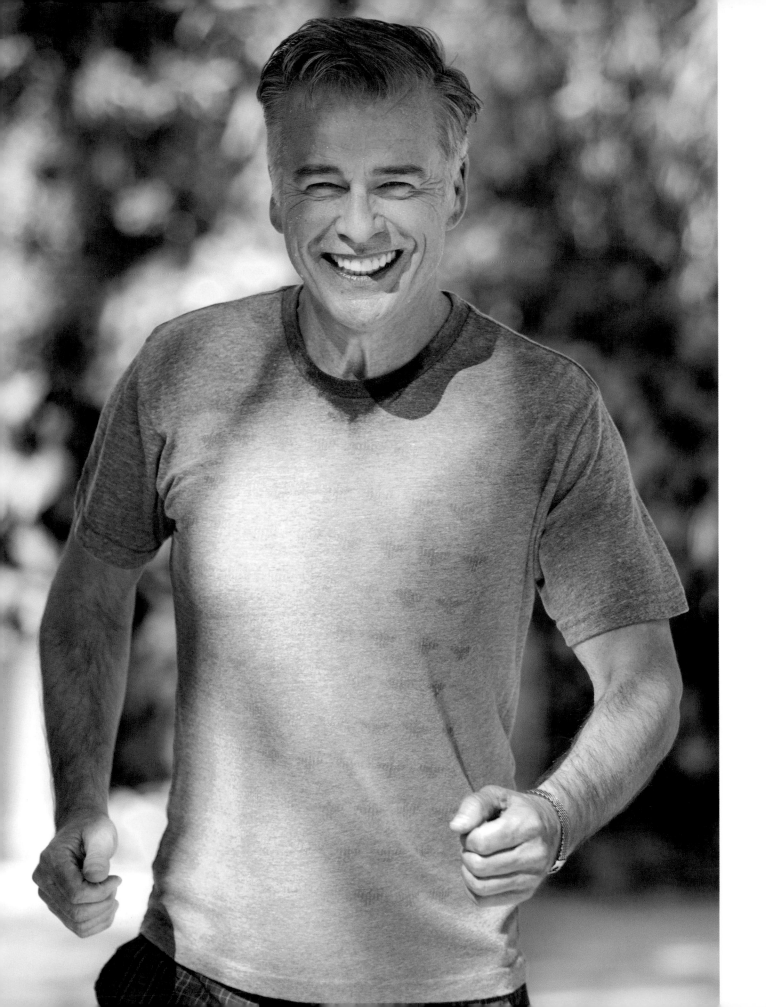

I do an hour of cardio six days a week. The elliptical glider is my passion other than walking. When I'm on the glider I feel like a kid running through the air. I do enjoy jogging occasionally, but I much prefer low-impact exercise. I'd rather go for long walks around my neighborhood even if it's raining.

I walk up to three to four miles a week.

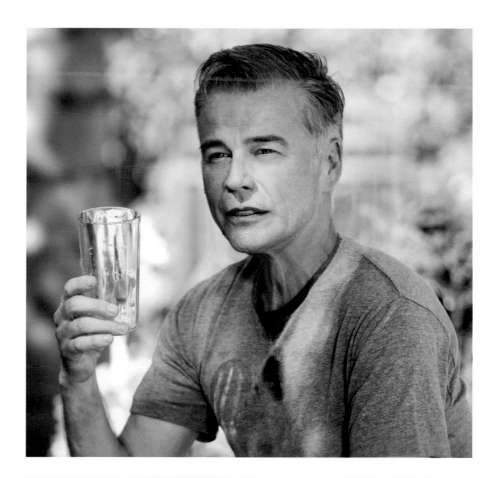

I like stretching because it's not only a great workout, but it also keeps you flexible.
—Ian Buchanan

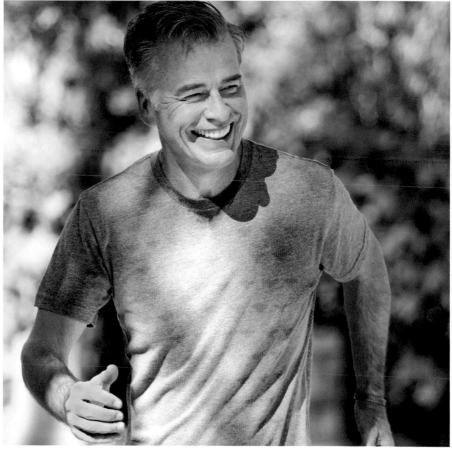

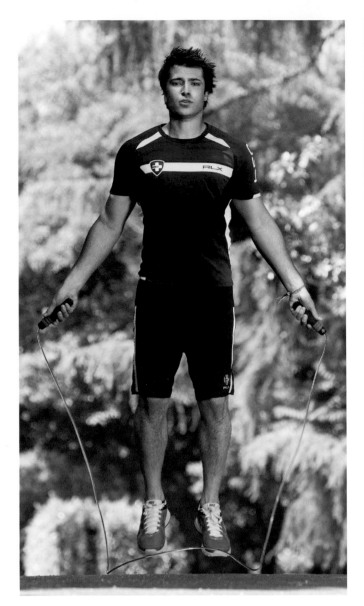

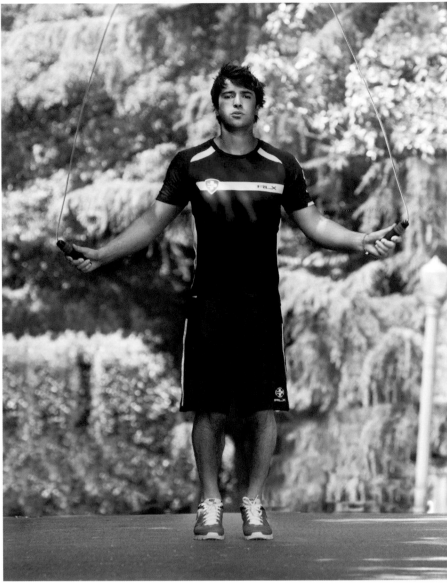

I try to stay on a strict diet and stick with regular exercise.
—*Freddie Smith*

Along with hitting the gym four times a week, I like to mix things up with jumping rope and hiking. I like to get out of the city to hike in places such as Topanga Canyon, Malibu Creek or Runyon Canyon. Hikes are great because it gets me out in the fresh air. Depending on the day, sometimes I'll do a nine-mile hike.

I've been working with a trainer because it helps to have someone show me exactly what to do so I don't hurt myself. And I can get maximum results. Occasionally, I refer to YouTube to see how to do certain exercises. You'll see results more quickly if you do exercises properly and you stick with it.

Take it day by day. Set two-week increment goals. Don't weigh yourself every single day.

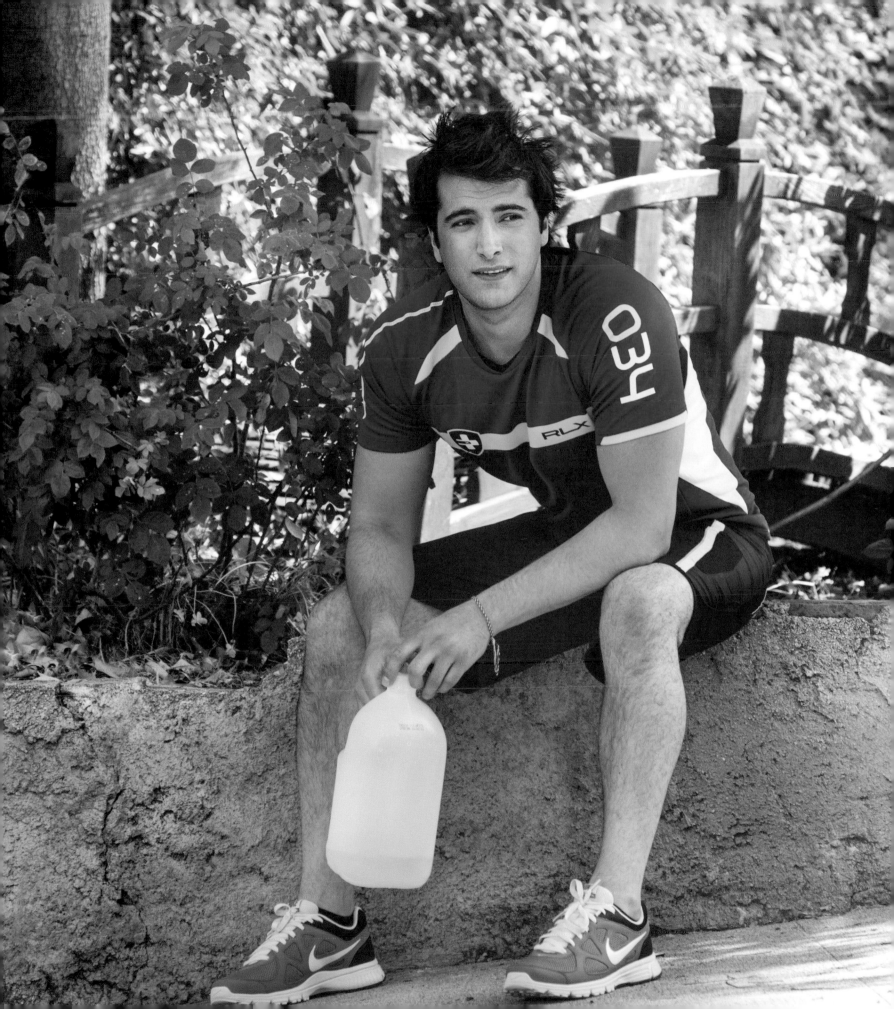

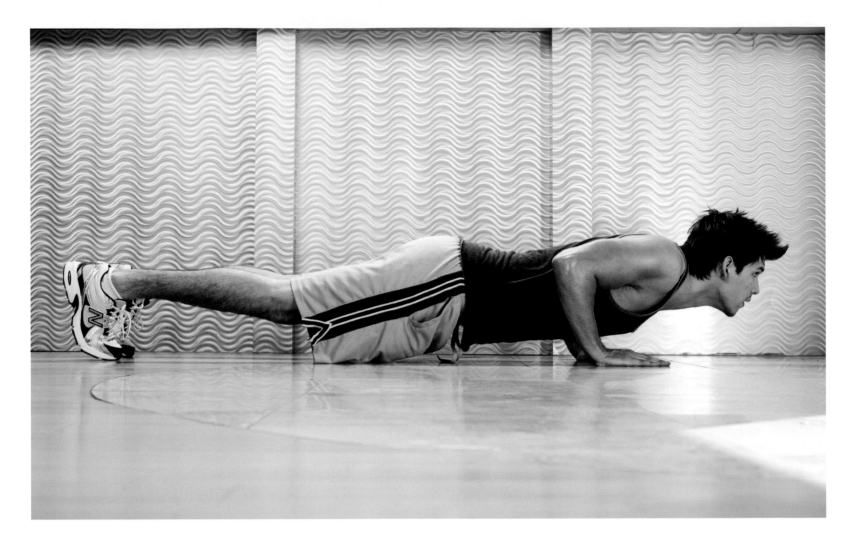

I try to get to the gym three to four times a week. As a warm up, one of my favorite exercises is a quick set of explosive push-ups. I do a lot of heavy lifting. I do what I call the "Brad Pitt" workout, which he did to train for the movie *Fight Club*. This routine consists of working out every single muscle group on different days. One day, I'll work out my chest and add an abdominal routine. The next day, I'll go back and work out my shoulders and jog for 30 minutes.

To change things up a bit sometimes I get a good overall workout in by rowing.

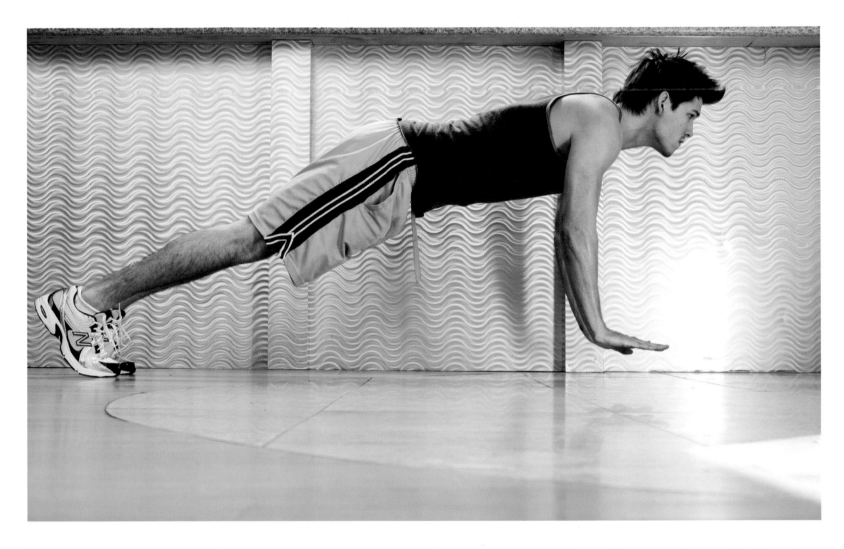

EXPLOSIVE PUSH-UPS CAN BE DONE ANYWHERE!

I'm not going to lie. Starting a new fitness and diet regime is going to be hell. The first week is hard, but not every week will be like that first week.

—*Casey Jon Deidrick*

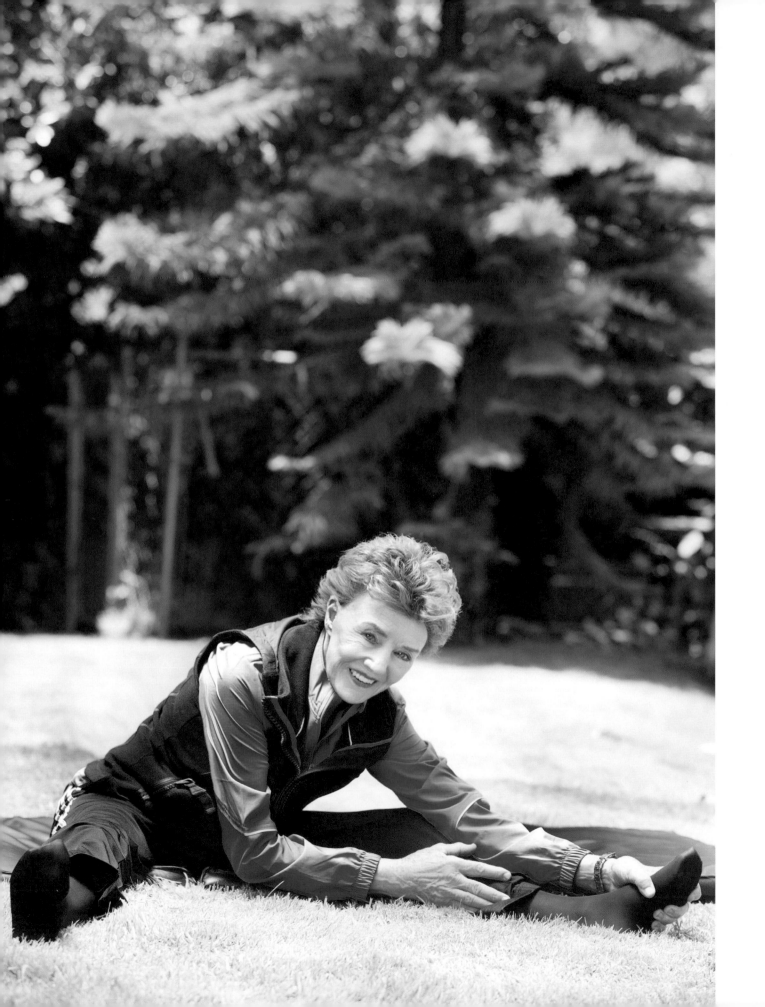

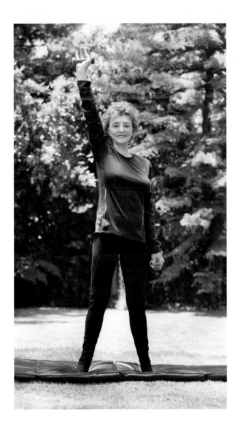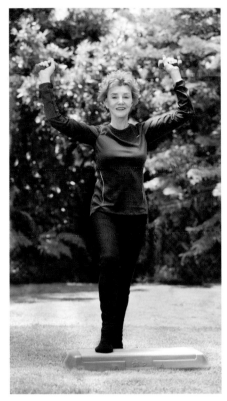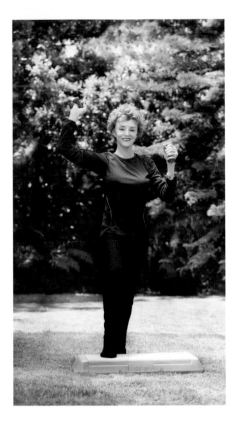

I lift small weights when I stretch. I have some unusual exercises that I do. One of them is for the sacrum. That's your bottom tailbone. A chiropractor's daughter came up with this rare but important exercise. You lie on your back with your knees bent. Then, lift up and down, which will stretch your lower back.

Stretching is so important. I think it's one of the most important things you can do for your body.
—*Peggy McCay*

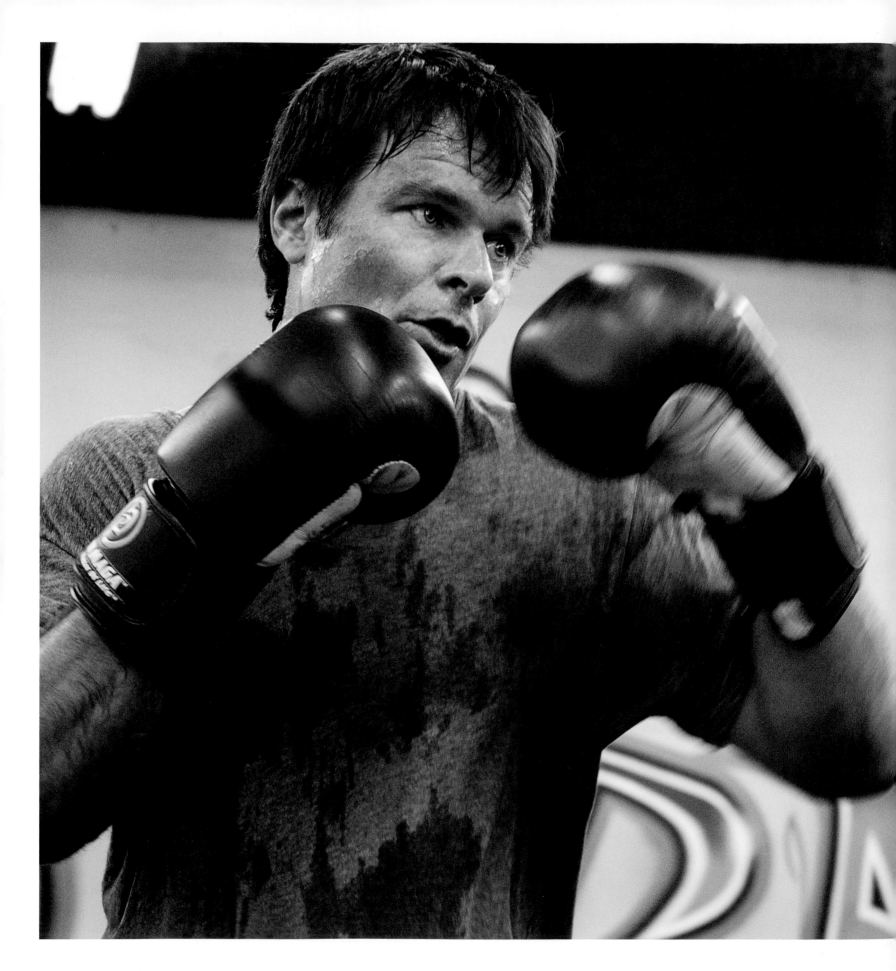

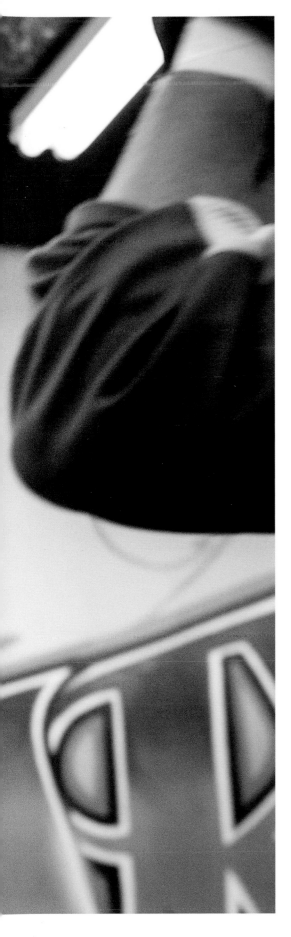

Boxing is a mental workout in addition to being a physical one. To box, you have to be relaxed. People may think that boxing is tight and violent, and, of course, it is violent, but more than that it's an art form. There's a rhythm to boxing, and you have to be relaxed when you do it. Otherwise, you'll expend so much energy it'll just drain you and not in a good way.

There's this kind of raw rhythm to boxing that I just love. I'm such a boxing fan. My idol when I was growing up was Muhammad Ali. I've always loved the sport.

I'll box for a while and then go to CrossFit or jump rope. I also take time off to let my body heal, which is a healthy thing to do.

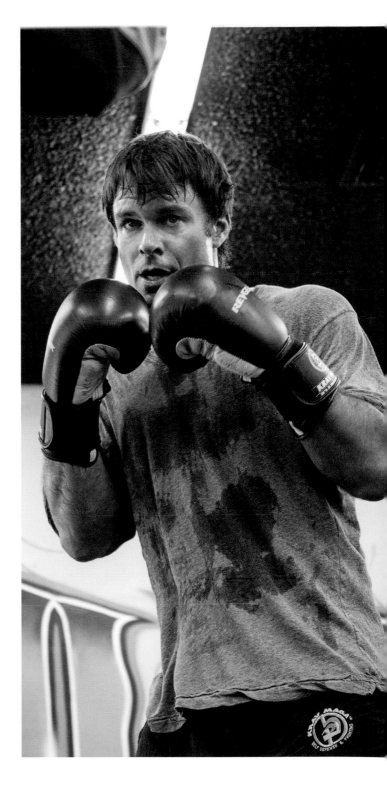

I'll switch my workouts every three or four months so I don't get in a rut.
—Patrick Muldoon

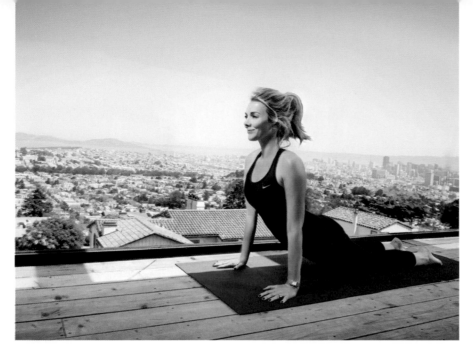

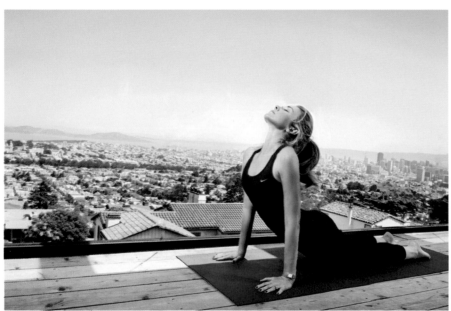

I do yoga twice a week, which isn't a lot, but when you have two kids and they're very young, it's not always easy to find the time.

There's something refreshing about doing yoga outside when the weather is nice. I feel more at peace and it helps if it's sunny out, but not too bright and there's a nice breeze in the air. I connect more with yoga this way.

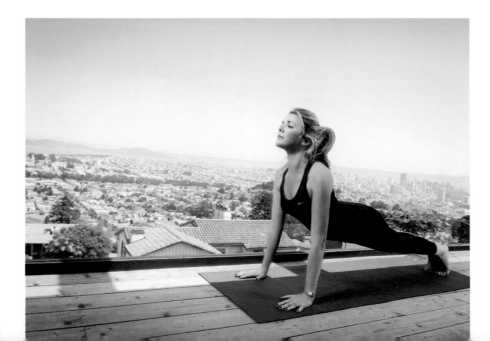

Yoga helps me feel more balanced. It's a great physical and mental workout.
—Christie Clark

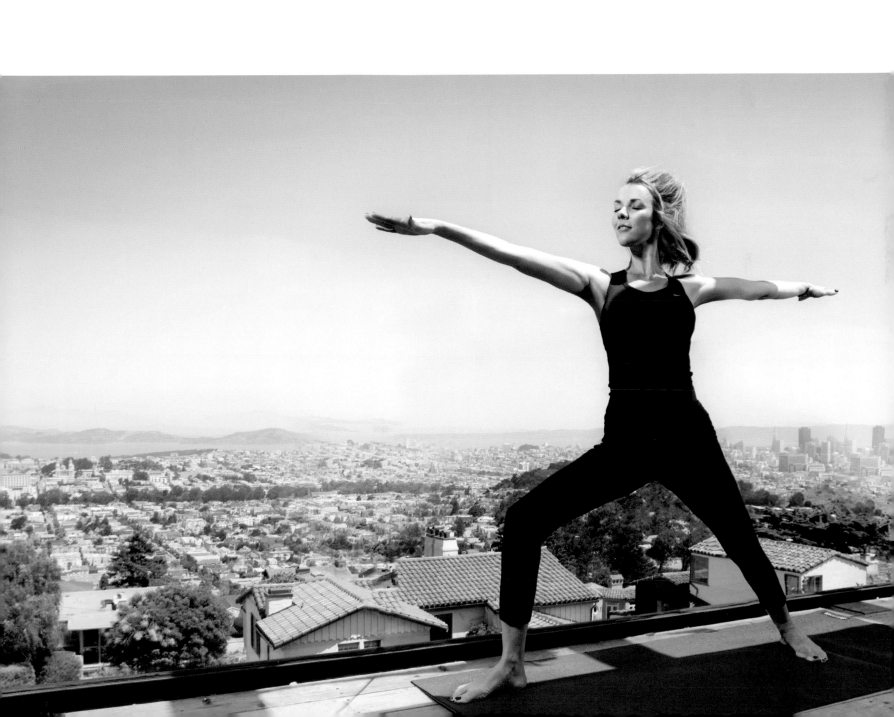

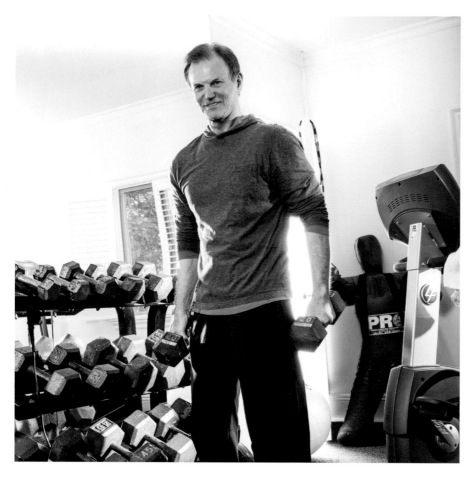

I work out four to five times a week. I'll do a variety of exercises, which keeps me from falling into a rut. My wife introduced me to Pilates and I do that twice a week. I read that a lot of professional football players, including a certain big offensive tackle, do Pilates. One player weighs about 230 pounds and I understand that he played football into his early 40s. He gives Pilates some of the credit to his longevity.

I was always so lazy about stretching, and doing Pilates and yoga force me to stretch. It feels good and makes your core strong.

For a cardio workout I prefer the treadmill at the gym and swimming on occasion. I belong to a few different gyms and I have weights at home as well.

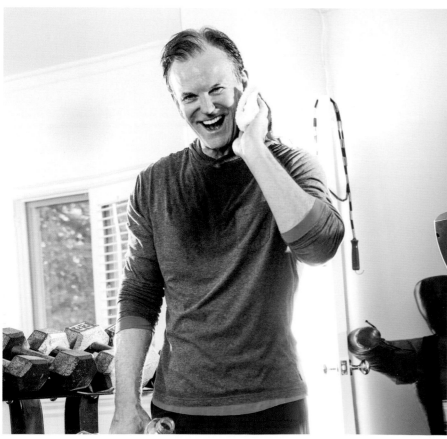

Weights are great for toning while Pilates and yoga are great for flexibility.
—*Josh Taylor*

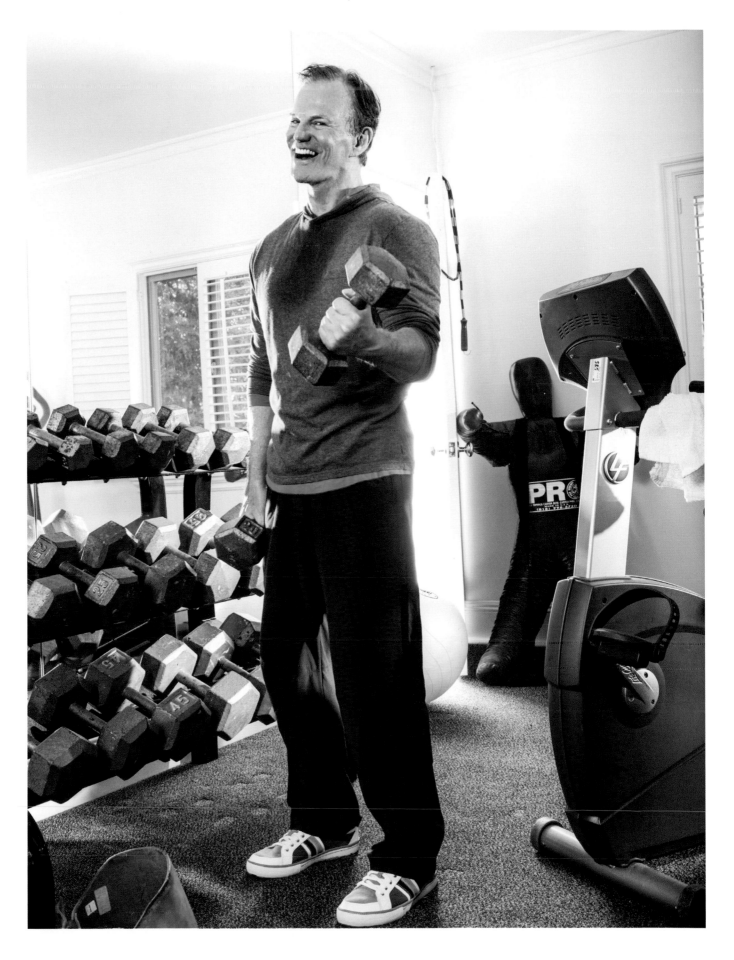

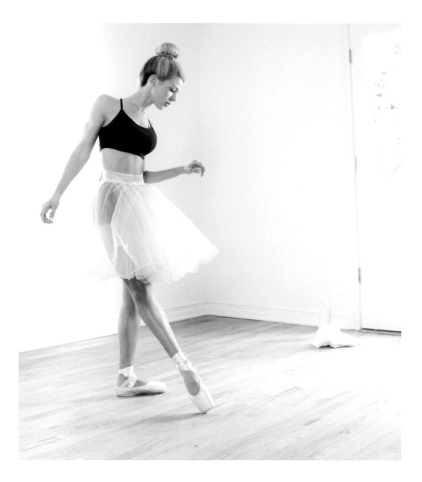
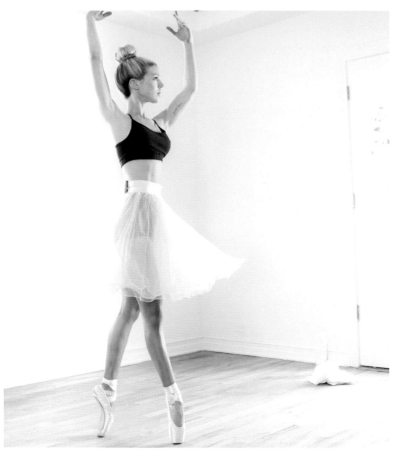
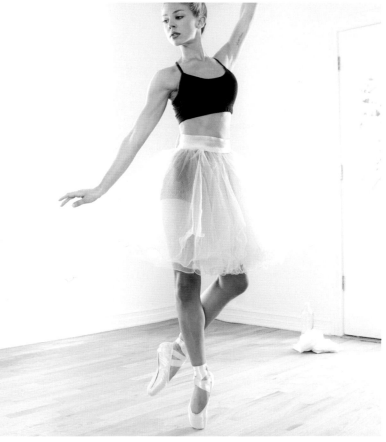
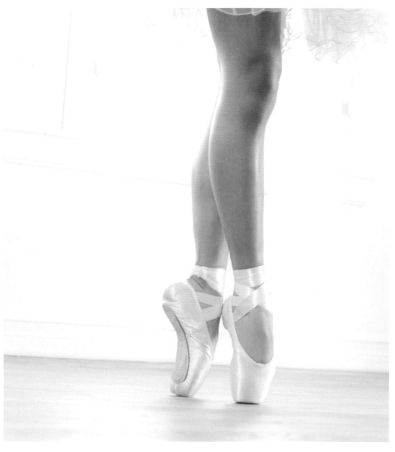

When I was very young, I started training to be a classical ballerina. Eventually, I realized I wasn't going to get as tall as I needed to be in order to pursue ballet on a professional level. Still, I have to say that dancing remains a passion of mine even today.

I grew up dancing and also horseback riding, and those are two things that I'll always do. It's not quite the same if you're not doing them competitively, but they are great ways to stay physically active. There are different dance classes out there you can take that force you to stay current. I take ballet classes in order to keep my technique up to date as much as possible.

It's really important to know yourself, your habits and what it takes to live your healthiest life.
—*Kate Mansi*

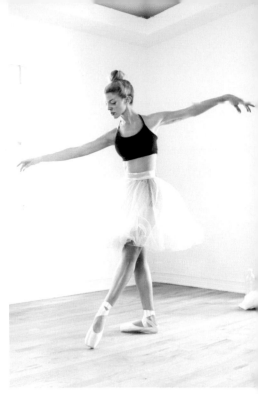

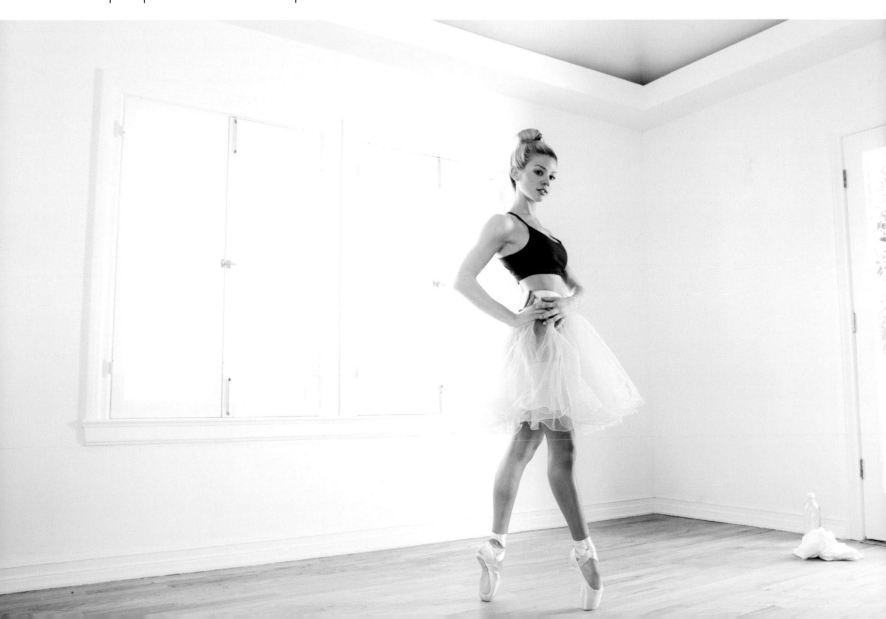

I love doing a great core workout. When you balance on a ball like this, you have to use a lot of the tinier muscles in your knees, calves and ankles. Keeping your balance on the ball involves constant adjusting so you're really working out those internal muscles.

You're working out your stomach and oblique muscles just so you don't fall off the ball. I'll do this for a while, which really warms things up.

I put the flat edge on the floor when I do this exercise, but you can reverse it and stand on the flat edge. Either way, you'll get a great core workout. If you don't have a balance bar, try using a broom stick.

People can have big accidents doing the littlest of things—like stepping off the curb the wrong way. Exercising and strengthening the smaller muscles in your body can help prevent injuries.
—Matthew Ashford

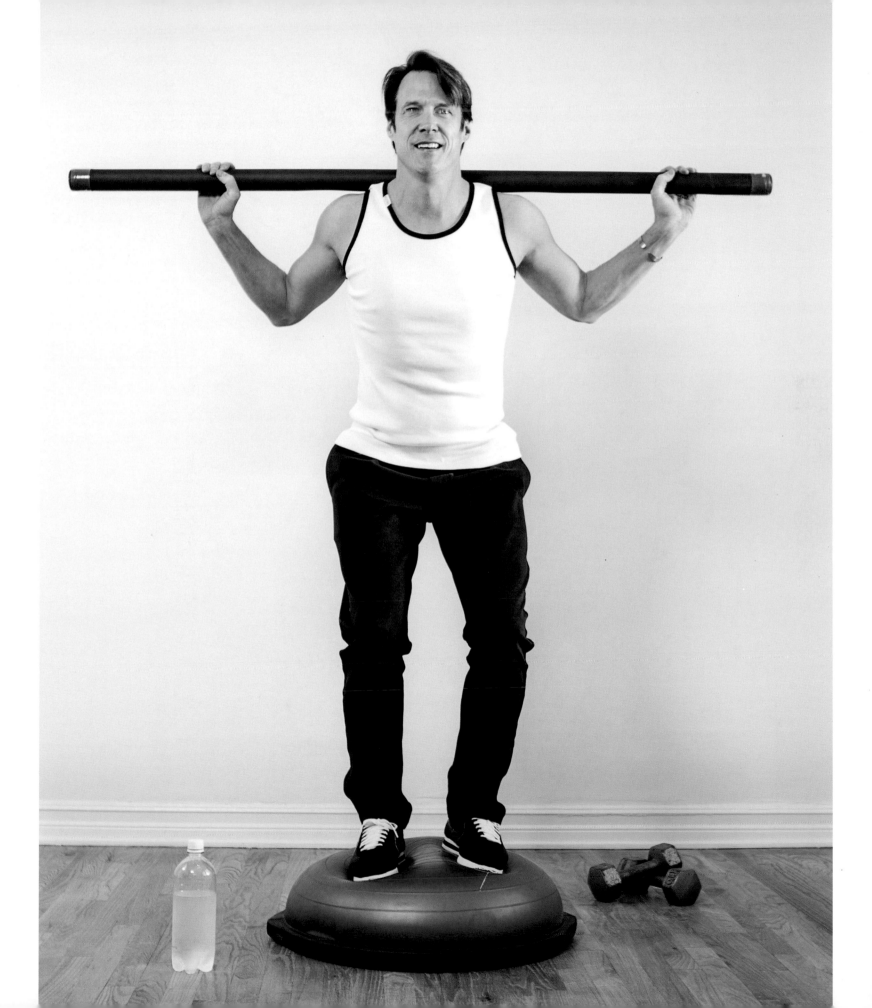

I live by the ocean. I walk. I run. I stretch. I also climb the stairs at the beach and I love to take swim classes. Swimming works for me because it's low impact. It's vital to find exercise that works for you.

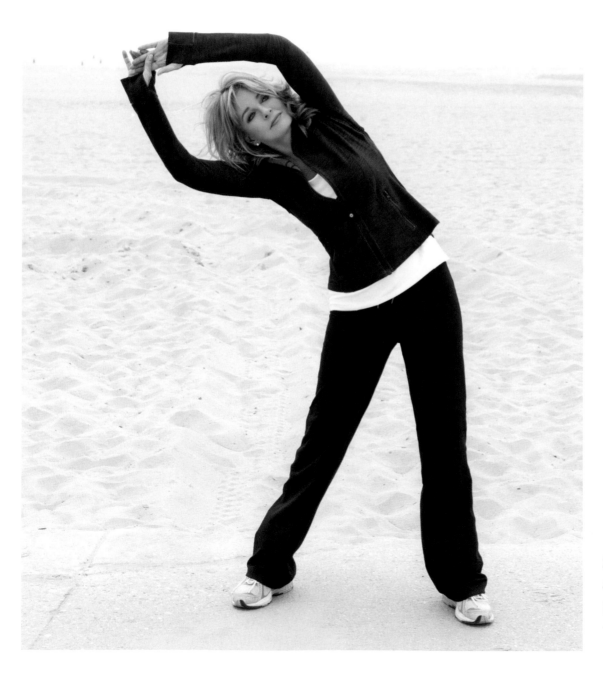

Staying active is an important part of my life!
—*Deidre Hall*

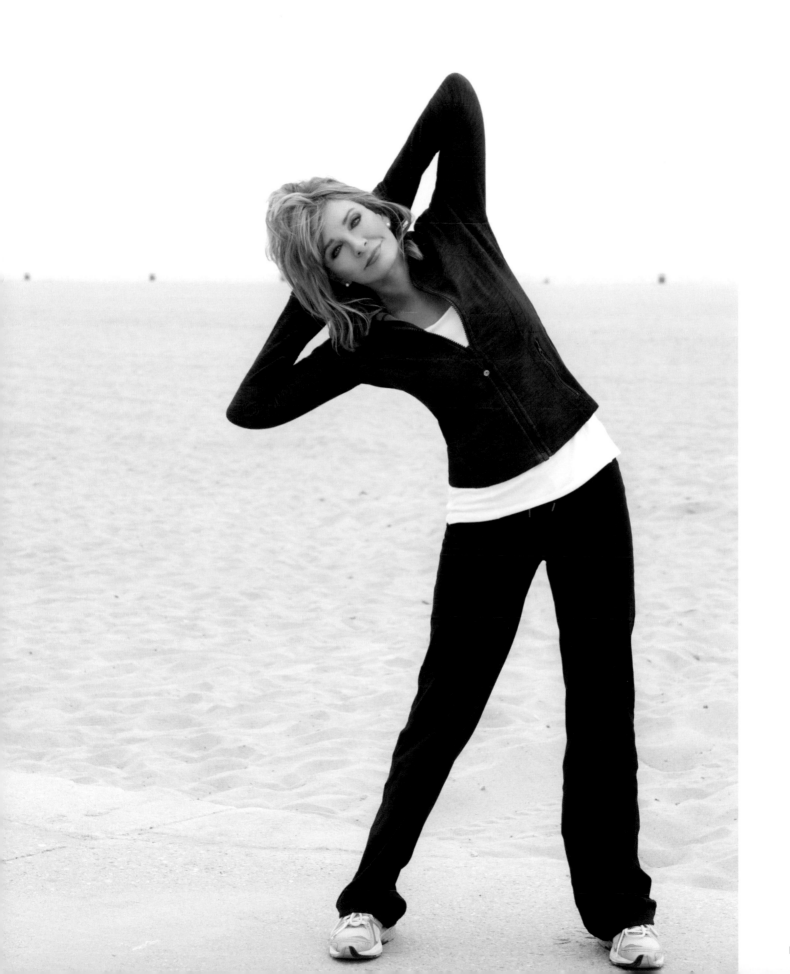

I enjoy working out on the elliptical machine. When I came back to *Days of our Lives,* I asked if it'd be okay if I put one in my dressing room and they said yes. Now, if I'm here for a long tape day or if I come in early to avoid traffic, I can do an hour on the elliptical.

I go to the gym to do TRX (suspension training, which is a pulley system that uses gravity and your own body weight). My husband told me about this and I fell in love with it after my first class. But, because of my schedule, I can't always commit to a class so I also have free weights at home.

It's fun to do activities with your children. I was at a water park with my son for 7½ hours not too long ago. We hit every slide—twice. Walking up all those stairs repeatedly was a great workout.

I try to do some form of exercise every day.
—*Eileen Davidson*

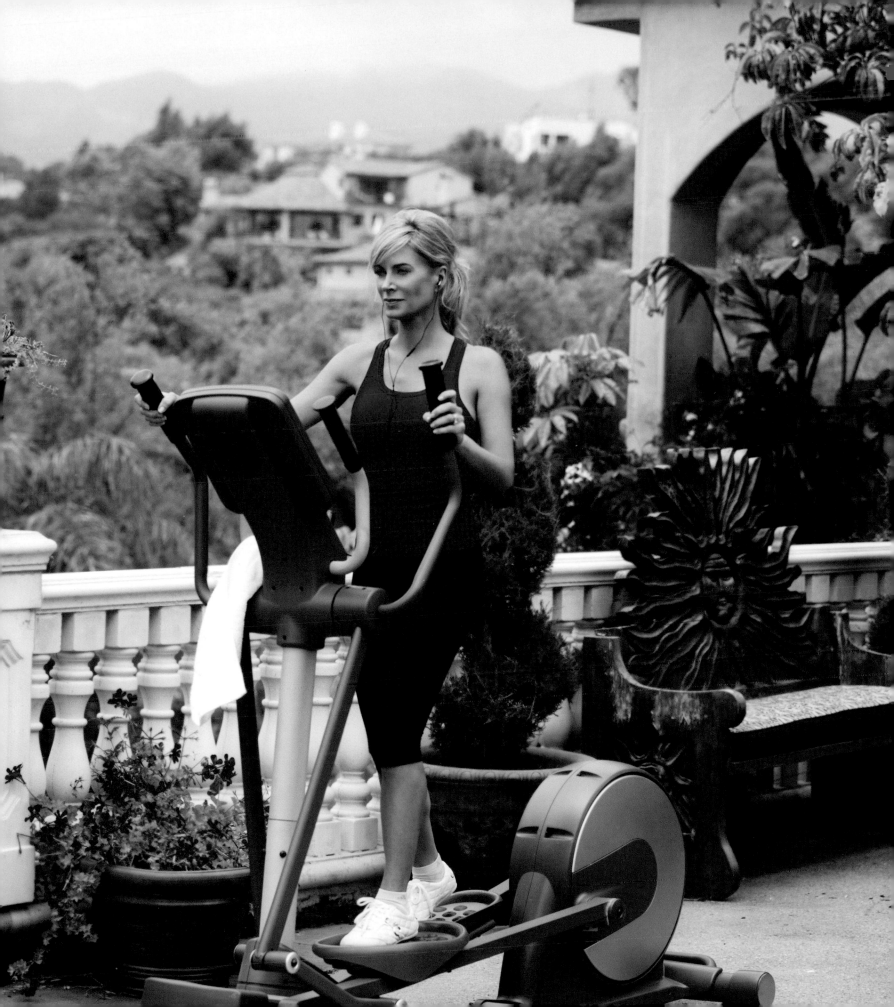

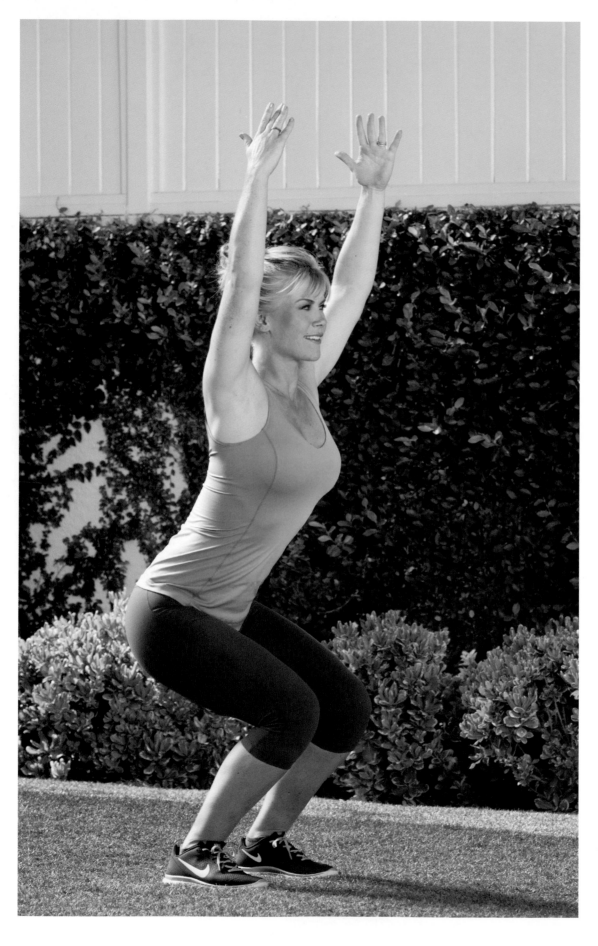

It's beneficial to do different types of exercise. I like to mix it up. I'll hike with my dog or take a basic yoga or spinning class. I'll work out anywhere from 40 minutes to 2 hours. I stretch every morning and night and I break a good sweat at least once a day.

Part of mixing up your workout routines is not only what you do, but where you do it. I like to exercise outside.

When it comes to exercising, find things that you like to do. Make working out enjoyable.
—*Alison Sweeney*

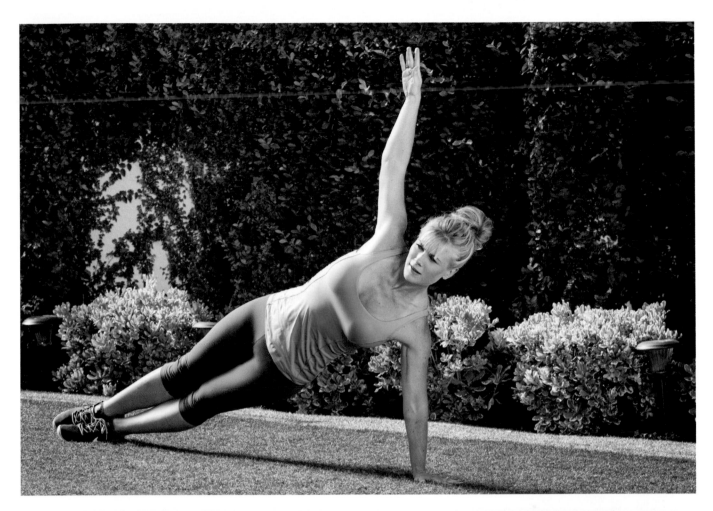

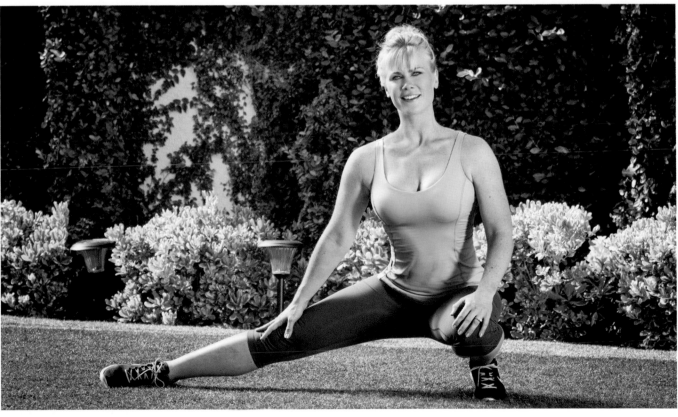

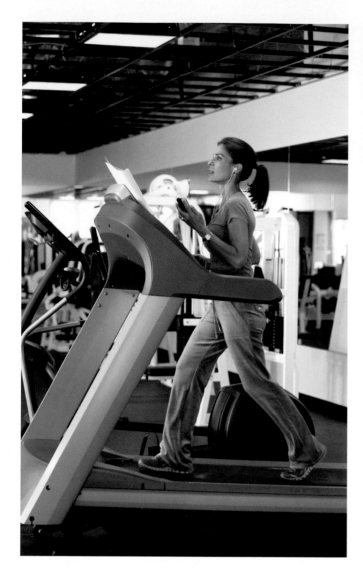 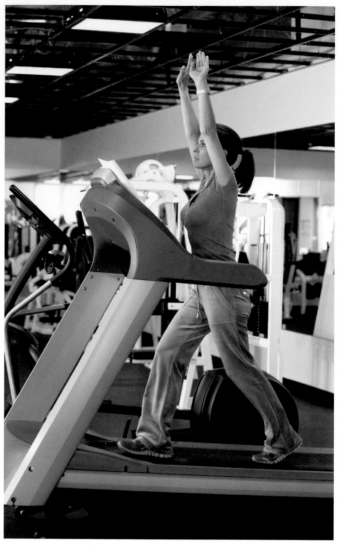

I start out slow and get my body warmed up. Then, I gradually increase my speed to burn more calories.

I like to do stretches while walking.

I listen to music that inspires me or I learn my lines while walking on the treadmill. This is my way of multitasking.
—Kristian Alfonso

I actually used to have a treadmill at home, but I found that it was just too loud for me. It was distracting to have it in the house so I gave the treadmill to a friend, who was working at losing weight. Now, I go to the gym either before or after work. There are days that I miss, of course, but I try to get there almost every day.

I'll walk on the treadmill at an incline. For walking, my top speed is 4.0 with an incline of 8. I walk a minimum of four miles. I work out by myself. Because of my schedule I can't be locked into something like meeting a trainer. I get in and out. I'll bring my scripts with me.

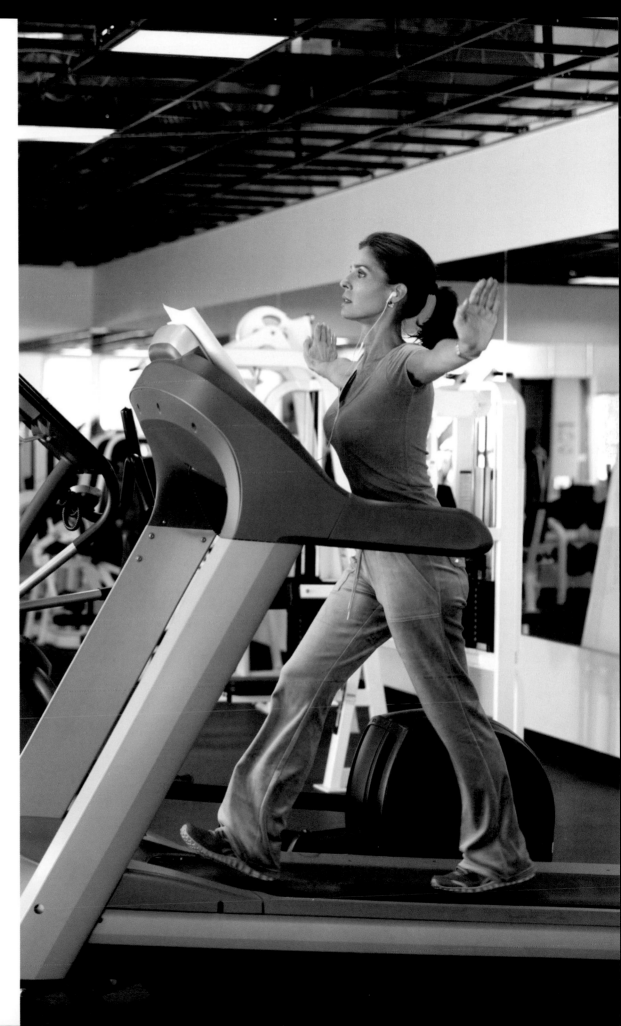

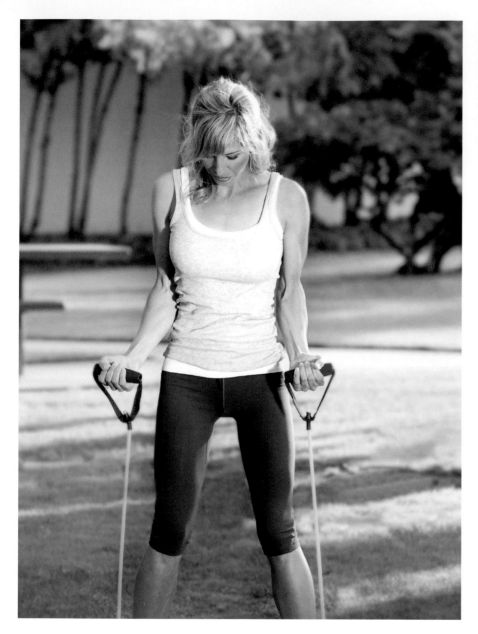

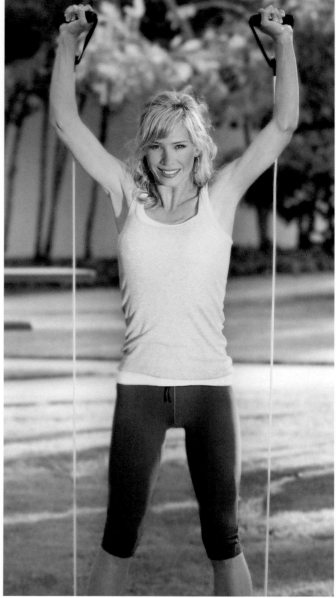

I was a gymnast for most of my life, and I continue to stay in shape. I don't lift weights at all. I prefer resistance bands for toning. They travel well and are inexpensive. I snowboard as much as I can on the weekends and I love doing yoga. I have a trainer named Jeff Phillips, who used to be on *Guiding Light*. I've known Jeff since I was 16 years old. He's an amazing trainer.

If you don't like exercising or if you find that you're just not doing it, find someone who motivates you. Stay active and get regular exercise each week.

—*Sarah Brown*

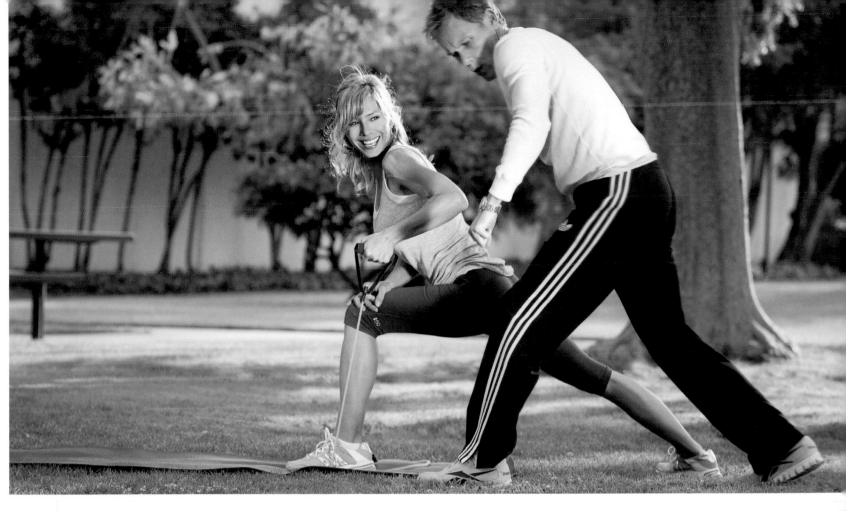
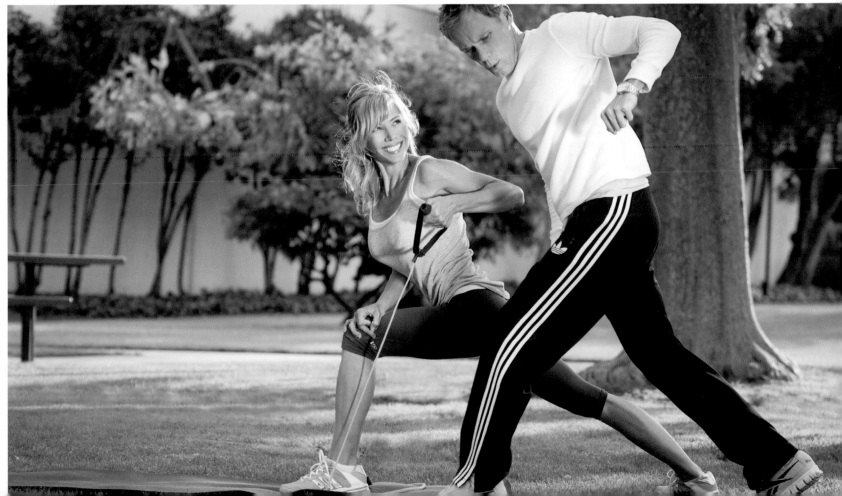

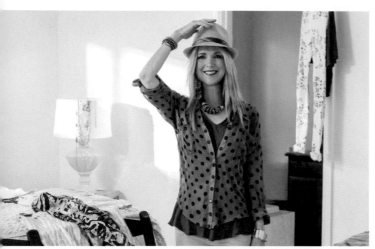
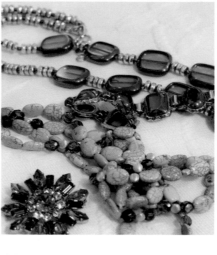
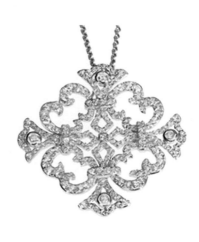
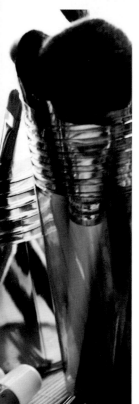
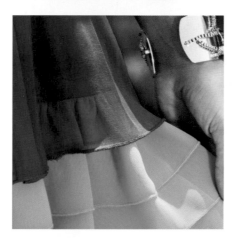
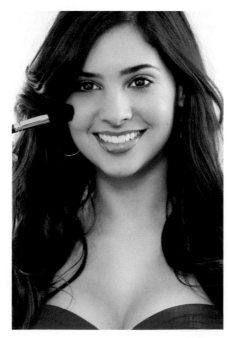
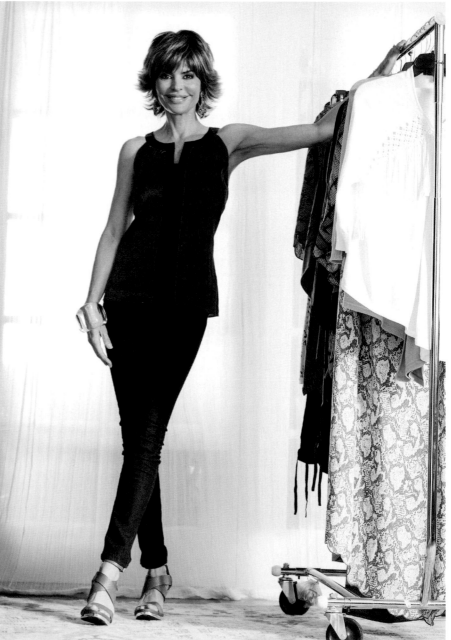

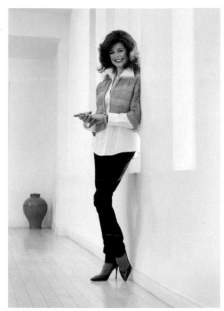
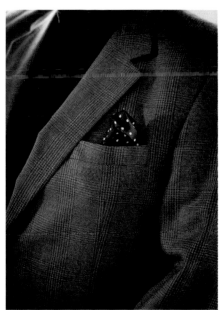
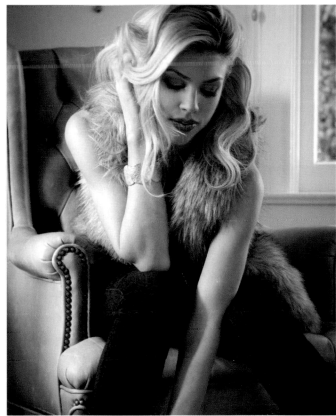
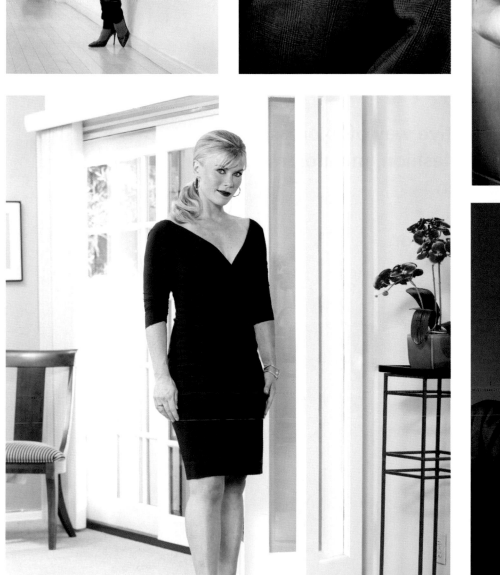
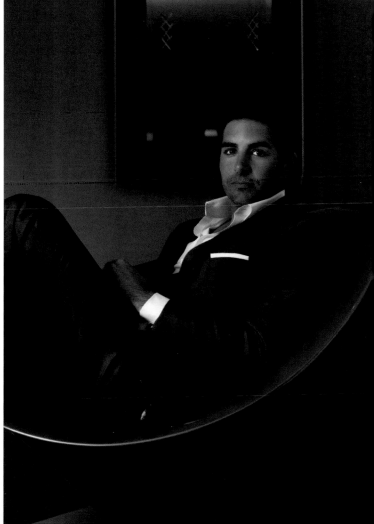

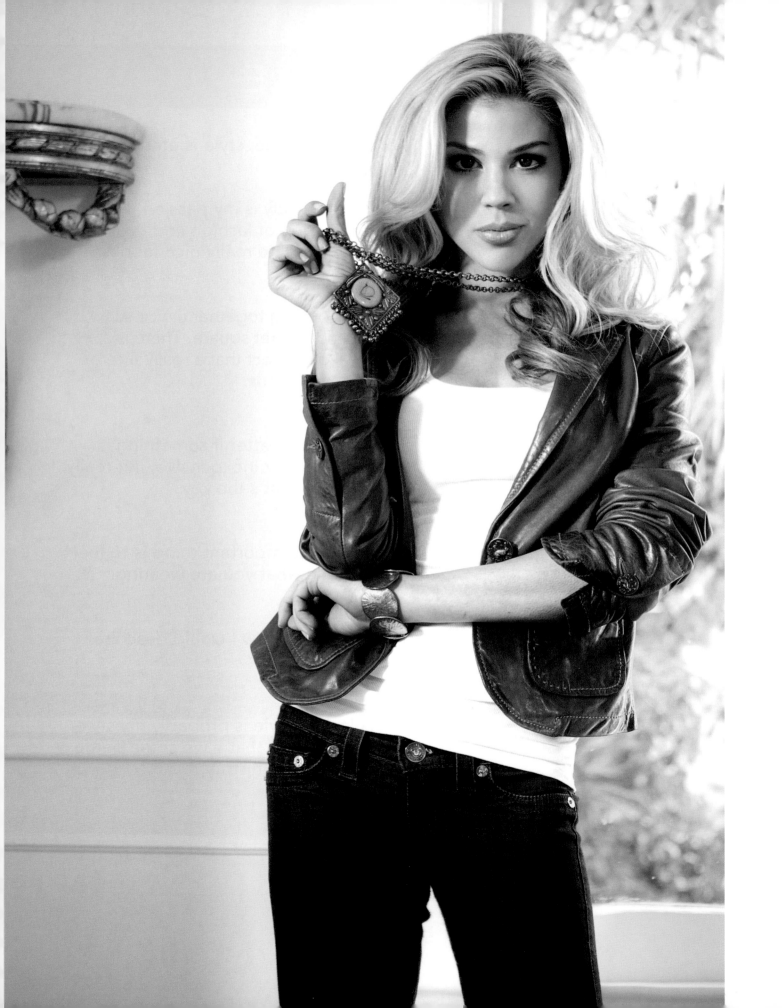

My own style is very different from Abby's. Abby has a very "girlie" style. She's very feminine and loves accessories, pinks and floral prints. I'm a bit more of a tomboy mixed with "Bohemian chic." I really enjoy taking chances and mixing things up. Nobody's ever described me as someone who follows the rules—like the one about not wearing gold and silver at the same time.

Shopping at flea markets and in vintage stores on the weekends are things that I love to do. I like finding things that are special and I find more one-of-a-kind looks there. As far as stores go, I like Urban Outfitters and Fred Segal, too.

A key for me is to build my look around one unique statement piece, either an amazing necklace or vintage jacket, and then add simple basics to finish the look.

The most important thing about style is to feel good about what you're wearing.
—Kate Mansi

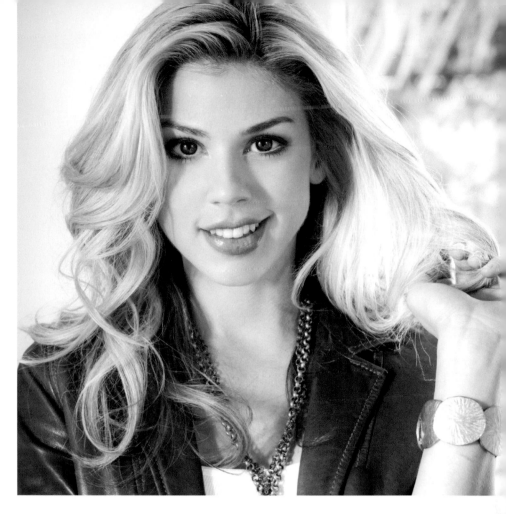

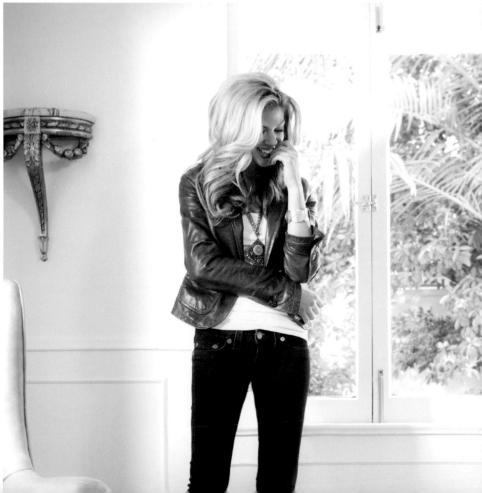

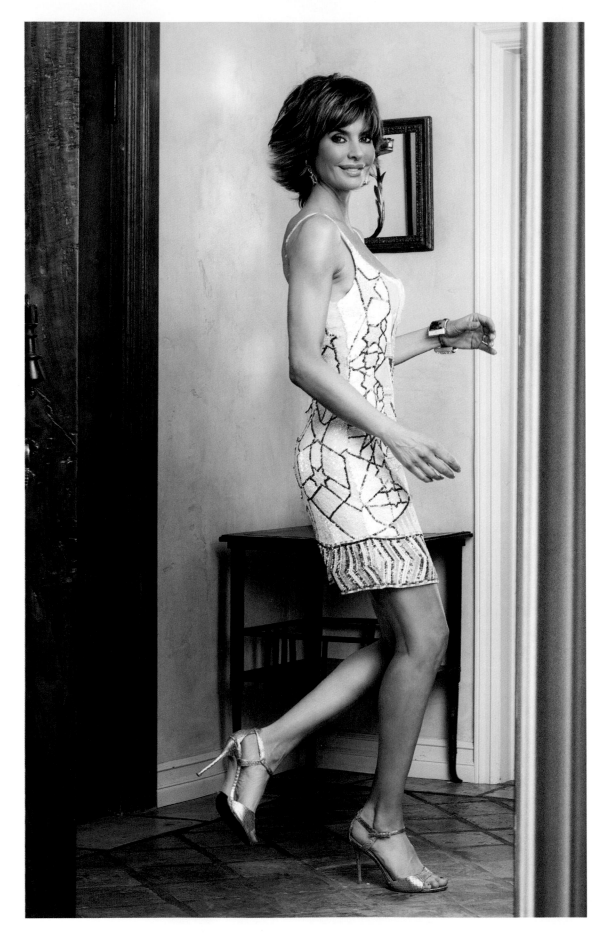

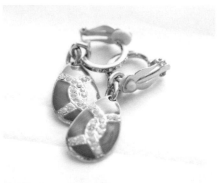

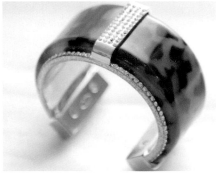

Fashion truly is my passion. I love the expression of it! Don't be afraid to go with bold accessories. They can make or break an outfit. You can look sexy at any age, it's just a matter of doing it tastefully.
—Lisa Rinna

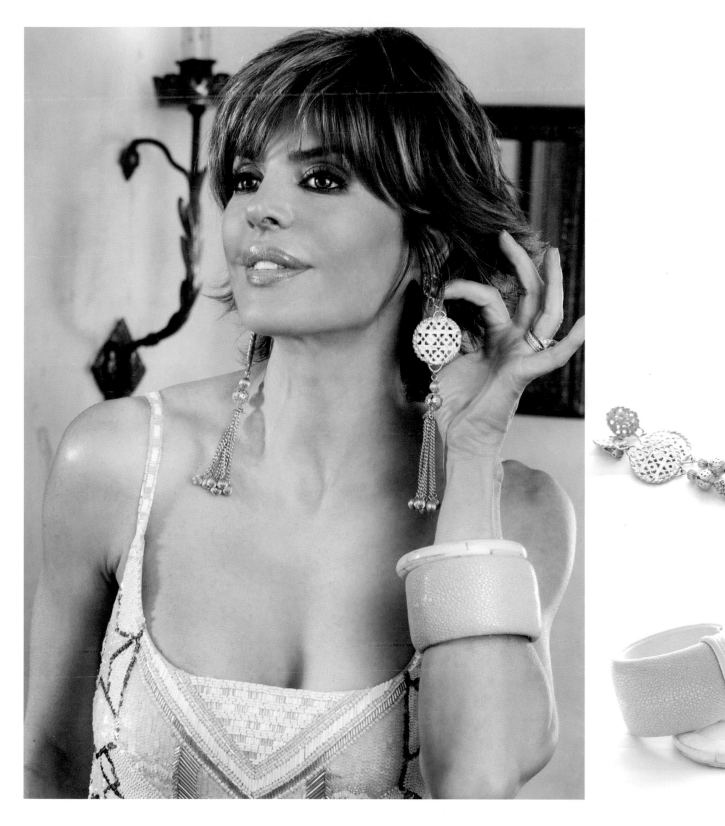

It's funny when you try to describe your own style. I would say mine is constantly evolving, but I like to think that it's always been simple, classic and chic. I know what I like: I enjoy really nice fabrics and things that are made well. My sense of style is always evolving.

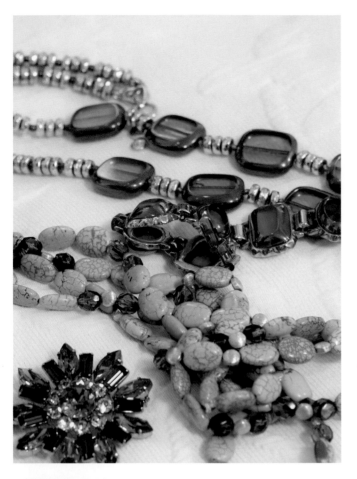

Perhaps it's because I've been so preoccupied with close-ups on television, but I believe in fashion that leads the eye to the face. I like earrings that have a little impact and face-framing necklines. Generally, I like solid colors. I was impressed by Audrey Hepburn, who advised wearing beige and black. Why wear anything else? Of course, she dressed in all sorts of colors throughout her life. She was slender and tall, two things I am not, but I took the beige and black part of her advice. That's a lot of what my own personal wardrobe looks like.

I've learned to love the color blue. My eyes are blue so I'll think, "Maybe a drop of blue in this outfit would be nice?" If you stick to a smaller color palette you're apt to make fewer mistakes.

The plenitude of cheap, comfortable clothing that exists is a constant temptation to keep adding to your wardrobe, but I think you'd do better to have fewer items in your closet that are of great quality. Wait until they've passed their prime and then move on from them.

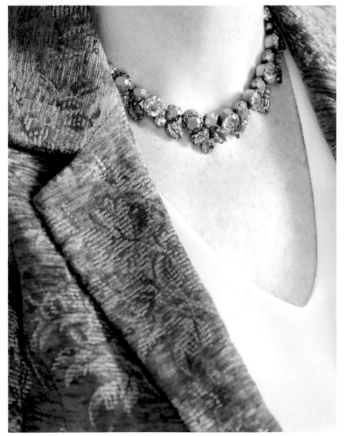

"It's a character flaw, an indulgence," Susan Seaforth Hayes says of her lifelong fascination with admiring and shopping for jewelry. But don't think the actress is out there breaking the bank as she adds to her eclectic and tasteful collection of necklaces, rings and bracelets.

"Susan is not a spendthrift," says Bill Hayes, her always-supportive husband. "She buys inexpensive jewelry and loves matching this to that. She gets great pleasure out of it."

"I do," Susan adds. "I feel very childlike when I open my jewelry packages. I love going on quests where I might find a wonderful old broach in Toledo and then realize it's a great match to some earrings that I'd purchased in Albuquerque ten years earlier."

"And," Bill says, "that broach will only have cost $2.50."

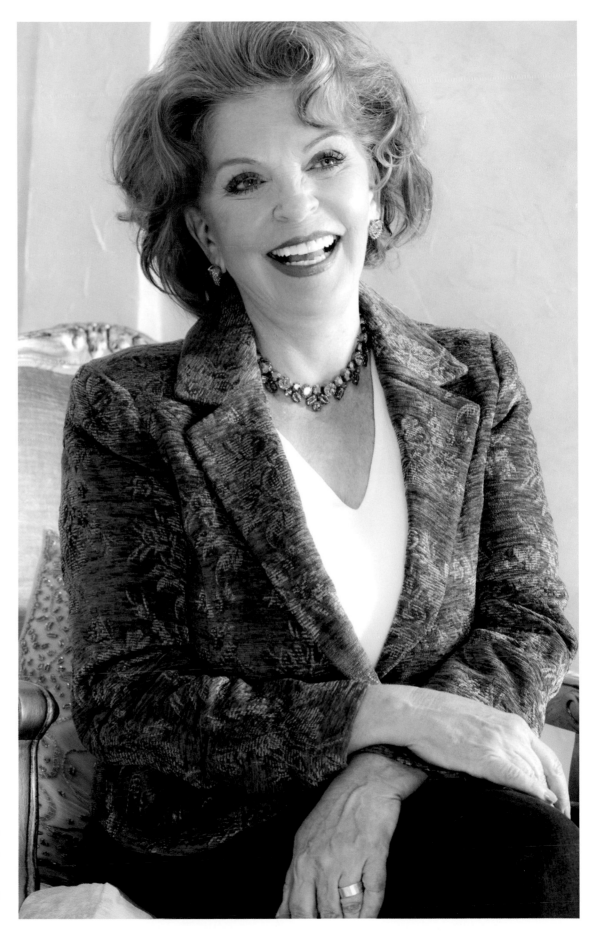

Try to dress for the times—and not like the time when you were 16.
—*Susan Seaforth Hayes*

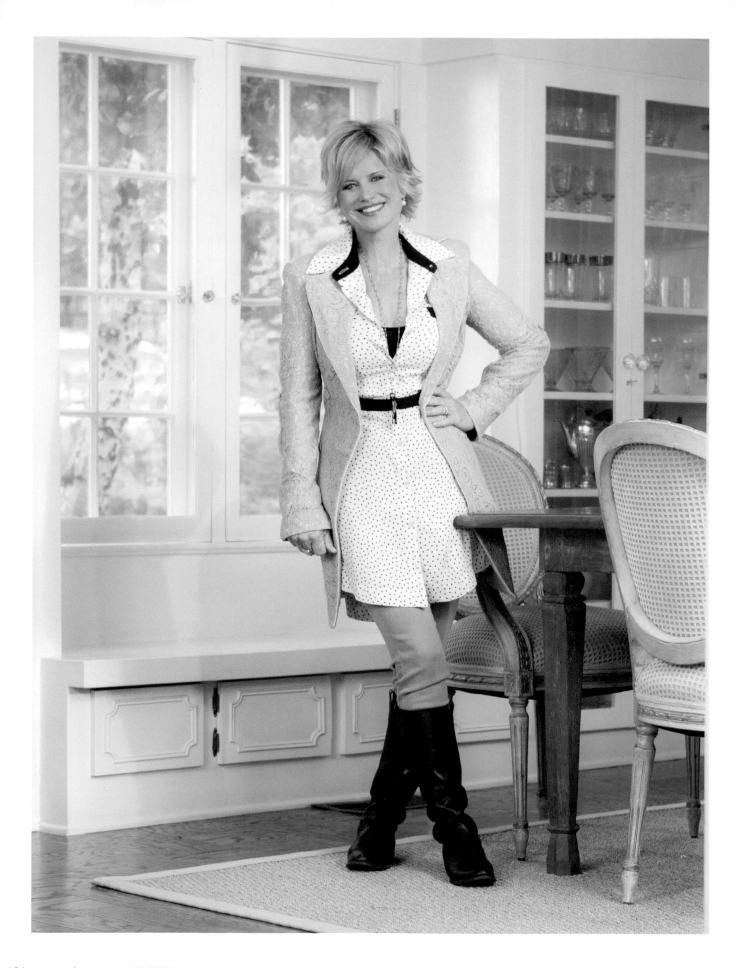

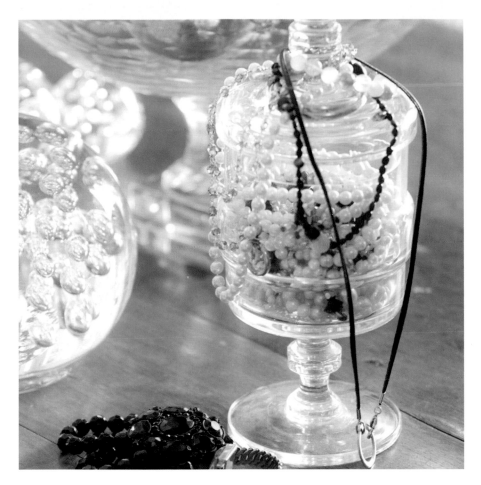

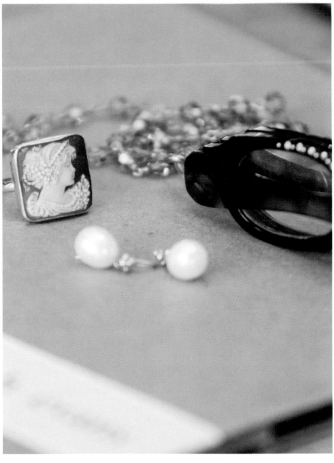

Layering can make an outfit look more polished. I love to pair a crisp blouse with a button-up vest, a funky skirt and a pair of riding boots—it's about having fun with your style!

My style is eclectic both in the way I dress and what I buy for my house. My home has so much stuff in it from swap meets and flea markets. I like to dress a little funky. My clothing style is more funky than it is classic.

I used to get things for my house at this giant swap meet at the Rose Bowl in Pasadena. I used to go there a lot, but now I don't have room in my home for anything else. If I run out of space for something I might put it in my garden.

I like funkier, more eclectic stuff. I'll wear a sweater vest with a jacket. I like it funky. I don't do a tight skirt and blouse. That's not my thing.
—*Mary Beth Evans*

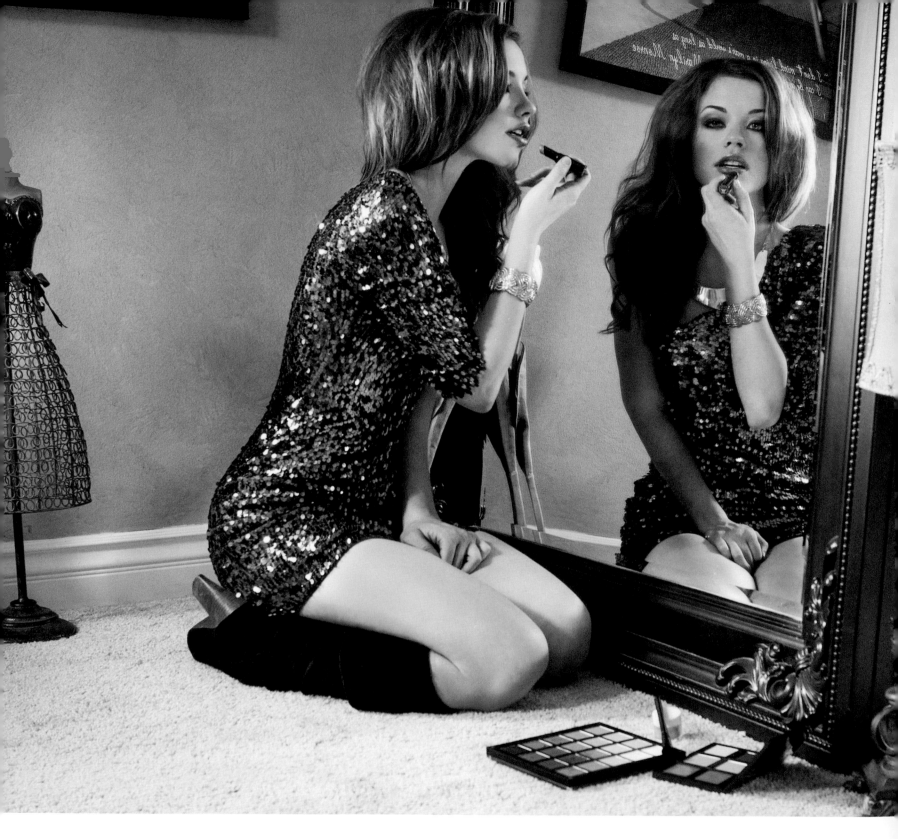

Less is more when it comes to makeup, but every now and then I like a smokey eye and a great red lipstick.
—*Molly Burnett*

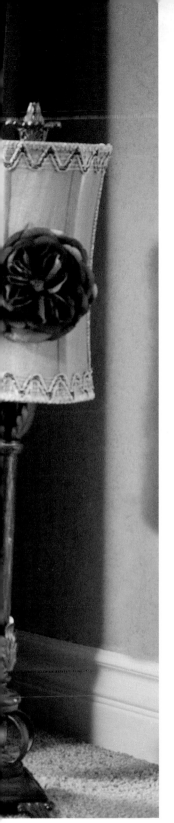

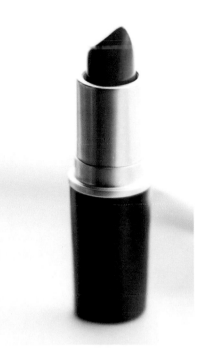

I'm a big fan of being comfortable when it comes to wearing clothes. I'm happy in jean shorts and a T-shirt or a beach dress. I also enjoy skinny black jeans and funky high heels when I'm feeling "girly."

When it comes to makeup, I love a light swoosh of hot pink blush! It makes me feel girly! I also like to line the top lid with a black liquid line, which adds a little "cat eye" for fun. I also love glitter—not outrageous over-the-top glitter, which I do save for some special occasions, but just a little sparkly glitter. Of course, this is all relevant when I'm actually wearing makeup, which isn't very often! Red lips are fun for a dramatic look for a special evening out.

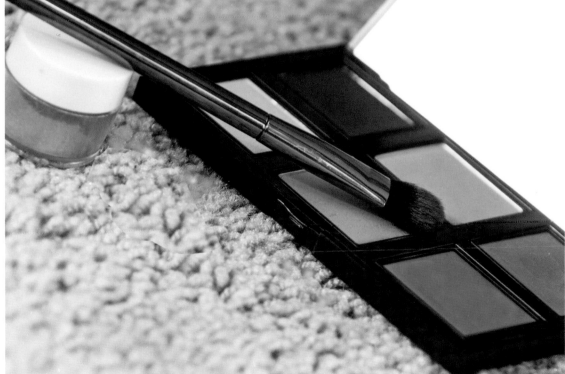

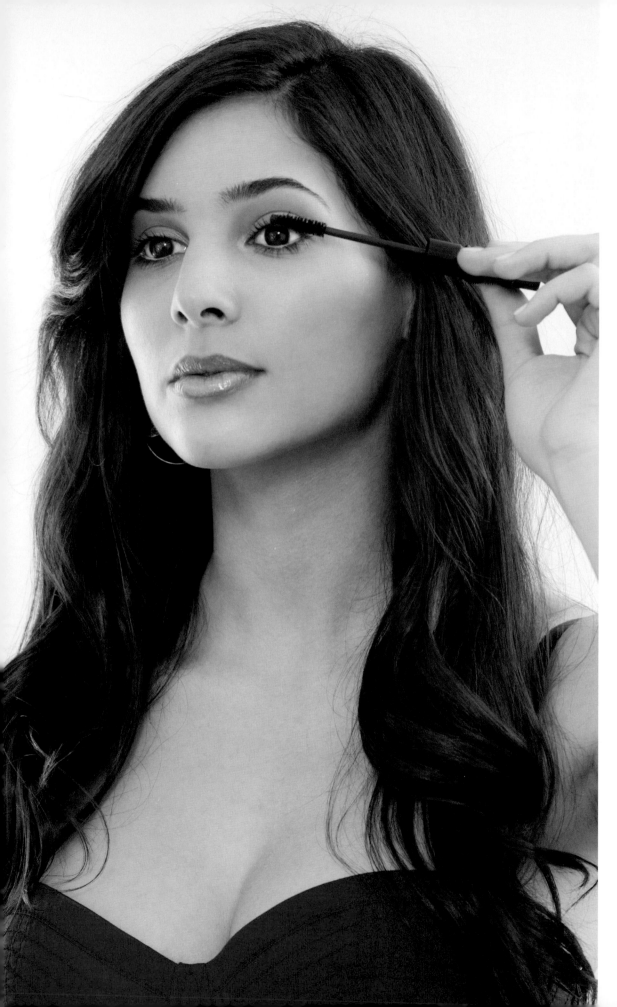

I embrace moisture. It does wonders for my face and makes my hair beautifully curly and defined.

—*Camila Banus*

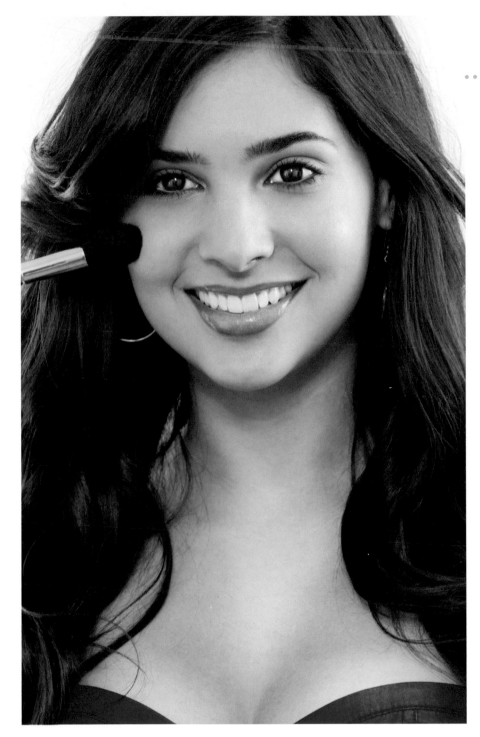

LESS IS MORE!

I've lived in both Los Angeles and in Miami and the styles of those cities can be similar, but I would say that L.A. is more "Bohemian." I definitely still have my Miami-style with me, which is dressing in really bright colors like fuchsia, orange and yellow. I'm a "beach baby," too. I love wearing sandals and linen clothing. I'll wear bathing suits under tunics. That's a very "Miami" thing to do.

There are times when I'll be going out to events and I try to dress a little like Kim Kardashian by wearing short, tight mini-dresses. It's fun! When I'm in L.A., which is a dry climate, I have to put a leave-in conditioner in my hair and moisturizer on my face.

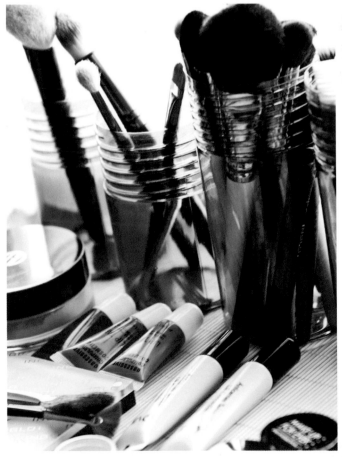

Tips for healthy hair and skin:
1. Wear only a small amount of makeup on your downtime.
2. Apply a scrub once a week and a toner to get oil out.
3. Once a month use a hairmask to lock in moisture.

MOISTURIZE!

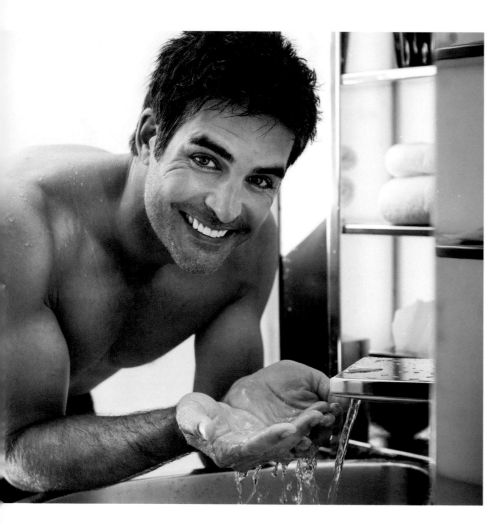

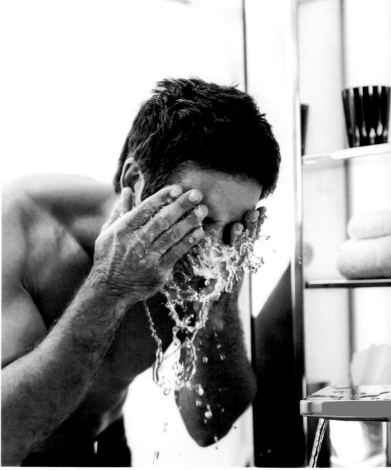

Skin care is important. I drink a lot of water, which keeps my skin clear. I also believe in washing my face with the right products. I moisturize daily and wear sunscreen, too.

I spend a lot of time outdoors and have seen the damage the sun can cause. Therefore, I always make a point to wear sunblock. If you are active, you must make sure it is sweat-proof.
—*Galen Gering*

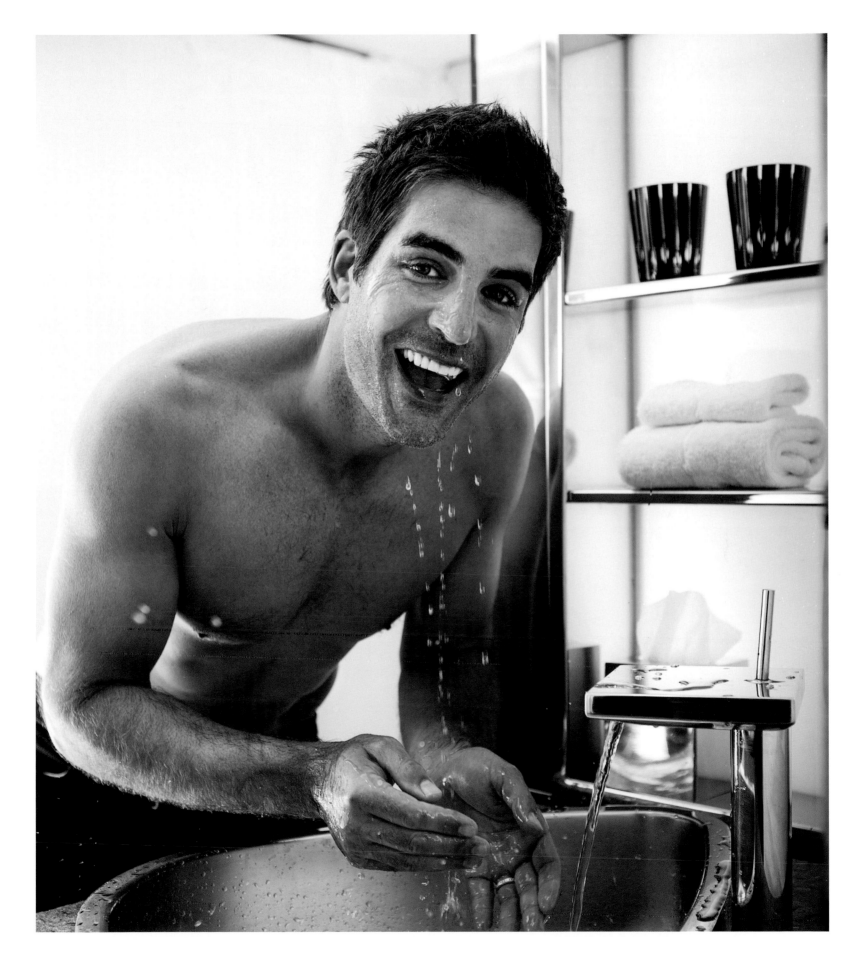

HAIRSTYLES

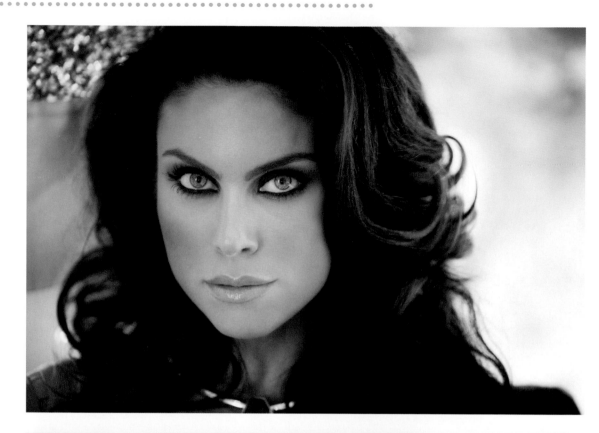

Nadia
Bjorlin

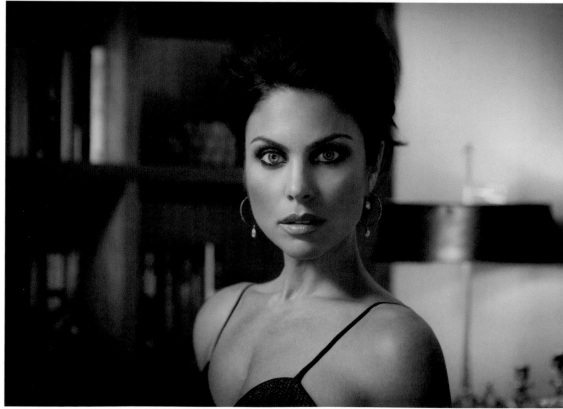

Down for day,
up for night!

Alison
Sweeney

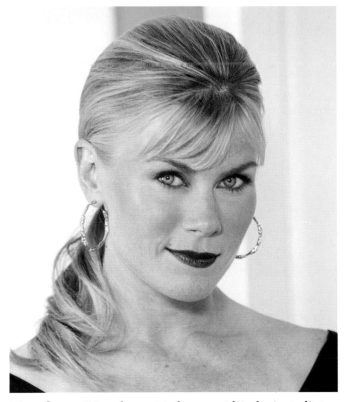

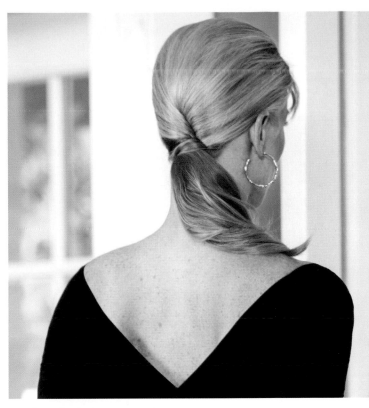

Tips from Matthew Holman, Ali's hairstylist:
Ali's side pony tail

1. Blow dry hair using volume spray.
2. Gather all hair to one side with a soft brush.
3. Twist hair at base and pin in place.

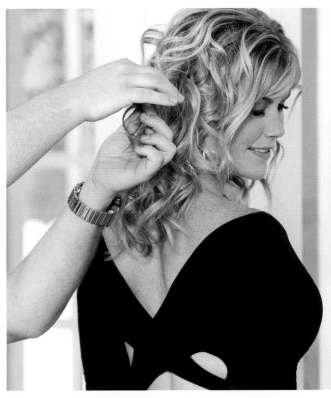

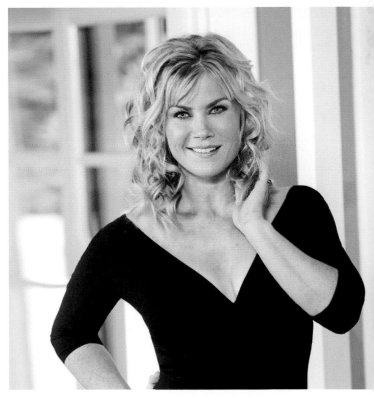

Ali's wavy beach look

1. Dry hair and create curls with hair wand.

2. Break up waves with fingers and finish with
   molding paste.

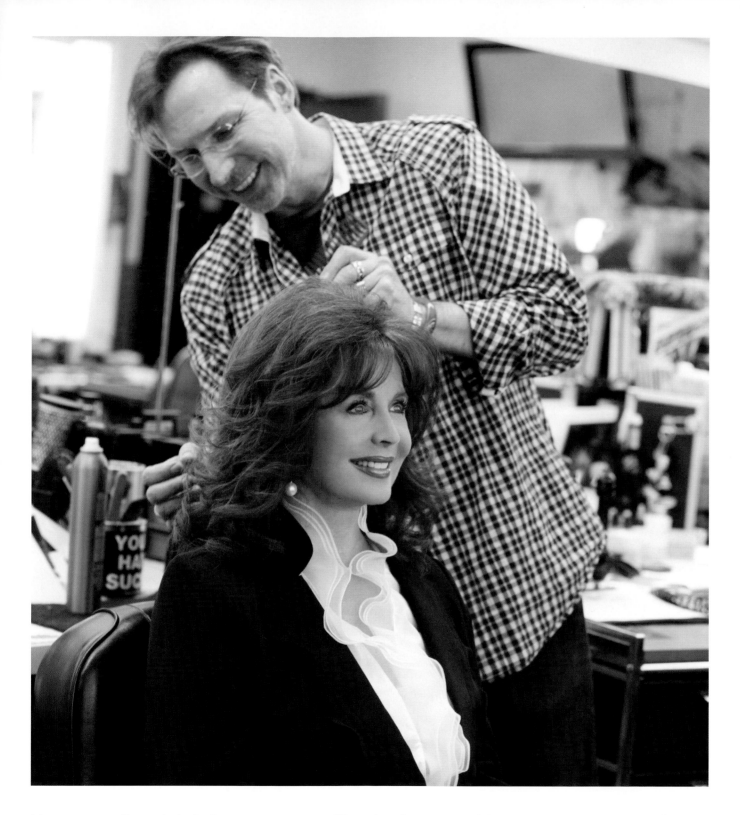

I have naturally curly hair, but not everyone likes that because it blows up on camera. I wash my hair with a cleansing conditioner, which doesn't strip my hair of its natural oils. I'll set my hair in curlers after I wash it and let it set on the days that I'm not working. That keeps it from getting too frizzy and curly. I don't use rubber bands to keep my hair together. Instead, I use clips.

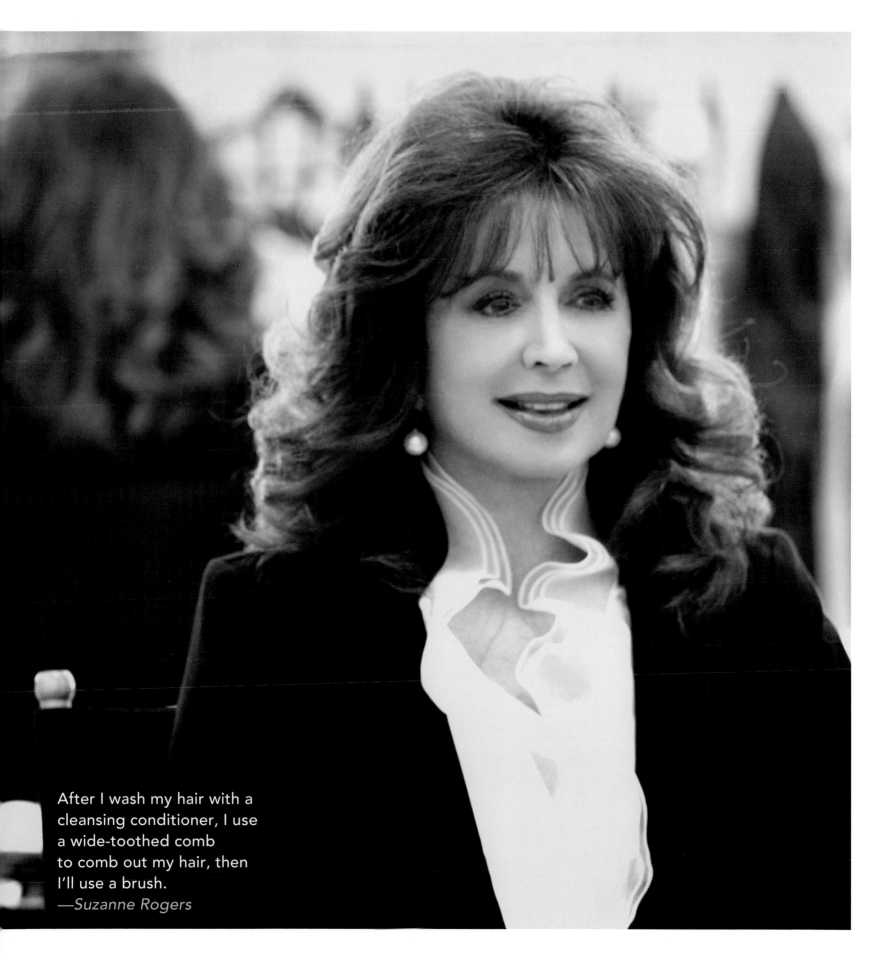

After I wash my hair with a cleansing conditioner, I use a wide-toothed comb to comb out my hair, then I'll use a brush.
—Suzanne Rogers

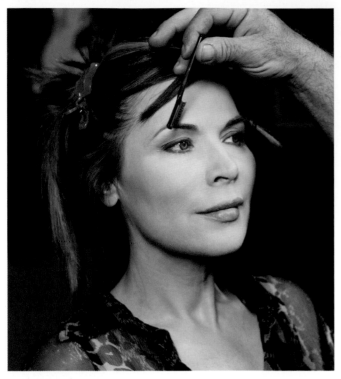

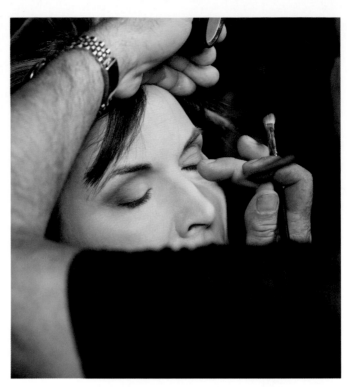

1. Start by shaping and enhancing the eyebrow with at least two colors of brow pencil for texture. Choose one color that matches your eyebrow and then go lighter or darker with the other color.

2. Add mystery by applying a deep dark shadow from your lash line to your eyelid and blend out.

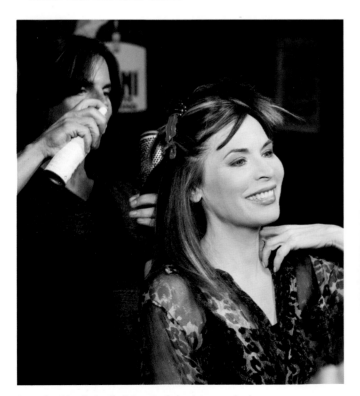

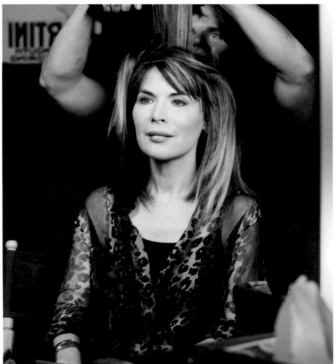

3. A simple "up-do" says nighttime and glamour.

4. Create intrigue by slightly veiling the eyes with wispy bangs. Lifting and teasing will add volume.

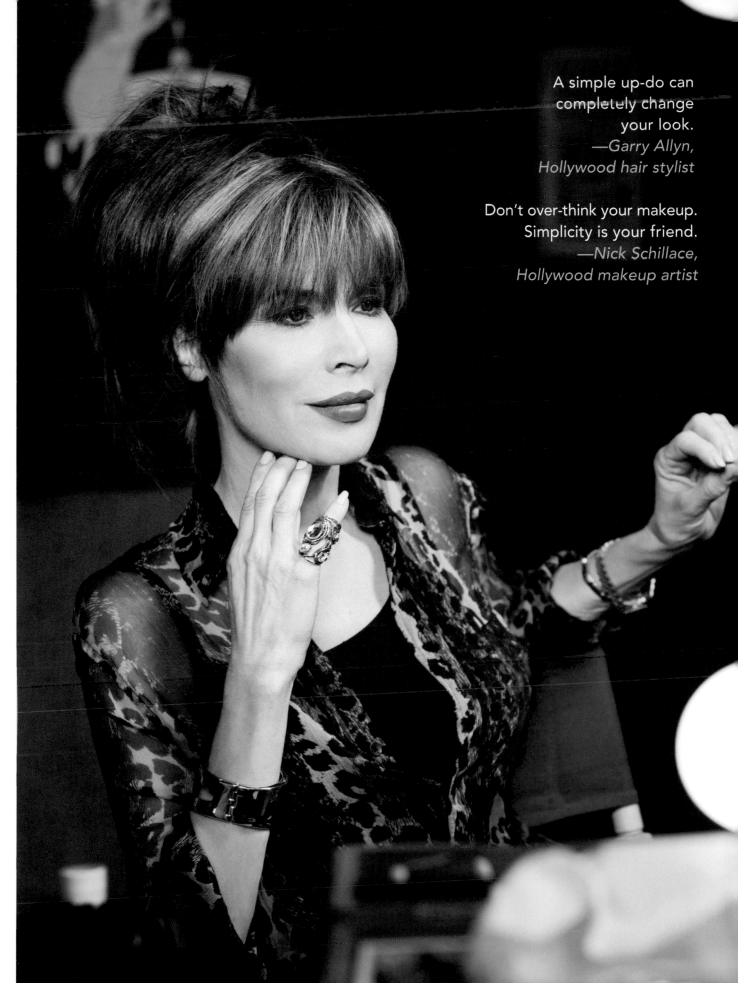

A simple up-do can completely change your look.
—*Garry Allyn,*
Hollywood hair stylist

Don't over-think your makeup. Simplicity is your friend.
—*Nick Schillace,*
Hollywood makeup artist

Lauren
Koslow

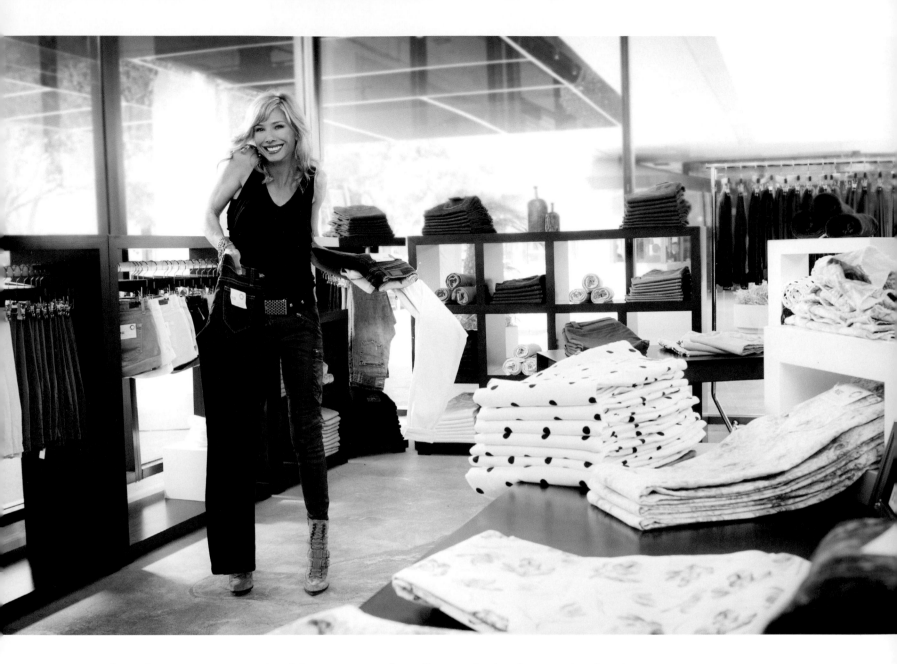

I'm a total tomboy in my everyday life, but I like to get dressed up when I go out somewhere fancy. My style is a cross between classic and simplicity. I don't like a lot of loud stuff. I like to be either in all black or all white or even polka dots.

I love great shoes and because I have so many I must have total organization in my closet. There will be organization! I have a

lot of great little shoe racks that I get from Bed, Bath and Beyond. It's not expensive, but they have everything.

If I'm not wearing something anymore, I'll give it away to charity. I don't save many things if I haven't worn them in a long time, but I do have this beautiful pair of Dolce & Gabbana shoes that are now considered vintage. I wore them out to dinner with my daughter, Jordan, recently and received some nice compliments.

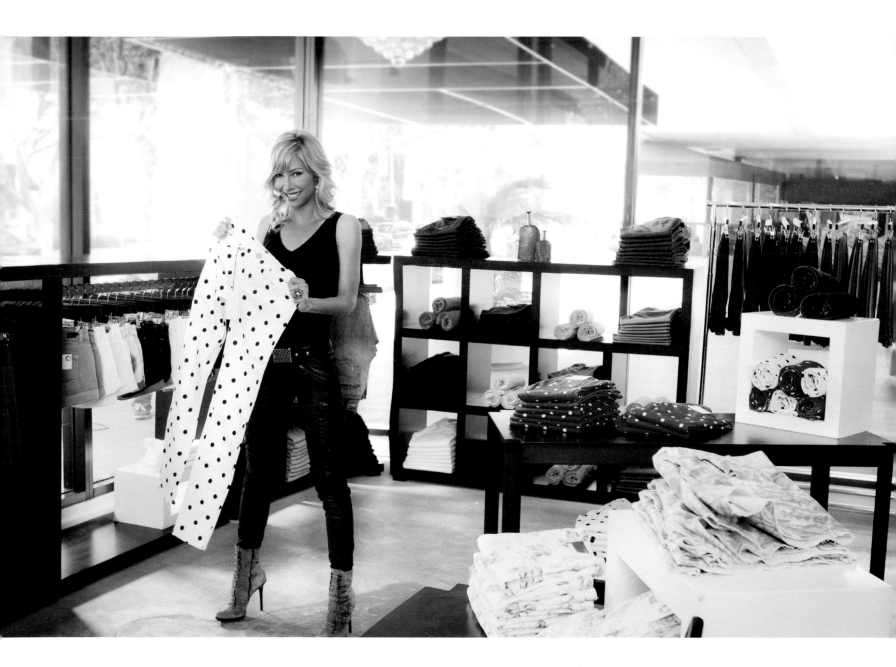

My style icon is Jacqueline Kennedy Onassis.
She showed how you could be beautiful,
put together and yet still be sexy.
She had such style!
—*Sarah Brown*

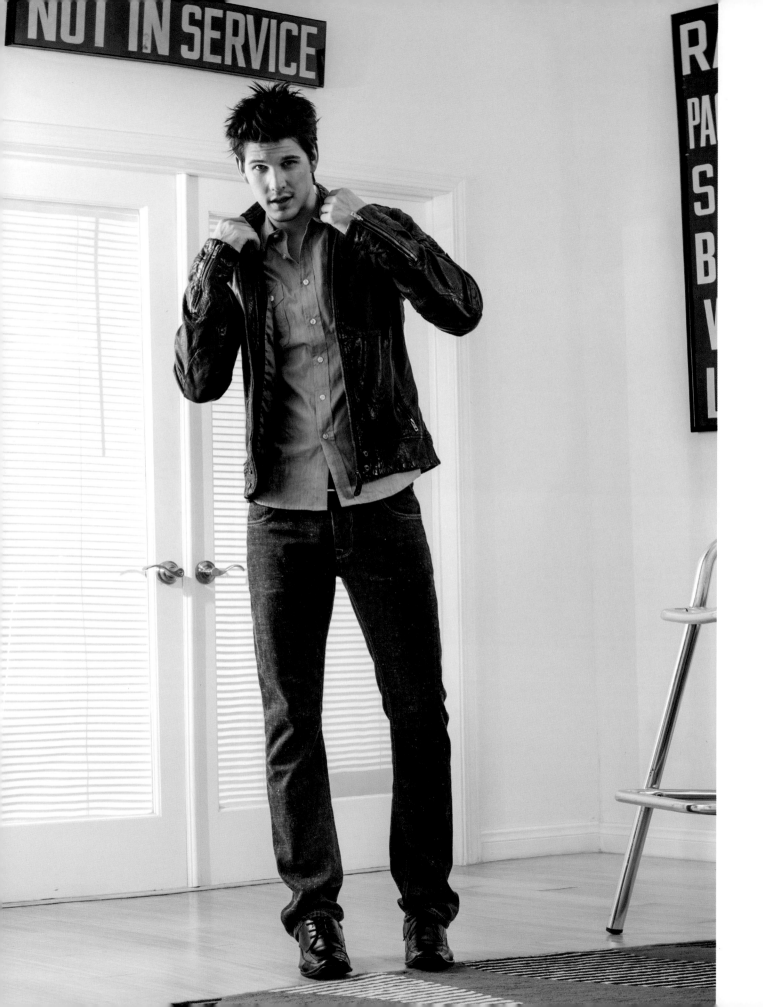

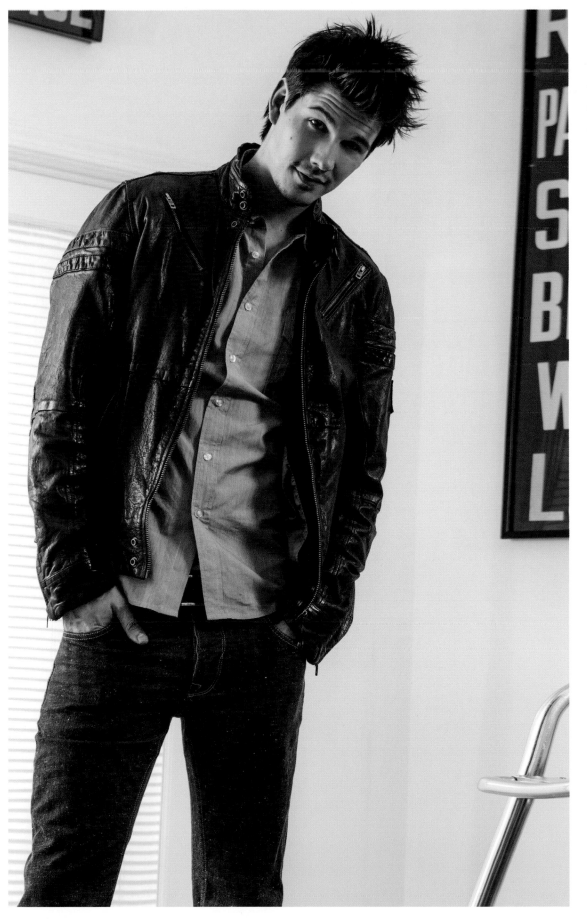

My style off-camera is pretty similar to what you see on-camera. I am not into flashy things or labels. There's a trend going around now with studded hats, shirts and pants, but that's too flashy for me.

I like black jeans, T-shirts and Converse sneakers. The splashiest thing I'll do is wear a leather jacket. I'm obsessed with leather jackets.

I feel confident when I'm wearing something that's simple.
—Casey Jon Deidrick

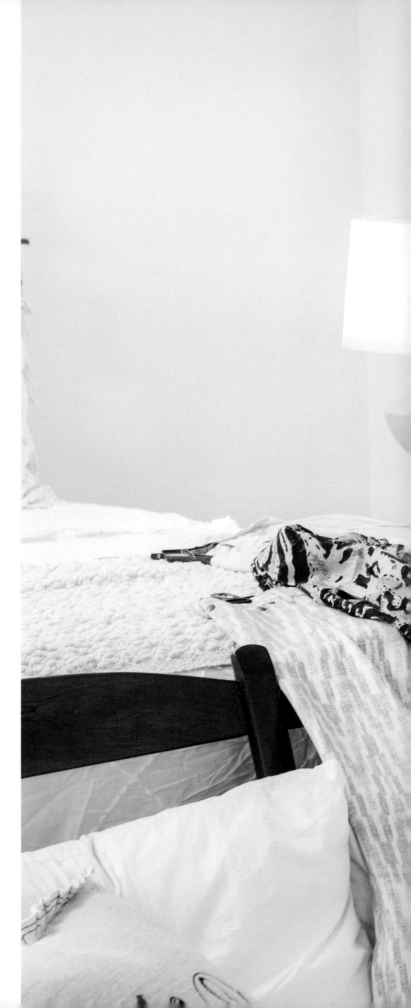

I asked Patrick in the *Days* hair department to describe my style and he said, "You're 'new millennium Bohemian.'" I kind of agree with that because I like to mix and match things.

People have said that I should have been born in the '60s because of the style choices I make. I'm teased because I don't often wear colors. I tend to wear blacks and creams, but when I do wear a color, I'll go for the boldest one I can find.

Rule: No more rules! Picking fun colors and mixing patterns is youthful and on trend.

I don't want to be the mom who dresses inappropriately for her age because that's just not good.
—*Melissa Reeves*

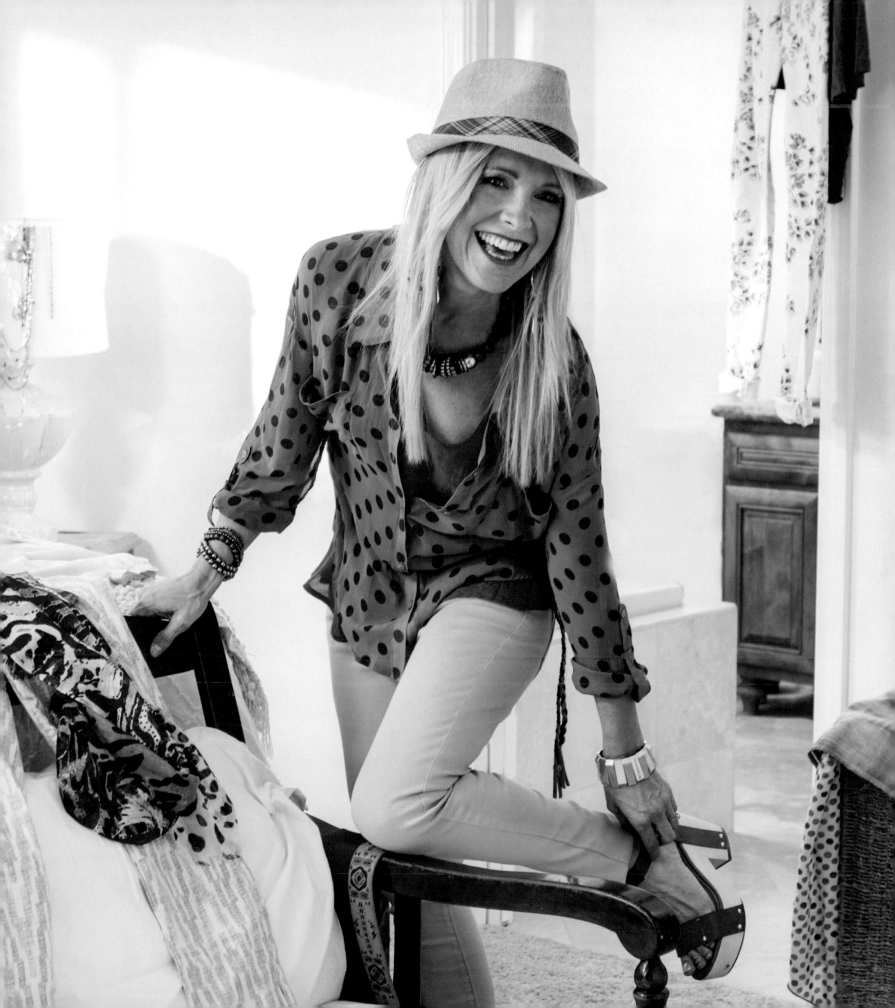

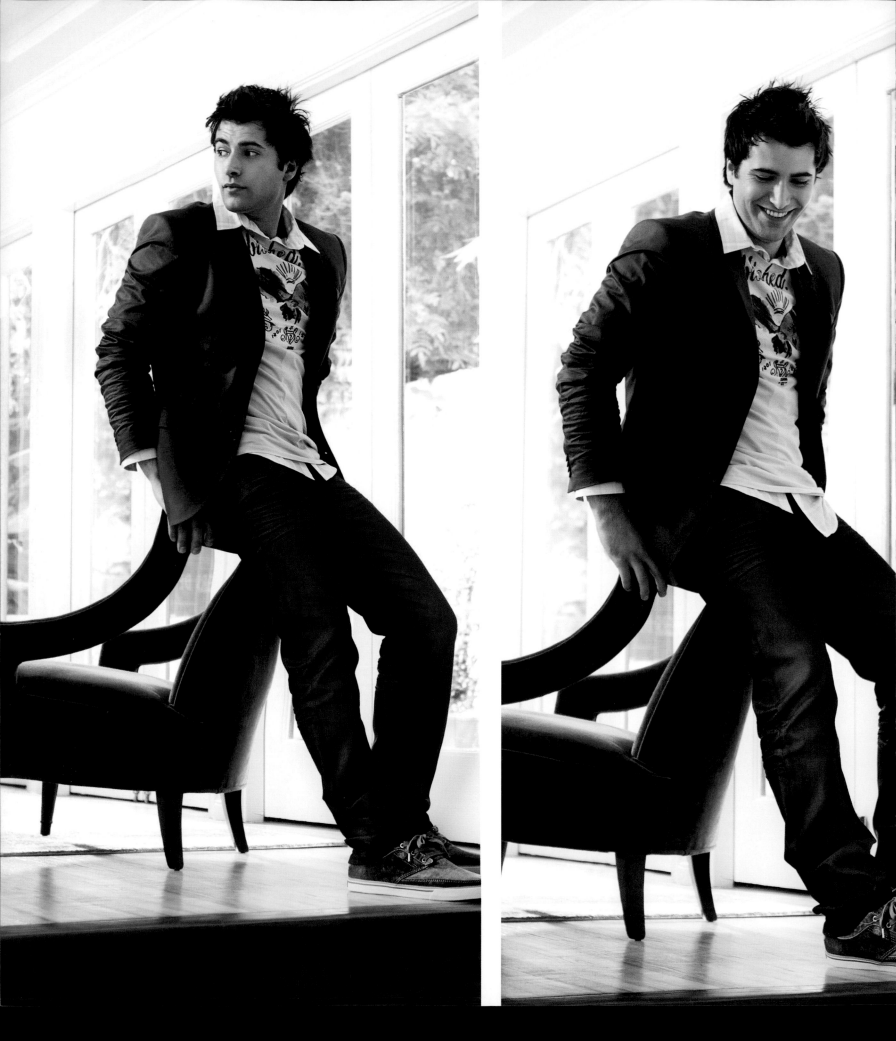

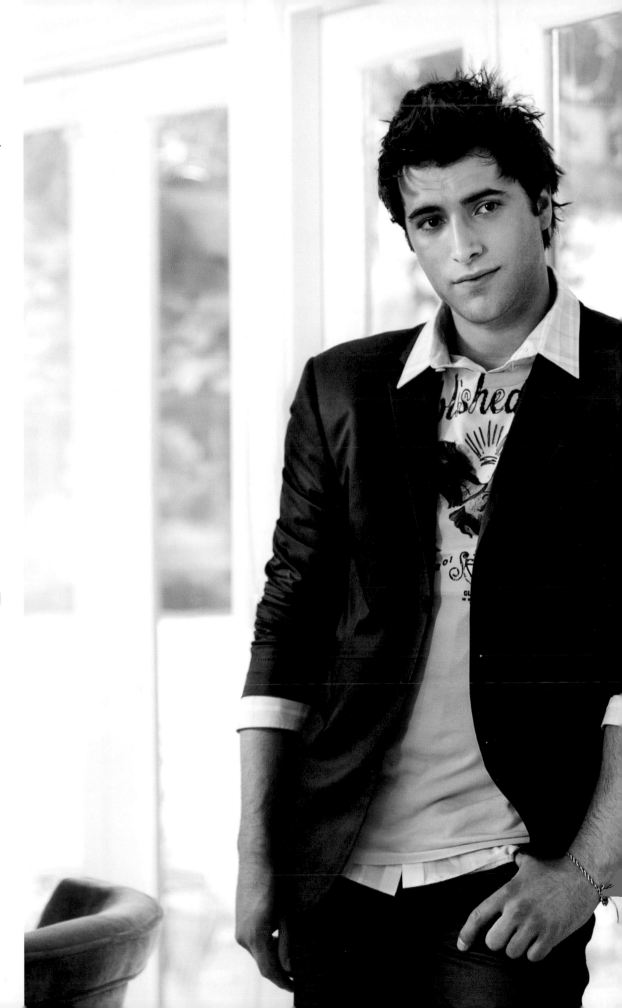

If you wash your hair every day with shampoo, it's much harder to style it. Most days, I'll just use hot water and scrub my scalp to get my hair clean. People will say about my hair, "Oh, he looks like he just rolled out of bed." But it actually takes time and effort to get it to look this way. Of course, I do wash my hair every day, but most often it's just with hot water. You know how your hair looks and feels after a day at the beach? That's how I like to have my hair. People will know when I've washed my hair with shampoo because then it'll just look weird. I've just discovered a great new conditioning shampoo that doesn't make my hair dry.

To dress up my T-shirt and jeans, I throw on a blazer and a great pair of shoes.

My style is "hipster."
That's when you say you
don't care about how you
look, but you actually do.
—*Freddie Smith*

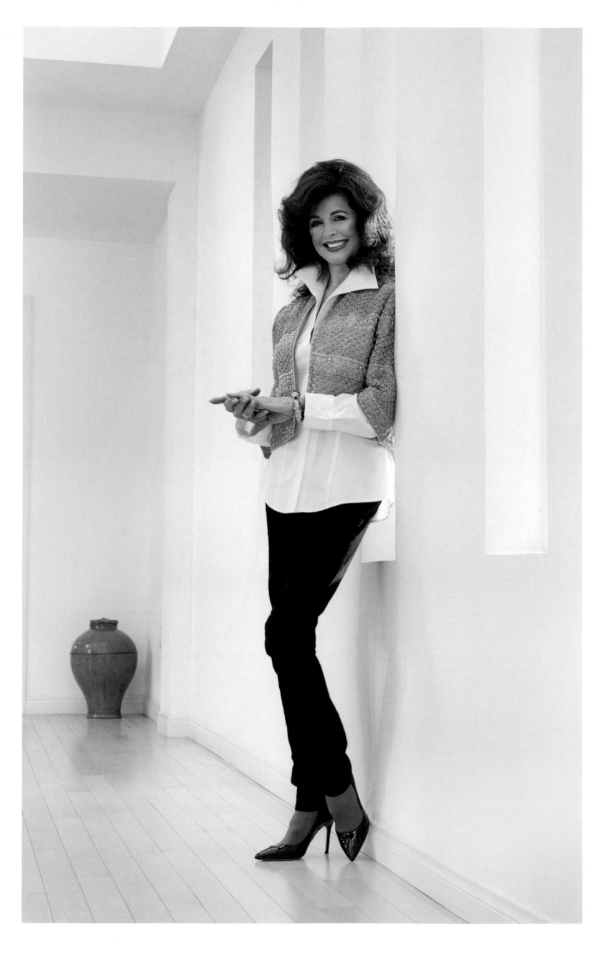

I believe that so much of your style and how you look is related to how you feel about yourself. My style is best described as very lady-like. I take my time getting dressed. I'll go back into my closet and look at different things as far as accessories are concerned. In the winter time, I wear slacks. In the spring and summer, I'll wear more dresses and skirts. I love wearing high heels. God made me a woman and that's what I'm going to be!

Style tips:

1. Take time to "feminize" your look with special accents, such as wearing high heels with slacks.
2. Keep a white shirt as part of your wardrobe because it brightens and frames the face.
3. Remember to edit the accessories you wear… less is more.

I love to feel pretty. "Pretty" is when I look in the mirror and I like the person who's looking back at me.
—*Suzanne Rogers*

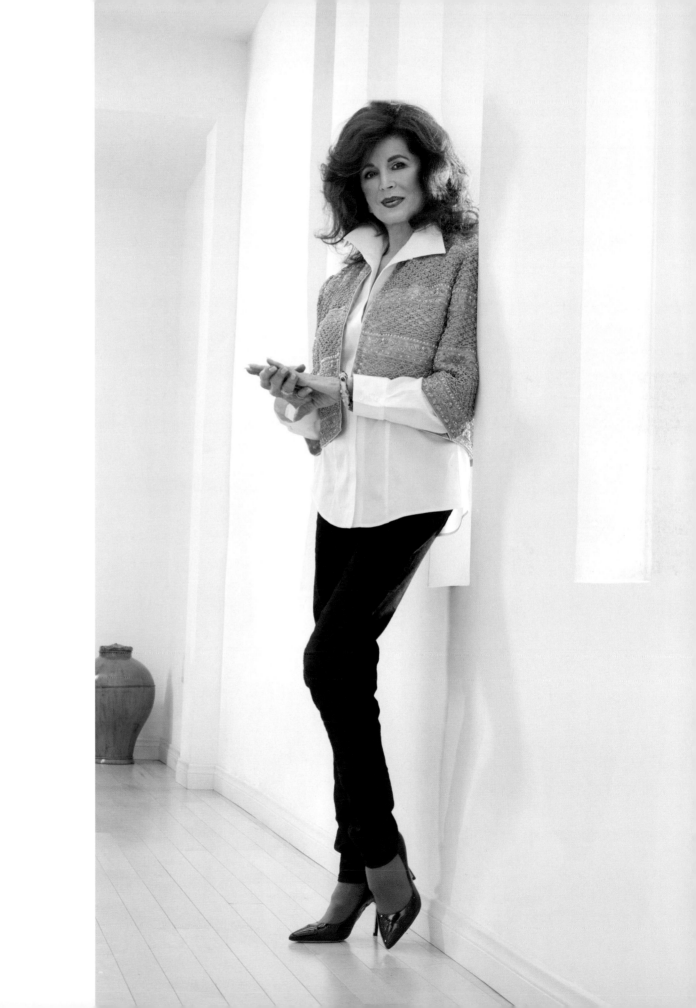

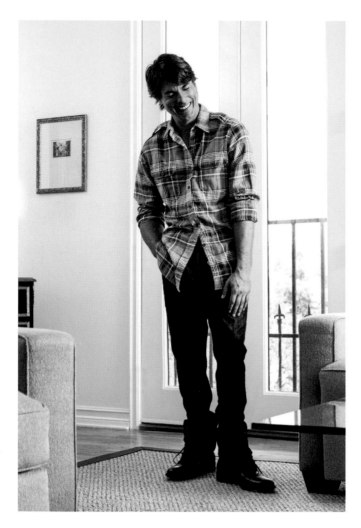

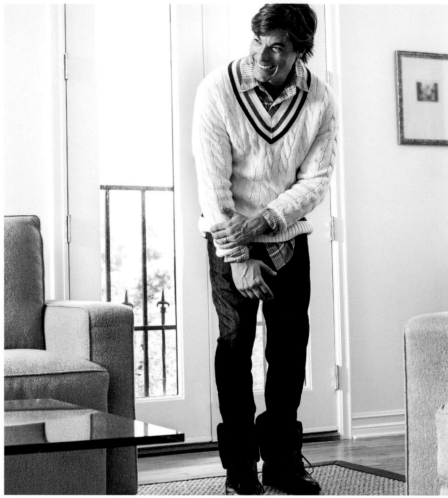

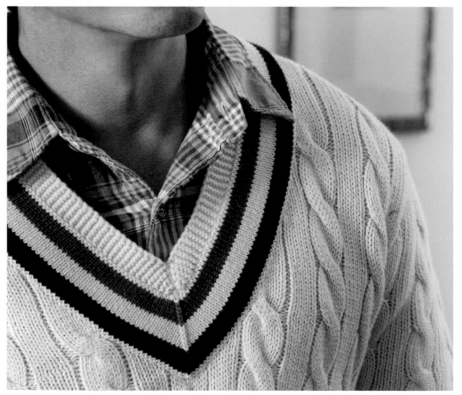

I tend to dress very casually when I'm not at work. My wife says that I dress like a 12-year-old—not like a 40-year-old. I like what I wear on the show, but I'm not sure that I'd go out in it myself. During the day, I'll wear a ripped-up T-shirt and a pair of oversized workout shorts. I don't have much fashion in my own life, but it's fun to have some at work.

Fashions change. I still have some skinny ties from the '80s and '90s that are now coming back in style. I like accessories—watches, necklaces and rings.

I actually love wearing suits and nice shoes if I'm going out at night.
—Bryan Dattilo

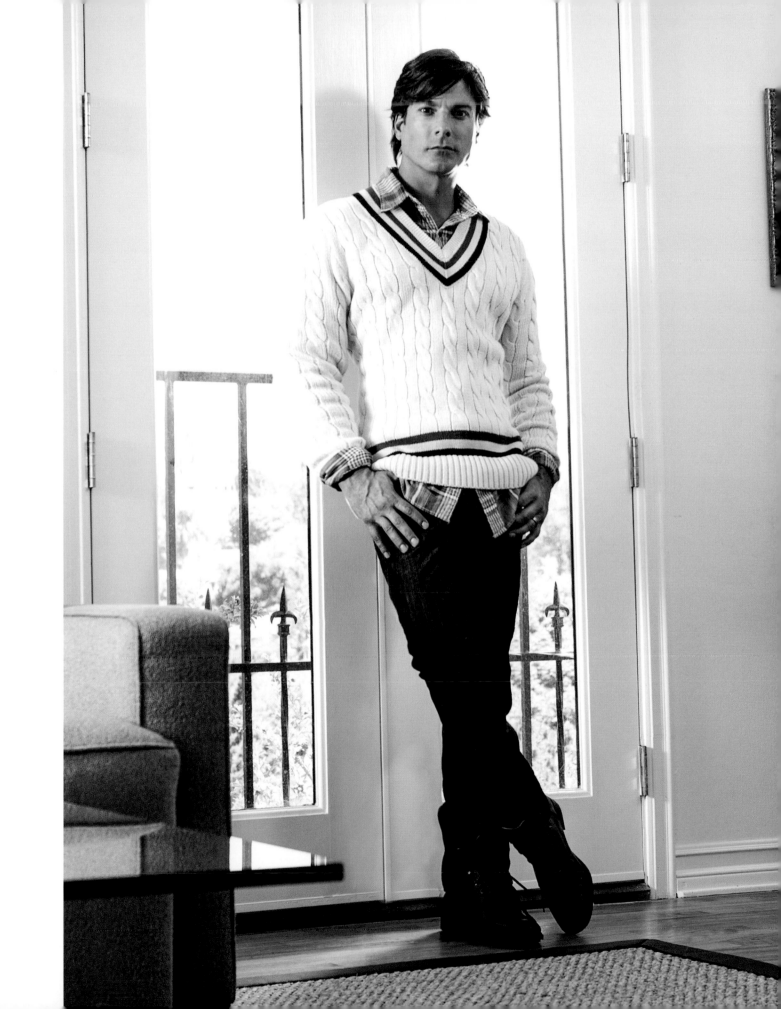

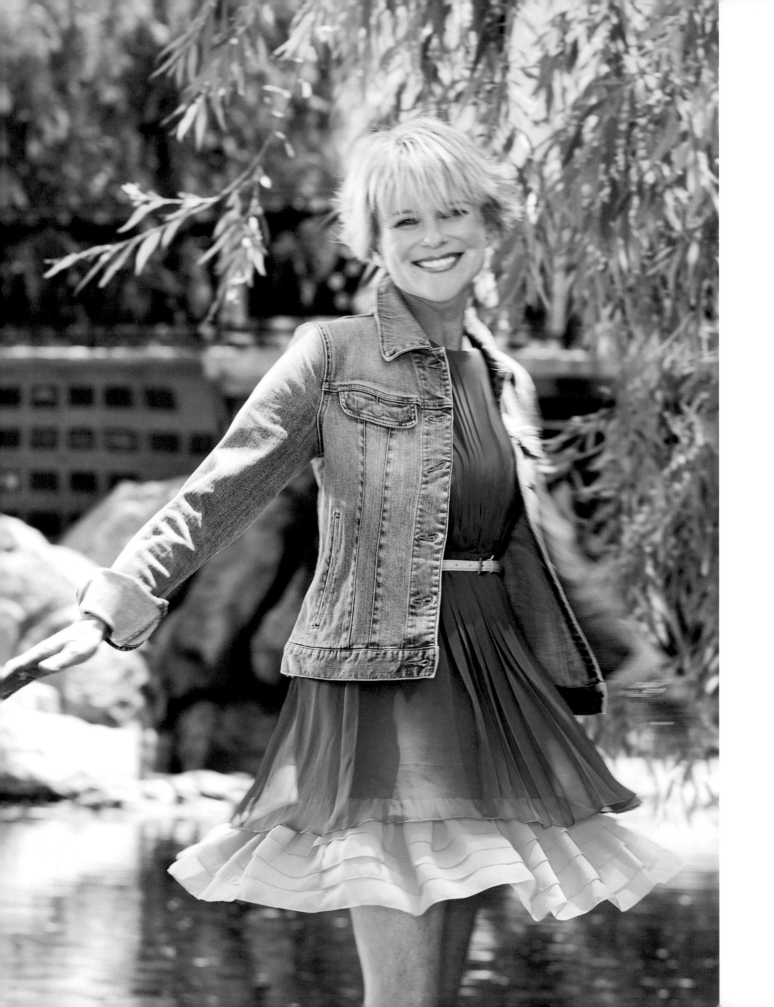

My style is comfortable and casual. Thank goodness there are designers out there who let me borrow their dresses for special occasions—otherwise I'd show up at the Daytime Emmys in a mismatched top and bottom!

My basics are soft, flattering jeans that I pair with vintage T-shirts and my favorite sneakers. When I dress for my day job, I wear comfortable separates such as a pair of basic black slacks with a variety of colorful blouses.

I have some really nice clothes that I wear to work at Rose Hills Memorial Park and Mortuaries, but my own personal style is jeans, T-shirts and jean jackets. I love sneakers and tennis shoes. I'd wear them 24/7 if I could. I'm not crazy about flip-flops unless I'm getting my nails done.

I've never been a "clothes person." A lot of times my outfits don't even match!
—*Judi Evans*

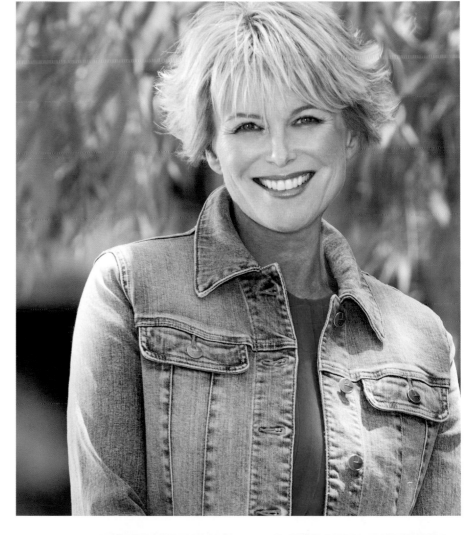

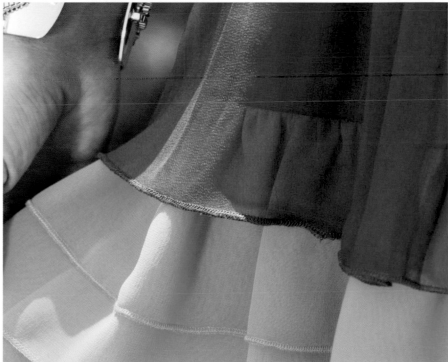

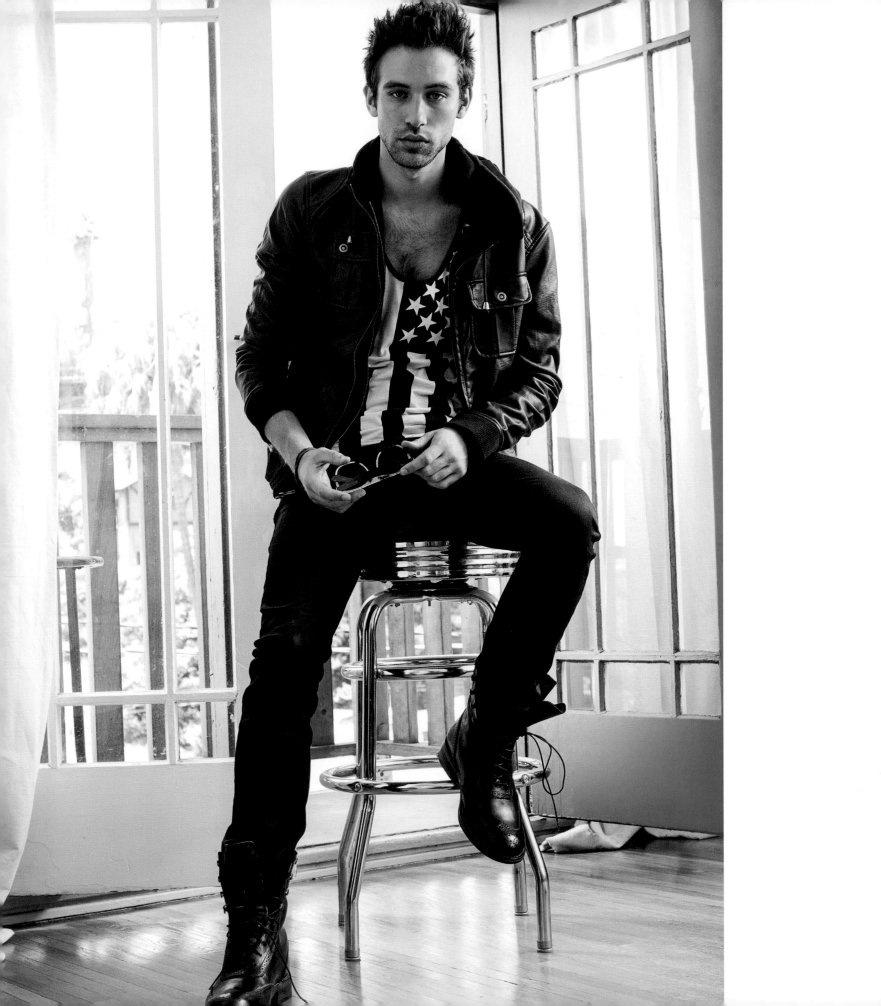

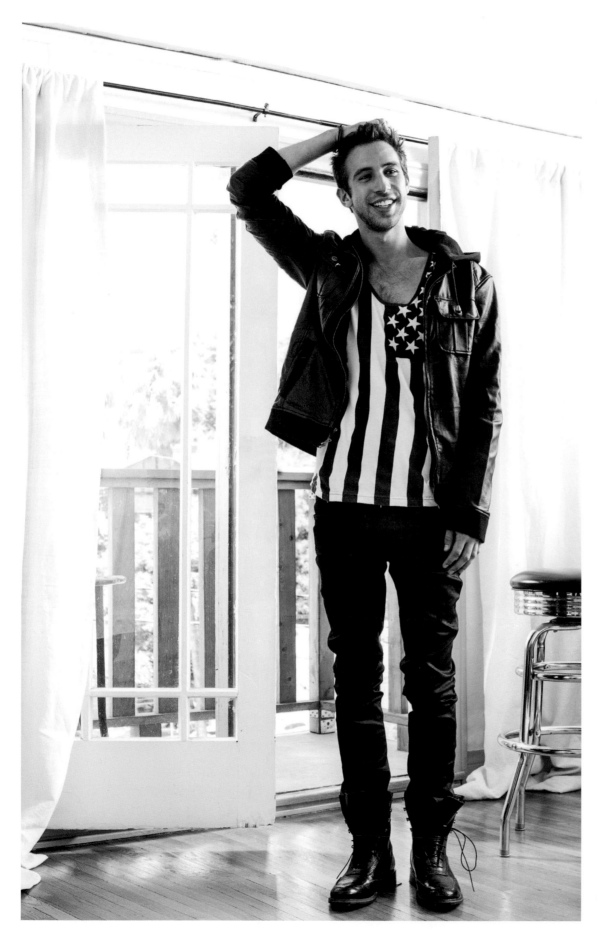

It's hard to pin down what you'd call my style. Sometimes I like to have a "rocker" look. You could call it a "Bob Dylan/indie" thing going on. I'm truly eclectic in many ways. I love music including hip-hop, rock and roll and classical. I don't turn my nose up at any kind of music. I'm interested in learning new things and in doing interesting stuff that influences my style.

When I was in Portland, Oregon, shooting a movie, I saw a lot of people wearing boots there. I realized I had to get some bad-ass boots—so I did. I still have them.

I'm a big fan of copying anything that I see that's cool.
—Blake Berris

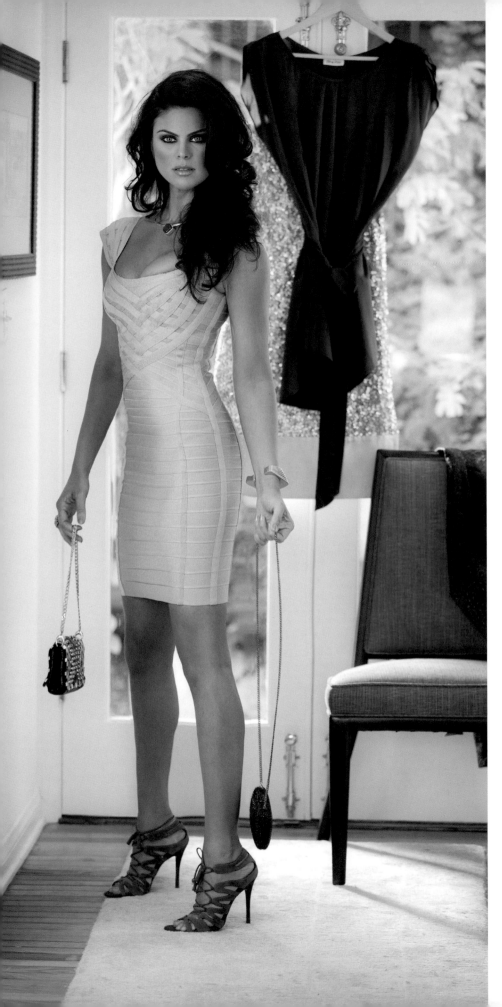

I'm not a "trendy" dresser by any means. The first words that come to mind when I'm asked to describe my style are "classic" and "feminine." I believe in wearing what's flattering to your body type. I veer toward classic, clean lines. I wear a lot of dresses. I love dresses. They're so comfortable. Jeans may be hugely popular, but I'm not a big jeans person. It may be my European sensibility, but dresses are much more flattering.

Here are some basics I keep in mind when I think about style and beauty:

1. Buy inexpensive clothes and have them fitted for you by your local tailor. You'll end up keeping clothing longer this way.
2. You can't go wrong with black.
3. Buy things that are timeless so they won't have to be recycled.
4. Feel that it's worth investing a little bit of money in something like a great leather jacket, purse or pair of shoes because you can end up having those things for years. I don't believe in buying something that you're only going to use a couple of times.
5. Costly items can be worth it if you wear them often. I can't live without my James Perse tank tops. They're flattering to my figure and make me feel good.
6. Carry blotting papers in your purse when going out. They soak up the shine and help your skin look refreshed. A similar paper that's used to cover toilet seats can be used in place of blotting papers. My girlfriends have laughed at me when I tell them this, but it works! They're cost-effective and they don't smear or smudge.

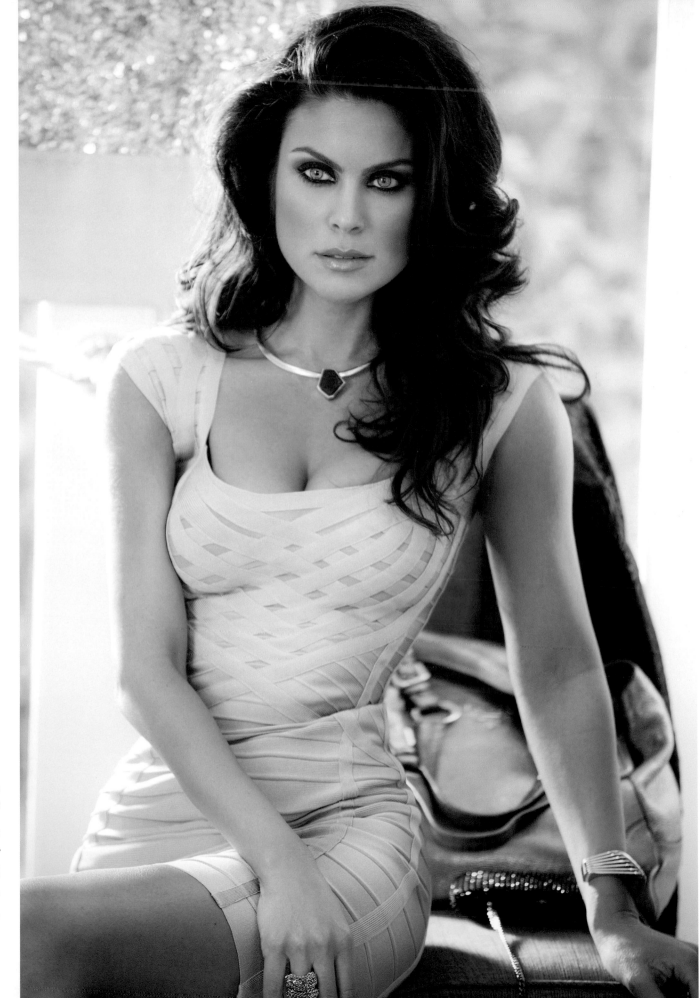

Don't chase trends, but if you find one that works for you, great!
—Nadia Bjorlin

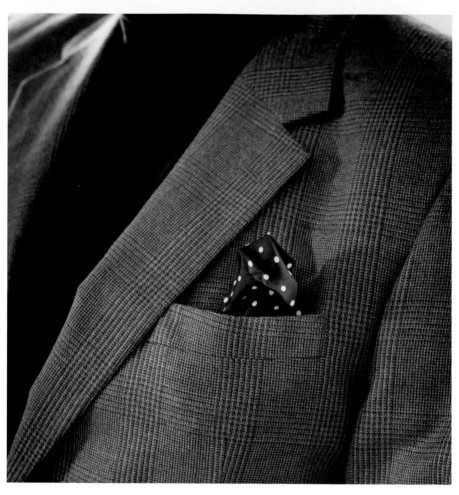

All my life, I've loved bright colors. When it comes to style I'm interested in warmth and color. I would wear nothing but bright colors all the time except for the fact that they're so bright that occasionally people around me will squint! So sometimes, I put on dark colors. My sense of style does not come from watching what other people wear. Susan and I come from a performer's point of view in that actors should always be a little more dressed up than their audiences.

Bill's look is classic. He is perfectly at ease in a tie and blazer. If there were a bowling alley in Salem, Bill's character would show up in a sports coat and tie.
—*Susan Seaforth Hayes*

When we go to the theater, I'll be the one wearing a tie and a pocket square.
—*Bill Hayes*

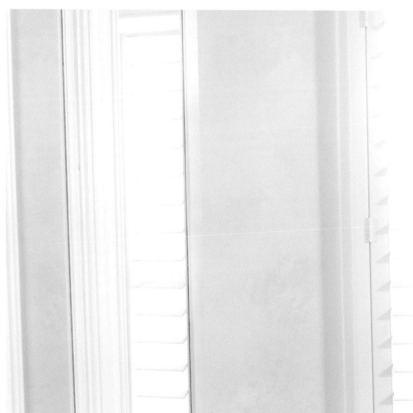

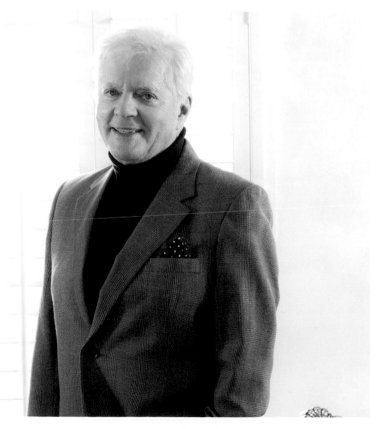

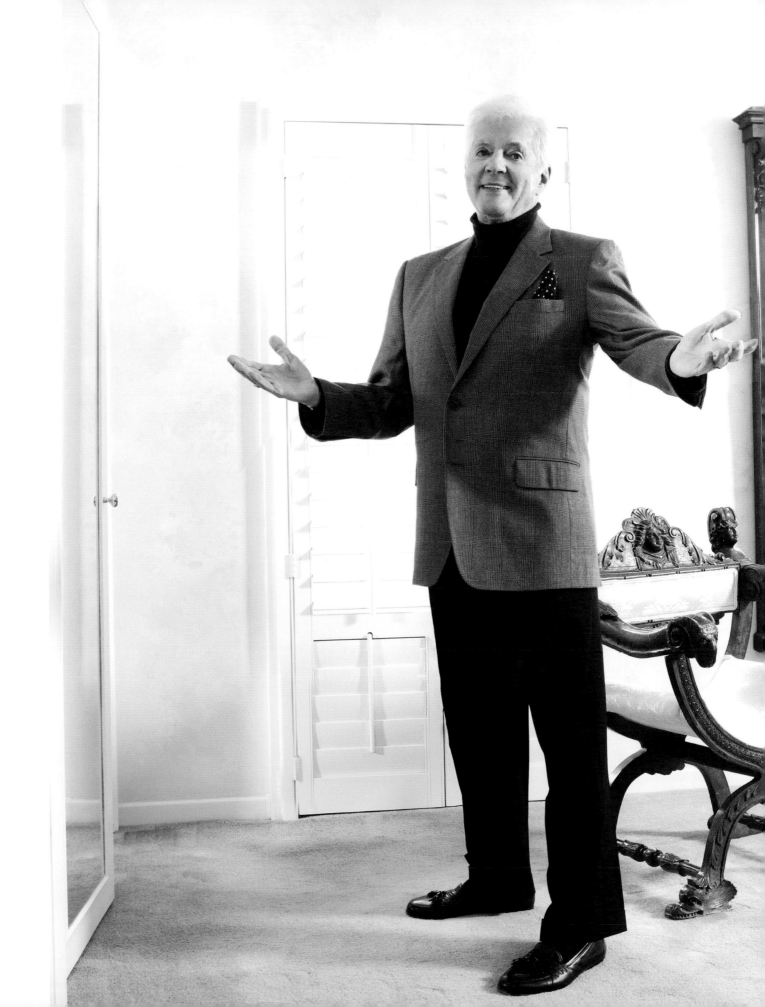

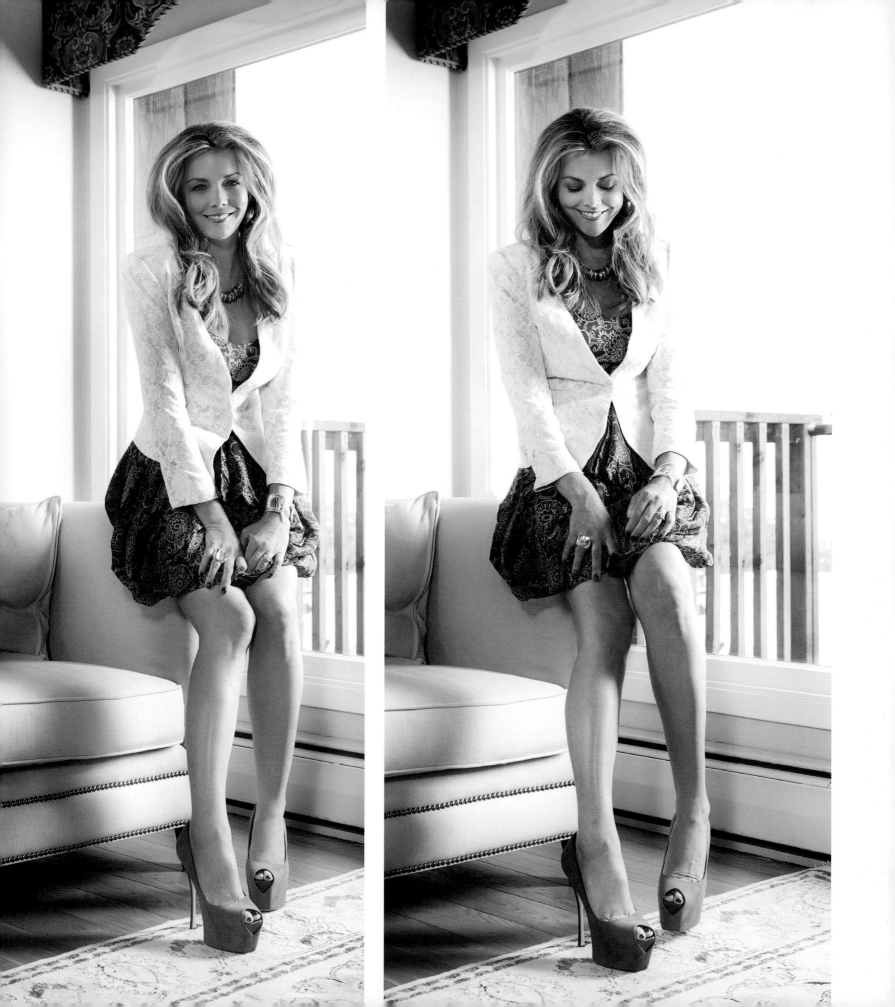

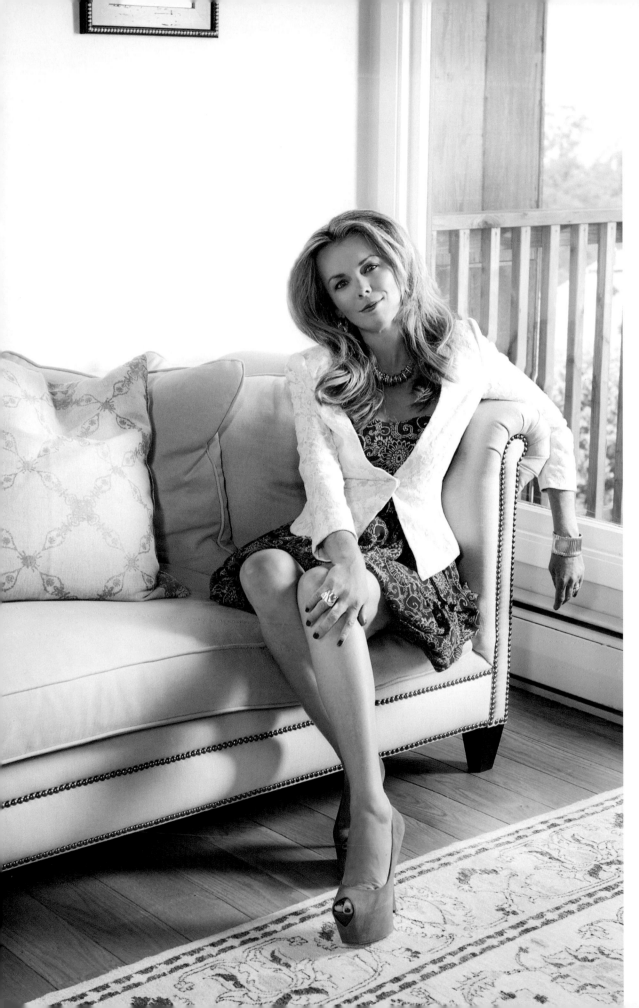

I have hips and curves like the ideal woman who lived in the 1950s. The *Mad Men* style looks good on me.

I like mixing it up, like wearing little black Victorian boots with a skirt that juts out.

I don't go shopping a lot, but I do frequent a specialty place that has fantastic high-end clothing at either a half or a quarter of the cost. If I go anywhere I'll go there. I have a lot of stuff from the past. I keep many things, but I do get rid of some stuff, too.

Three staples in my wardrobe:

1. A classic cashmere cardigan
2. A comfortable pair of maroon-colored boots
3. A beautiful turquoise necklace that I got on my honeymoon in Greece

I would describe my style as "edgy Mary Poppins."
—*Christie Clark*

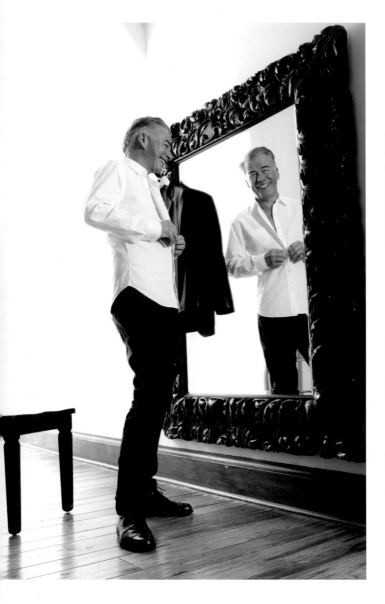

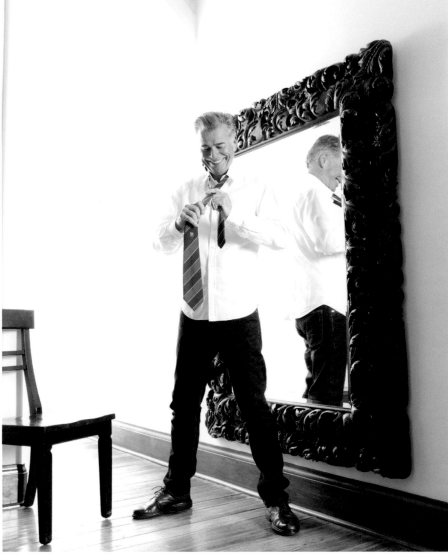

I don't know how I'd describe my style. It definitely changes. There was a time when a man would never wear brown shoes with a black suit, but now that's the style. I used to have a very simple routine when I'd go out: I'd make a martini, then shower and shave and I'd be dressed within 30 minutes. But that's not my routine anymore. I used to like getting dressed up more than I do now. It's funny. I look back at some photographs and ask, "Why did I wear that?"

Since my characters have always been sharp dressers, I've often thought about buying some of my wardrobe from the shows I've been on because they have been custom-tailored for me.

I've been around clothes so much of my life—I tend to gravitate toward what works and what's comfortable.
—*Ian Buchanan*

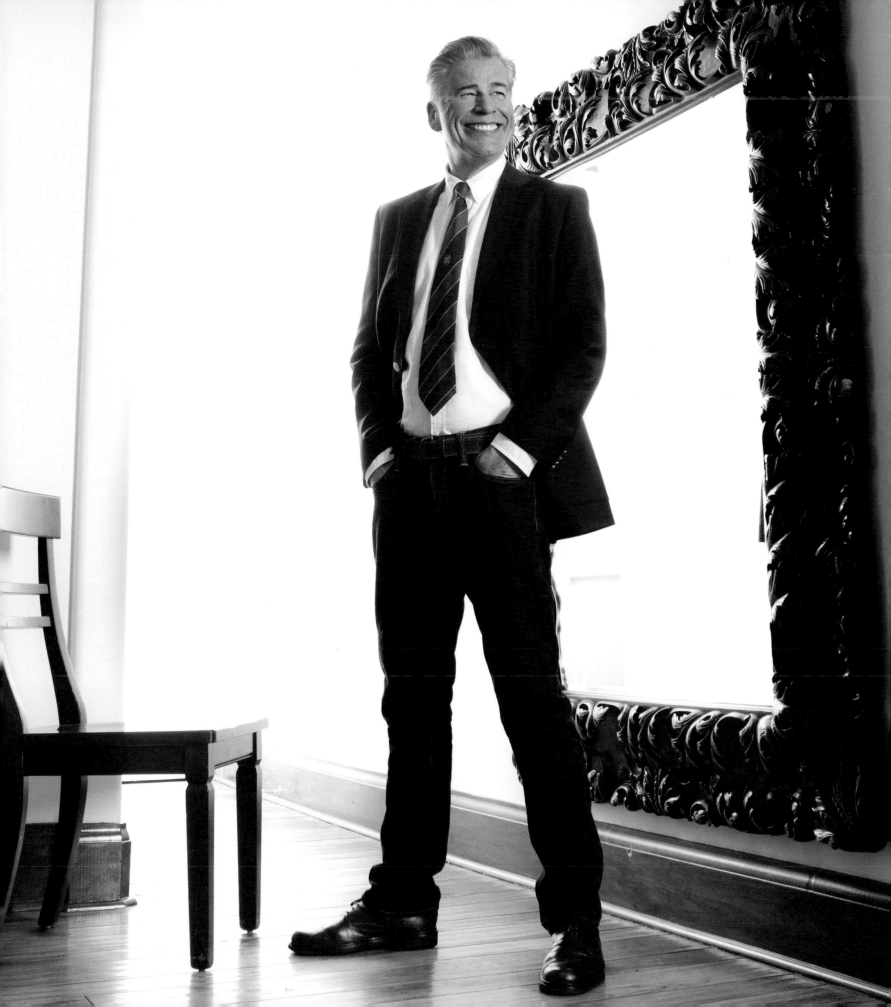

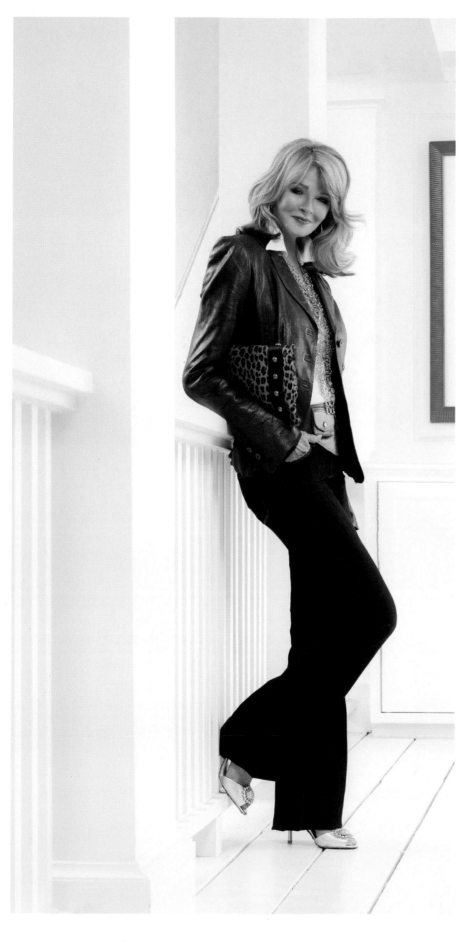

I think I'm younger, far less cosmetic and more active than my character, Marlena. When I go out and travel to women's conventions, I'm so tired of hearing, "You look so much younger in person!" I watch the show and I don't think I look my age on the show. When people see me, they see Marlena and they feel that they are in a safe place, which I think is what we're all hungry for—finding that safe place.

I've met thousands of people coming through book signings and at fan events. Marlena has become something of an icon. I get to play that person and, as a result, I get the residual effect of who she is on-camera and what she means to people.

A fitted blazer is key to a more-polished look while a fuller-cut, "boyfriend" blazer provides a more casual flair.

I tend to dress younger than Marlena does.
—*Deidre Hall*

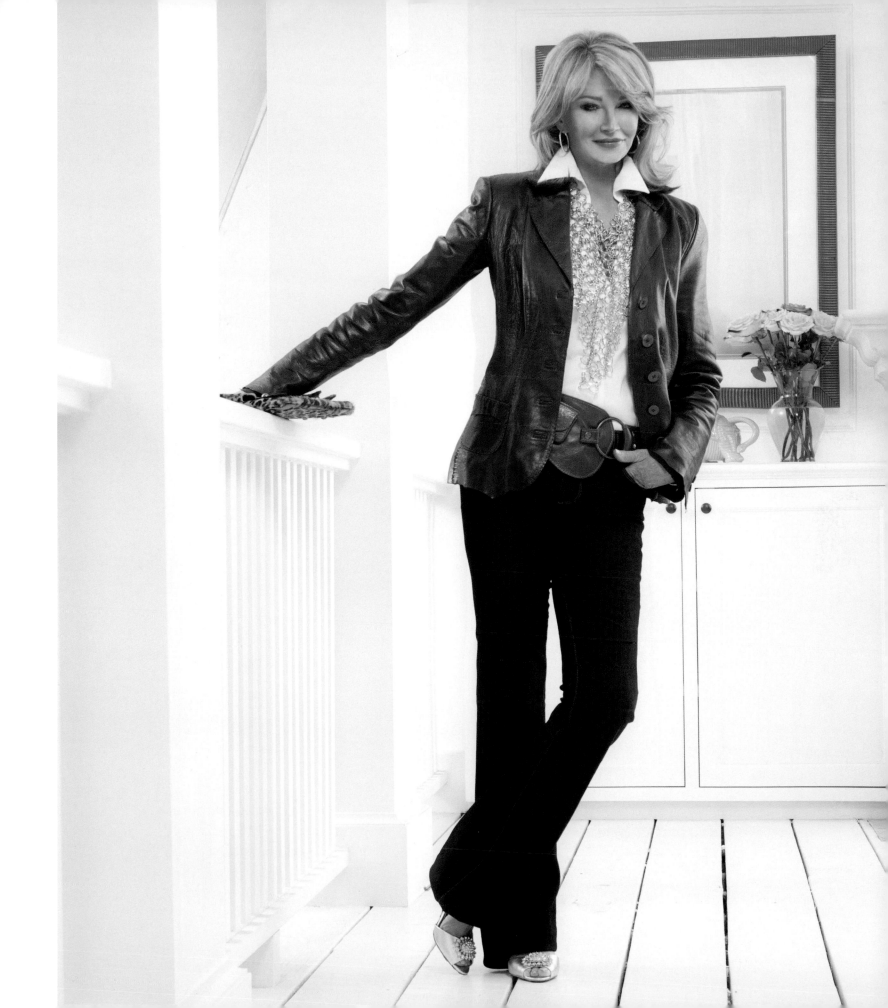

While I appreciate and admire Stefano's wardrobe, it's not my day-to-day style. You won't find me at home in a suit and tie. My style is much more eclectic—it definitely suits whatever mood I may be in. My idea of entertaining is to have a group of friends over for martinis, then gather around the dinner table with a great bottle of wine and probably an Italianate meal. It's not a formal environment—we are there to laugh, talk and have fun!

Style tips:

1. Cut and fit are key to a beautiful suit (I recommend investing in at least one expensive Italian suit that will last for years).
2. You can't go wrong with a well-tailored, button-down white shirt.
3. Good-looking shoes are important, but comfortable shoes are key!

There is much more laughter coming from my home than you'll ever witness coming from the DiMera mansion.
—*Joseph Mascolo*

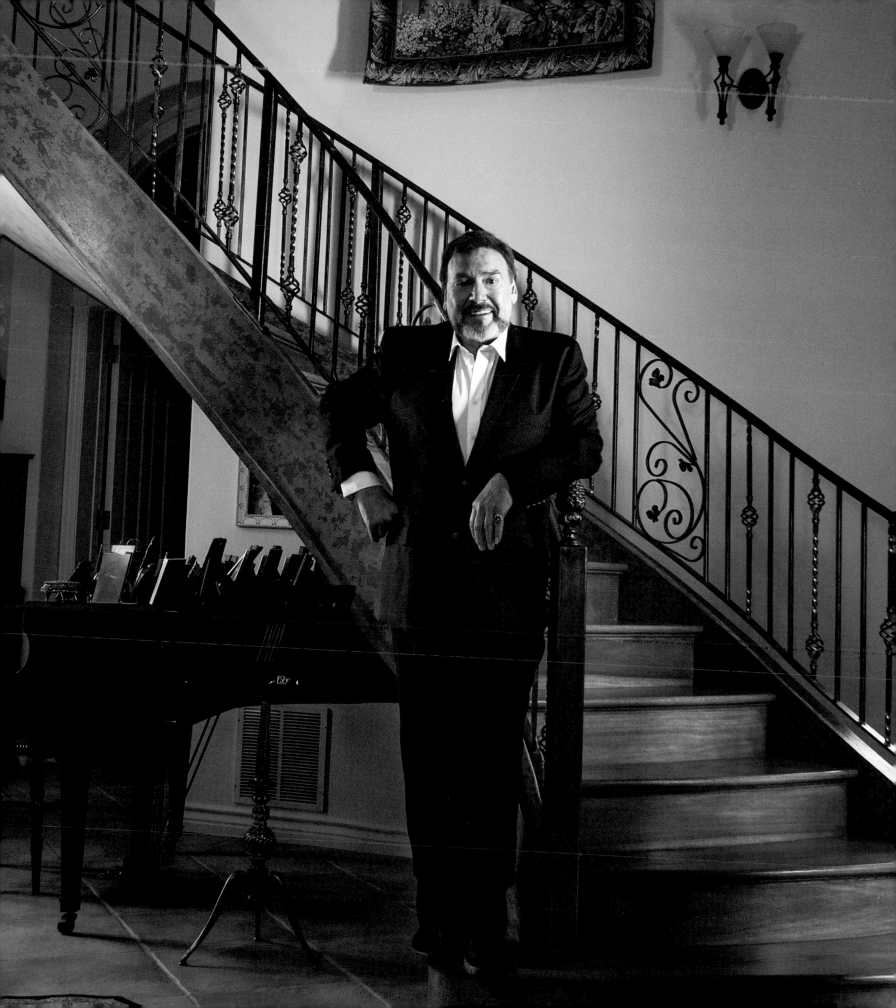

I adore Issey Miyake, a Japanese designer. He makes designs that can fold up as small as a scarf! He's amazing and is well recognized, but he's also completely original. His use of fabric has never been duplicated by any other designer. He's an artist and I know when I'm wearing his designs that I'm wearing the work of a true artist. That makes me feel proud and good! There's nothing ordinary about what he does. Looking at his designs is like looking at a meteorological display!

I like designer clothes!

I am not afraid to stand out in a crowd. I like things that complement me.
—*Peggy McCay*

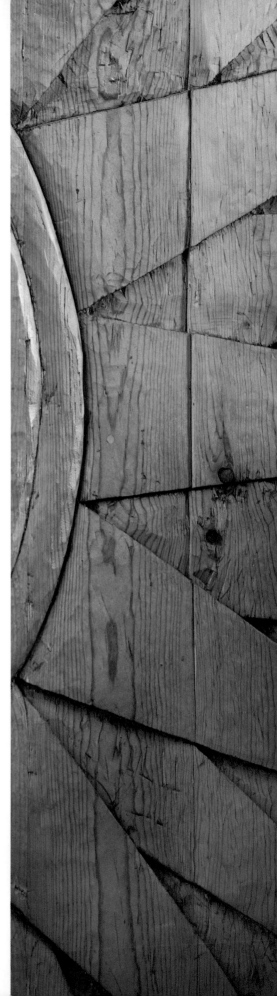

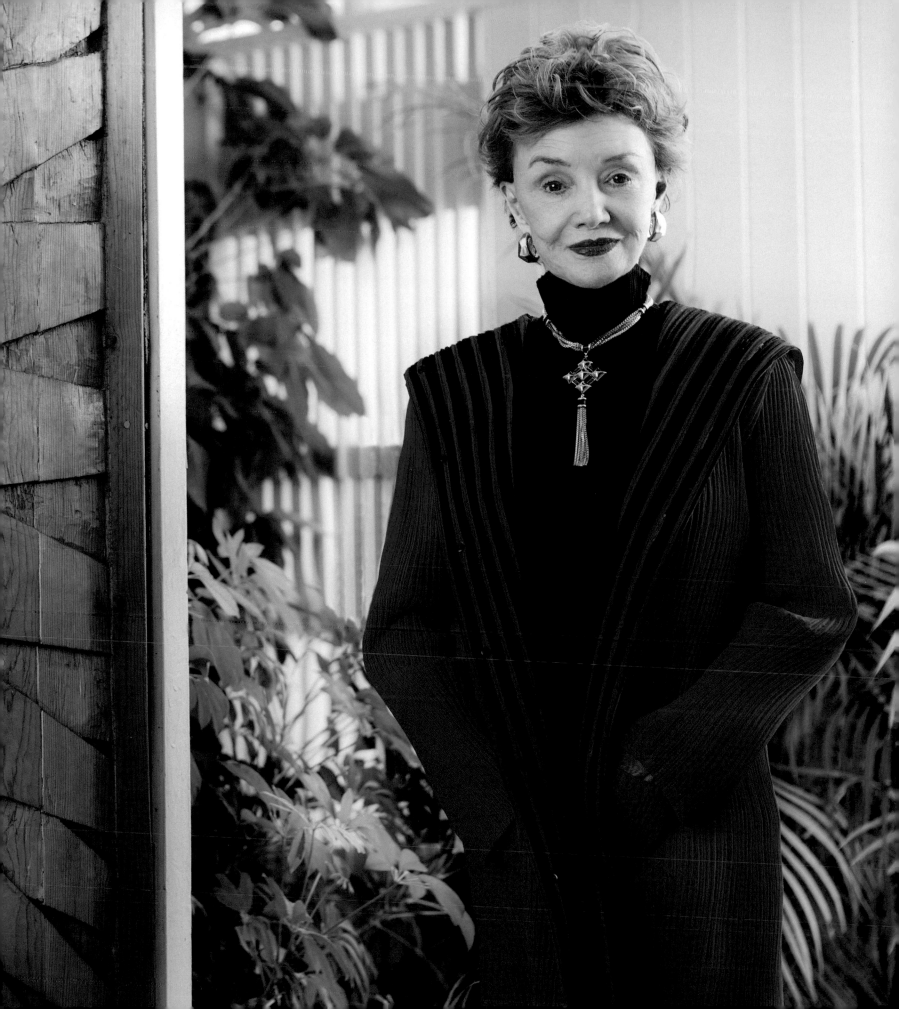

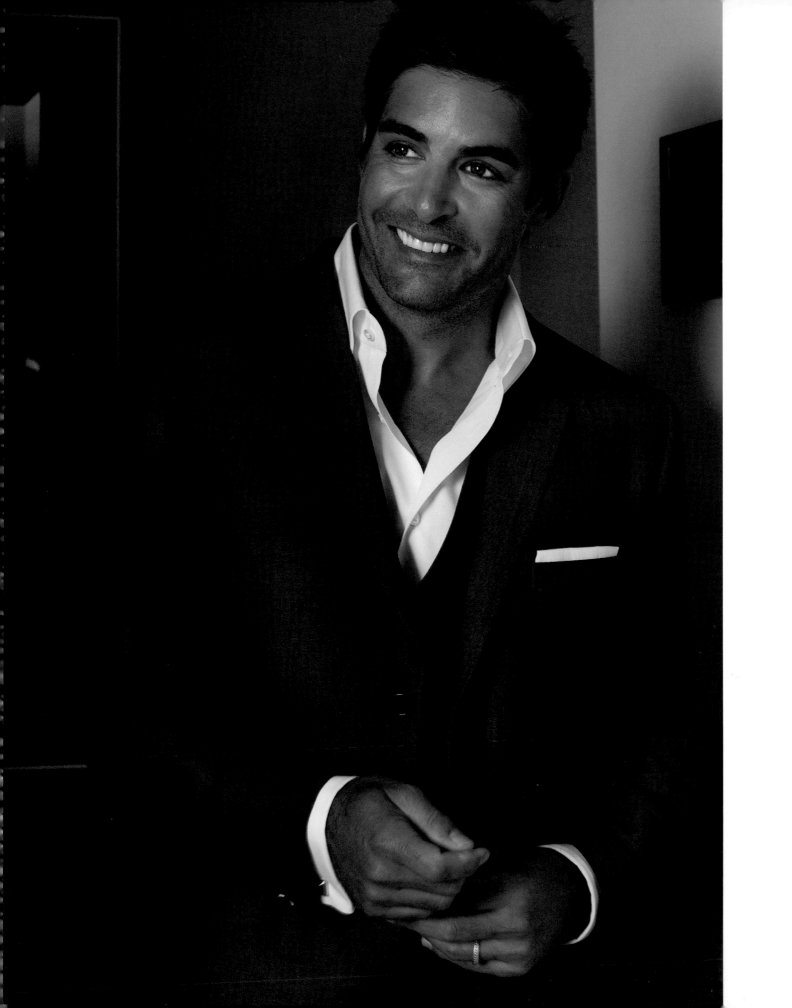

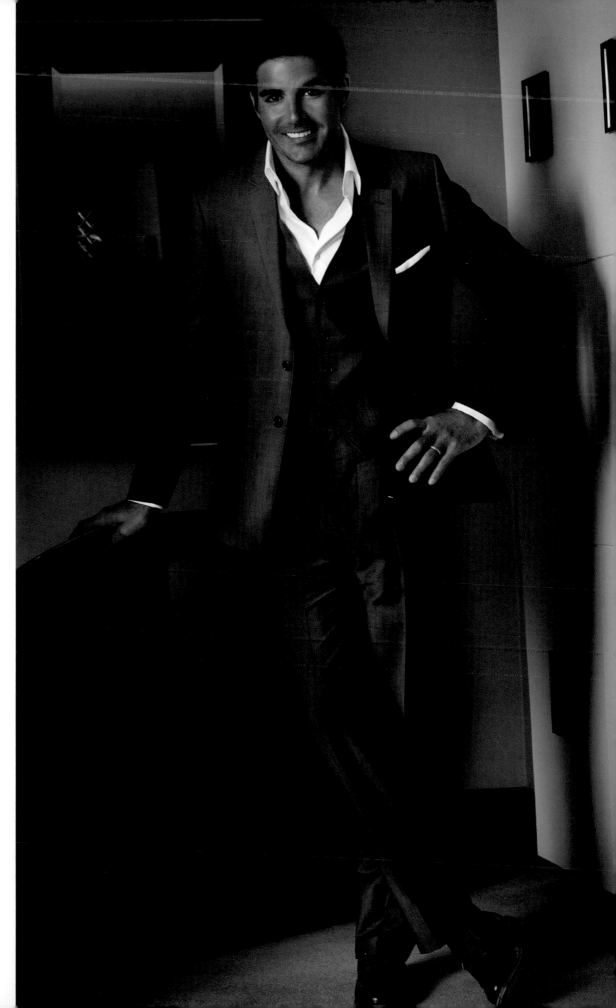

My style is laid-back and very easygoing. What I wear around the house depends on what I'm doing. Usually, I'll wear jeans and T-shirts. I'm very casual. I actually like wearing suits more than I used to. They're fun.

When you wear a suit, people look at you more. They notice the way in which you carry yourself. I like putting together a nice suit and shirt with a pocket square.

I'm pretty casual at heart, but putting on a nice suit and getting decked out from head to toe can make an evening special. Plus, people look at you differently, especially my wife. And that's a good thing!

—*Galen Gering*

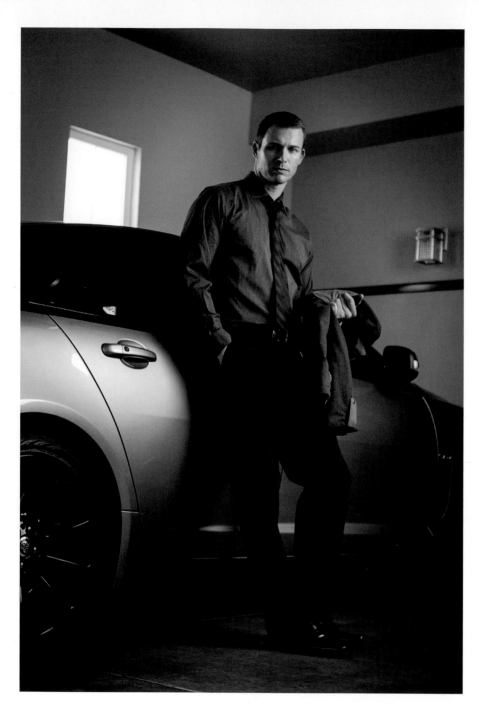

My style is actually very comfortable. I'm not a "fashion forward" type guy and I don't follow trends. My role as a parent has helped me with that. I'm at a point where feeling good has trumped looking good.

Having said that, I don't think the clothes you wear necessarily fully dictate your "style." Style is about how you hold yourself and how you're going to present yourself.

I'm a jeans and T-shirts type guy, but I'll often go out and buy the most expensive jeans and T-shirts I can find because the most comfortable ones are usually also the well-made ones, and, therefore, they're the most costly ones.

Clothes should not define you. I feel and perform my best when I'm wearing comfortable outfits.
—*Eric Martsolf*

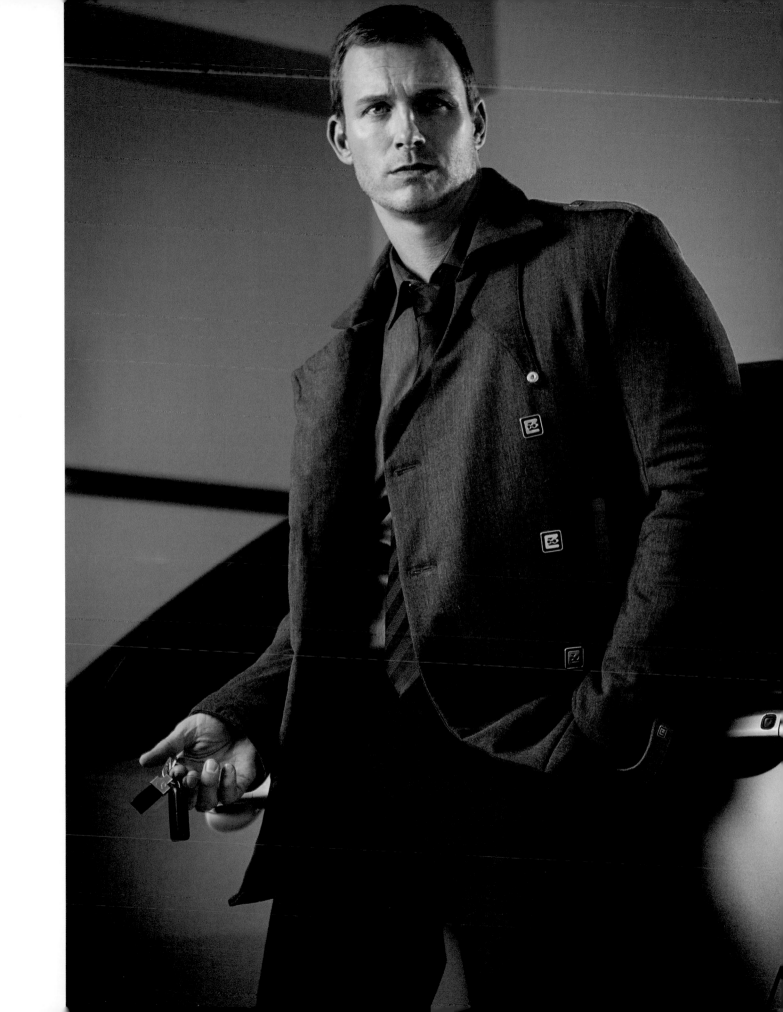

THE LITTLE BLACK DRESS

Fashions come and go…
trends can fade overnight…
but the little black dress is eternal.

· ·

Ideal versions of the little black dress (LBD) vary from person to person. Not all LBDs are short in length or are made of the same fabric. Sometimes the LBD can even be replaced by the little black suit or pant suit.

It was fashion icon Coco Chanel who first felt that every woman should own an LBD. In fact she was so passionate about it, she once said, "Really, they [women] are so badly dressed, I will put them all in black to teach them good taste."

Coco would be happy to know that for the past 80 years women have gladly hung LBDs in their closets. Provided that the design of an LBD isn't too offbeat, the dress can last for years. Properly accessorized, they can be worn for almost every occasion. While others may make a fashion faux pas wearing something that's considered "hip and trendy," the LBD is perfect for every occasion, running the gamut from conservative to sexy. It's a timeless choice and, therefore, foolproof.

The women of *Days of our Lives* wear their own versions of the little black dress with style and confidence.

When a little black dress is right, there is nothing else to wear in its place.
—*Wallis Simpson, Duchess of Windsor*

One is never over- or underdressed with a little black dress. A woman can never look bad in a little black dress, they can always trust that look.
—*Karl Lagerfeld*

Audrey Hepburn advised wearing beige or black—why wear anything else?
—*Susan Seaforth Hayes*

You can't go wrong with black.
—*Nadia Bjorlin*

I look for something short and sexy that's comfy and ageless in a little black dress. You can wear it during the day and then dress it up for an evening event by changing shoes and adding jewelry.
—*Eileen Davidson*

There are some things a woman should limit in her wardrobe, but not the little black dress. It will never go out of style!
—*Kristian Alfonso*

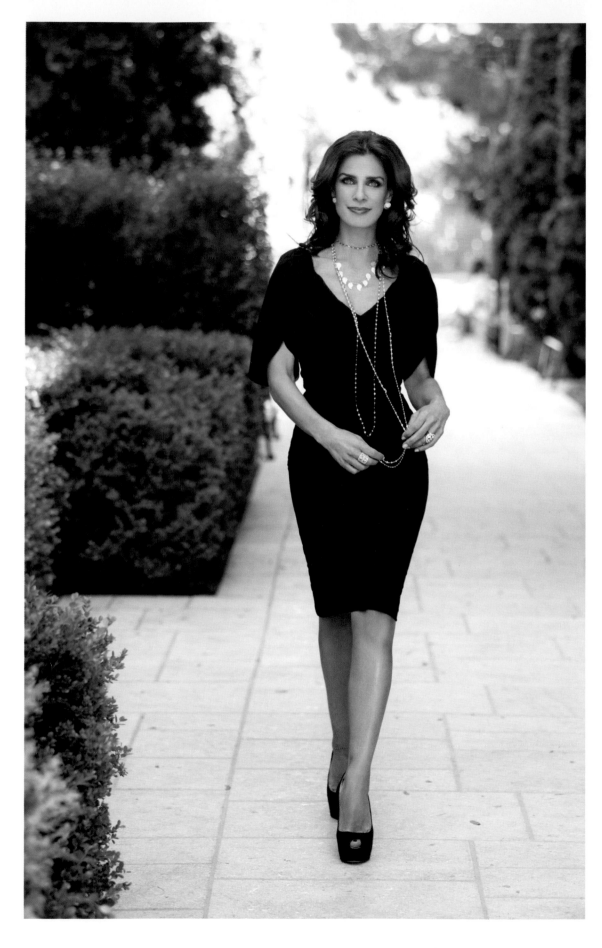

What makes this LBD special are the sleeves and neckline—elegant and classic with a modern twist.

The perfect little black dress.
—*Kristian Alfonso*

This classy LBD looks even more feminine with the addition of a ruffled, high-collar blouse.

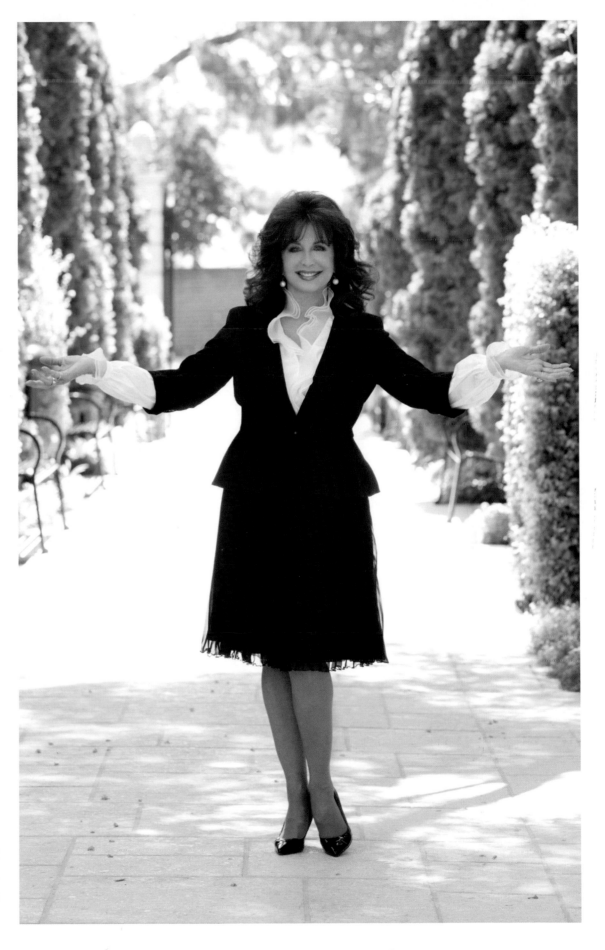

The perfect black suit with a white blouse.
—*Suzanne Rogers*

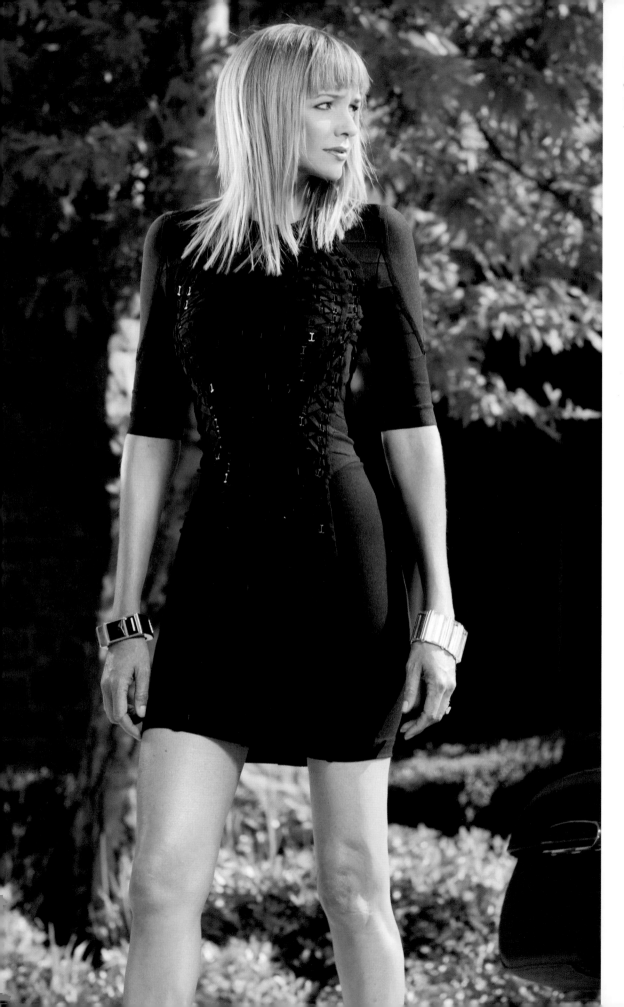

I may have no idea who designed certain things, but I definitely know what I like.
—*Arianne Zucker*

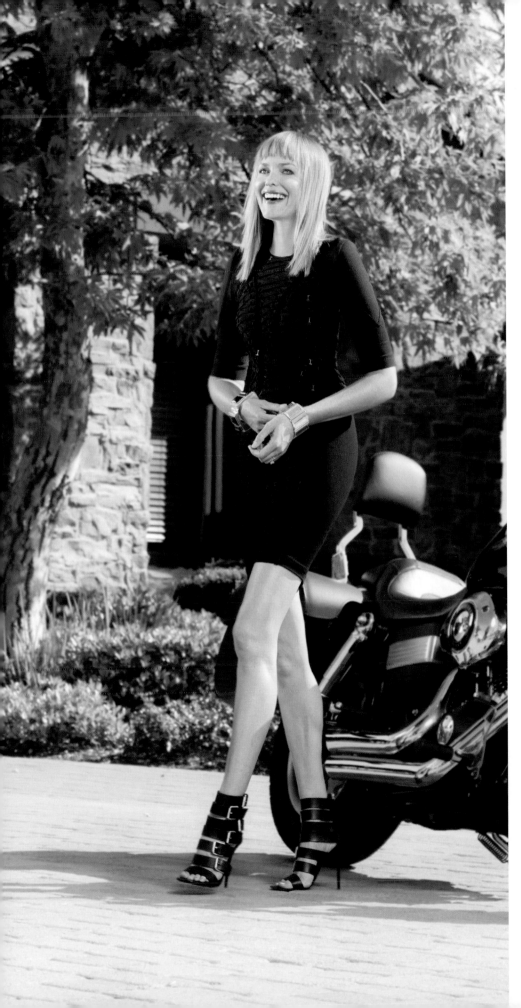

My style definitely varies. I'm a Gemini so there are definitely a few of us in here! It's fun to get dressed up and go out, but mostly I'm a jeans, T-shirt and leather jacket girl. I love a hot pair of boots, either flat or with heels.

When summer rolls around, I'll wear cute dresses. My outfits are simple, but at the same time they're put together well. I learned how to do that from being on *Days*. I love shoes. If I spend money on anything it'll be shoes and purses. I'm not a shopper or obsessed with labels. I like quality and I want to be able to keep things in my closet for a while, but not overdo it.

People have looked at my closet and asked, "Where are the rest of your things?" I tell them that's it. I'm living with my husband and we share the closet space. I'm really very simple. If something comes in, then something goes out. When I realize I haven't worn it in over a year then out it goes, unless it's vintage or from my shoe collection.

The perfect edgy black dress with killer shoes…a sassy look.
—*Arianne Zucker*

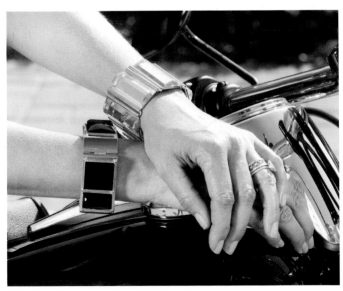

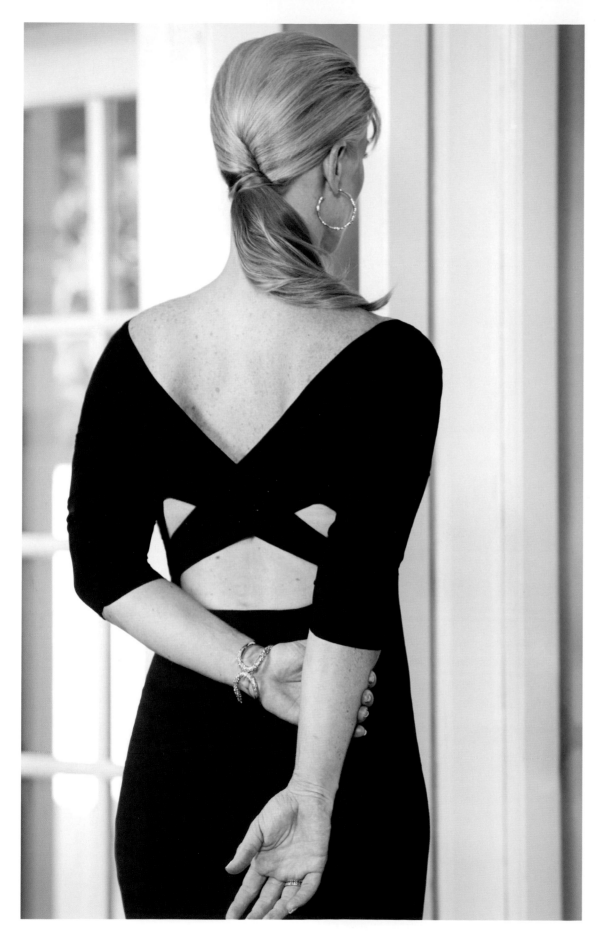

Little black dresses with different necklines are always great because you can dress them up or down for a completely different look.

I always look for a black dress that meets the following criteria:

1. Flattering to the figure
2. Doesn't wrinkle easily
3. Proper length for both standing or sitting

The perfect black dress with a beautiful crisscross design on the back.
—*Alison Sweeney*

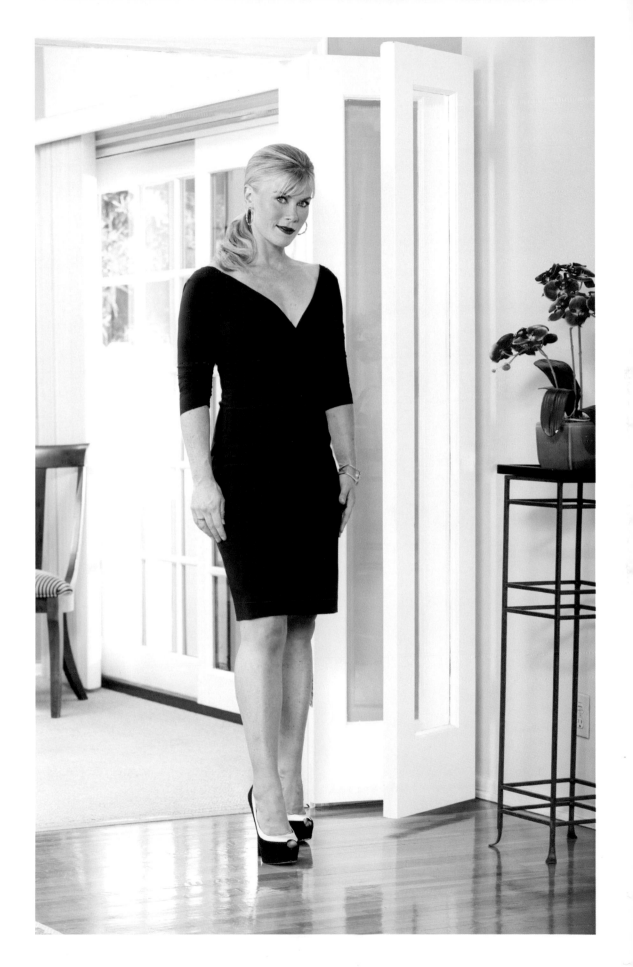

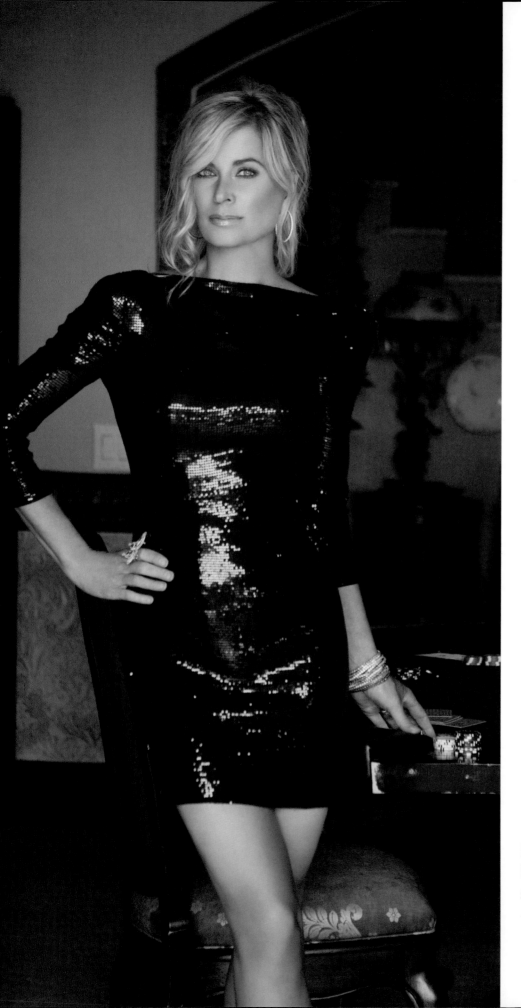

My idea of the perfect
black dress is simple,
sleek and sexy.
—*Eileen Davidson*

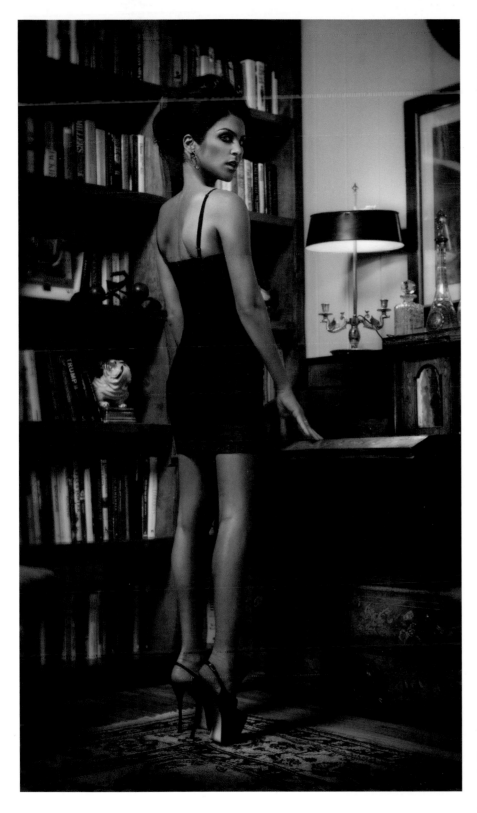

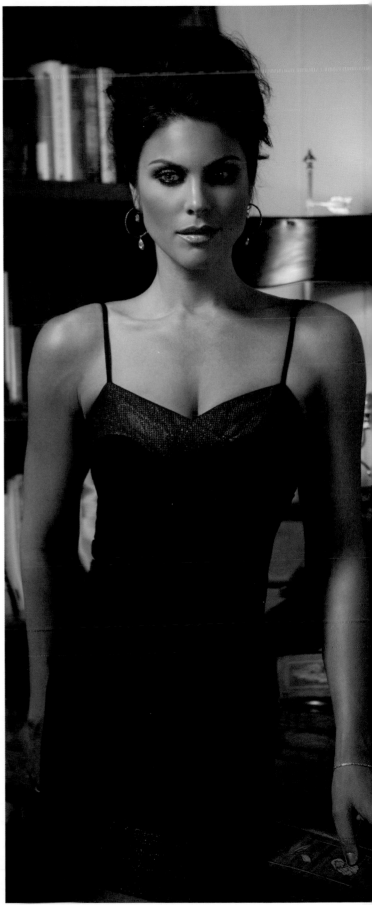

I love to spice up a
little black dress with a
great pair of heels.
—Nadia Bjorlin

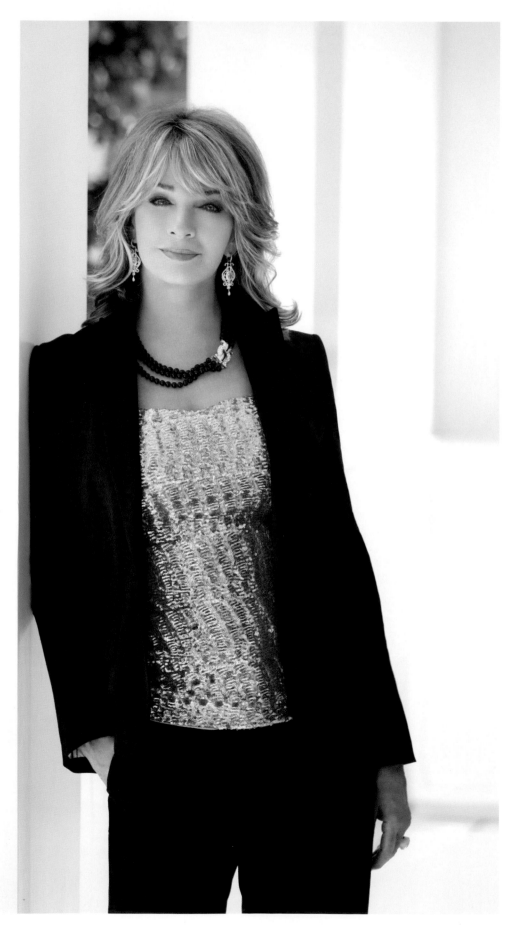

The most important aspect of the LBD is that it must be both flattering and feminizing.

An alternative to the LBD is wearing a simple black suit with a special top.
—*Deidre Hall*

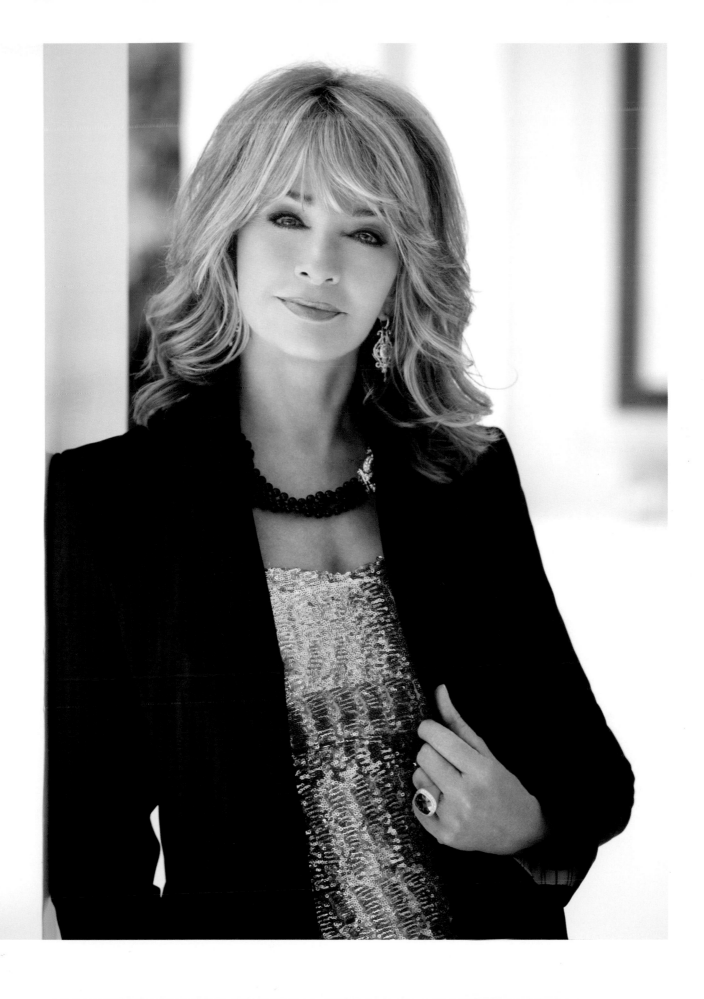

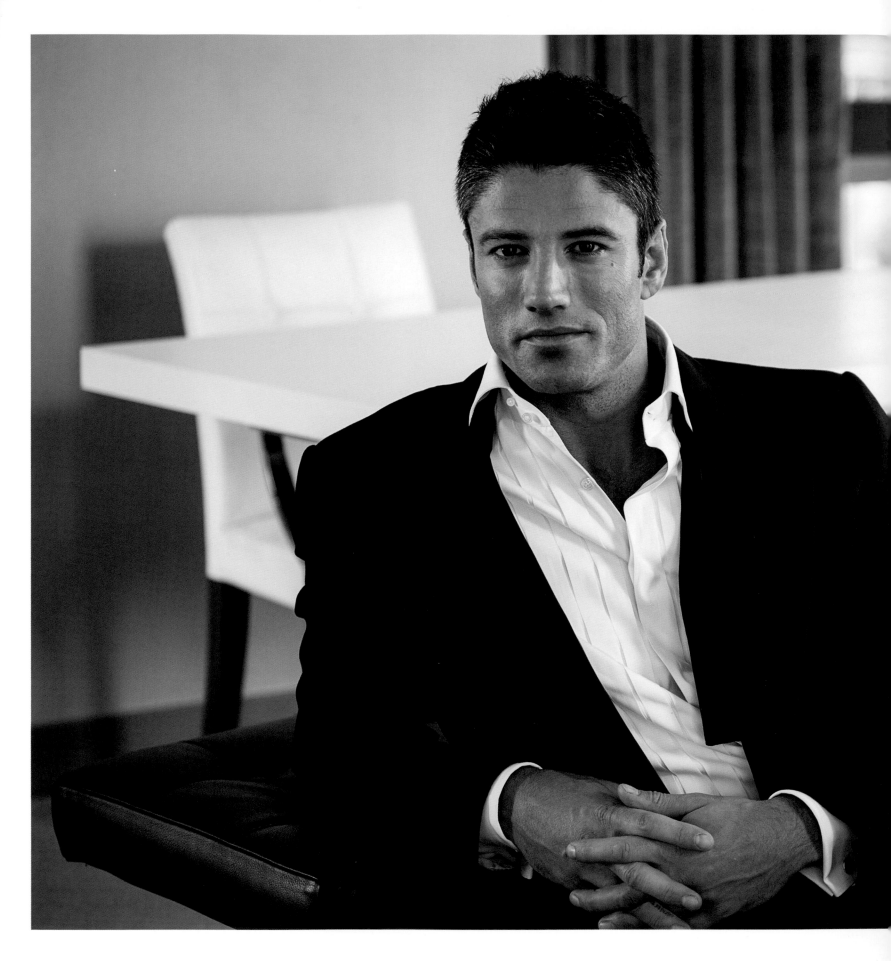

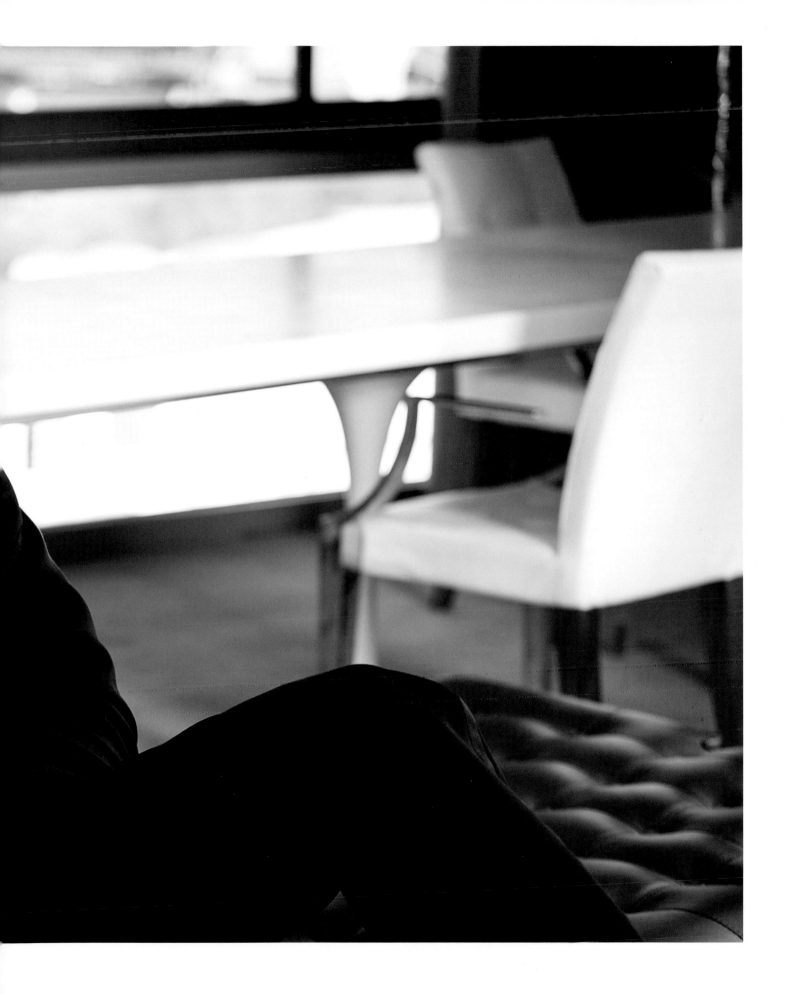

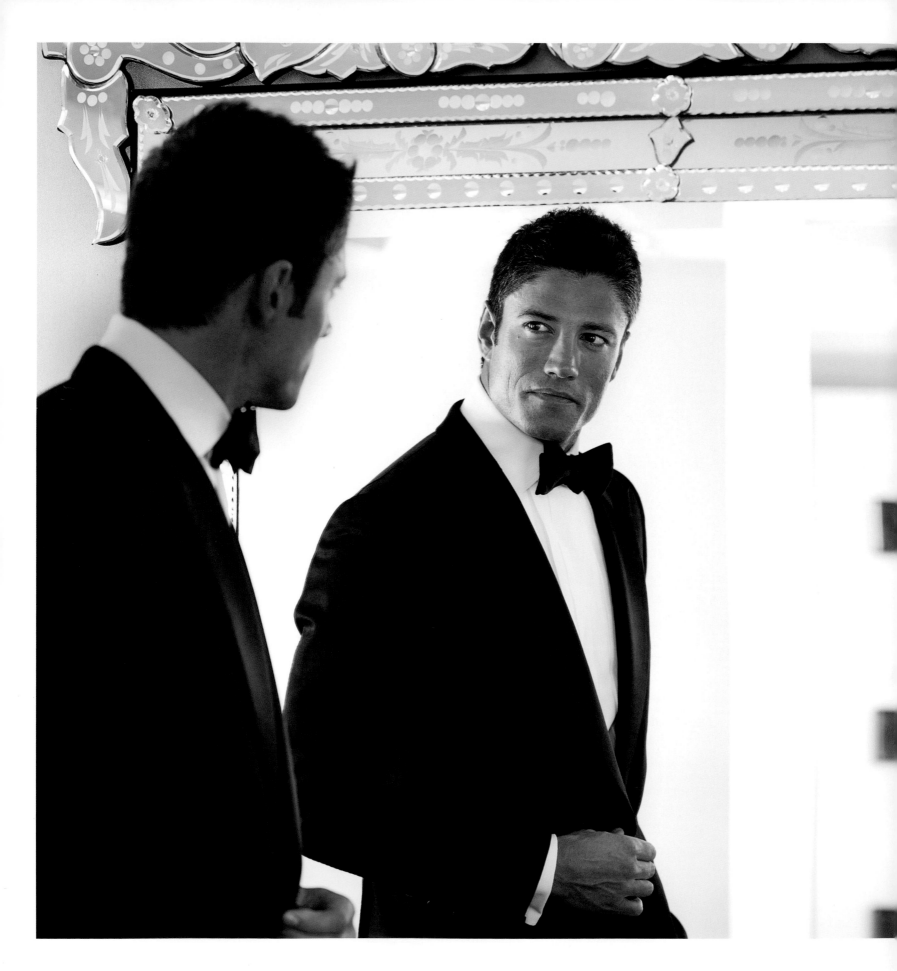

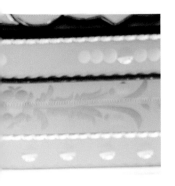

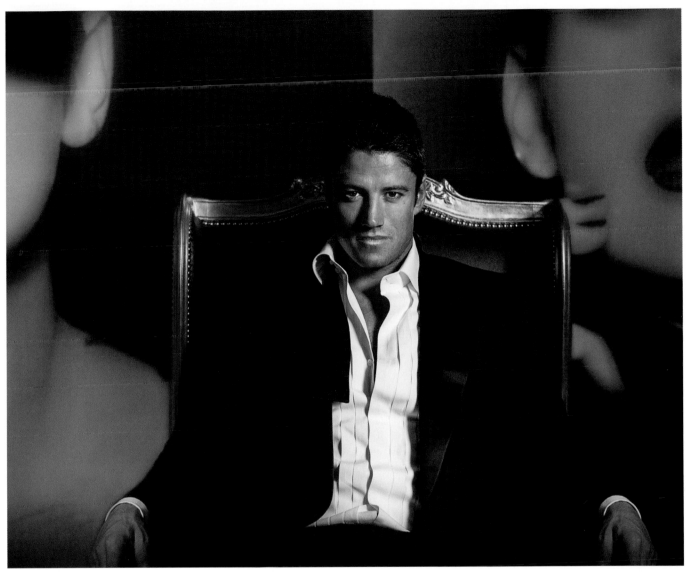

I don't know how I would describe my style. I wear a lot of clothing from a variety of British designers, although I recently purchased a gorgeous jacket from a famous French designer. Recently, for a very special event, I obtained a beautiful tuxedo from American designer Tom Ford.

I prefer to wear whatever is comfortable. I have a pile of T-shirts that are littered with holes that are very comfortable.

I enjoy the ritual of getting ready. Attention to detail is key.

Don't be afraid to go for a more polished look.
—James Scott

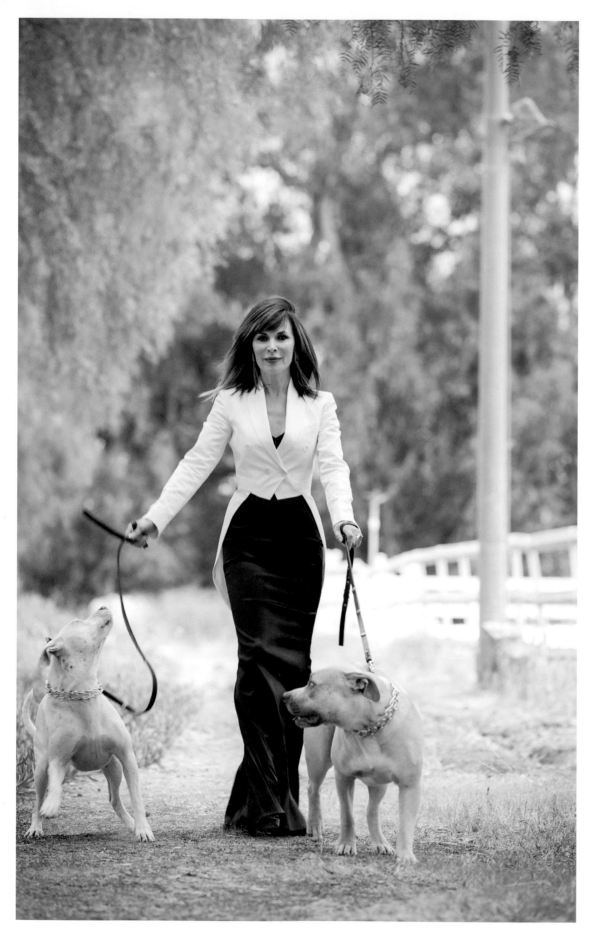

I'd have to say my style is adventurous. I've always loved fashion. I trained as a costume designer in college. That definitely has contributed to my personal sense of style. Along with a love of fashion, I have a love of history and of fashion costumes. All of these elements combine.

I love theatrical dressing. There are so many historical references in costumes. There's a similarity between Lauren and Kate's style of dress.

I'm always thinking of character in terms of style, as well. What would Kate wear when she's going through a particular crisis in her life? I dress very differently when I'm away from the studio. When I'm on the farm I have work clothes—jeans, T-shirts, that kind of stuff.

It is important for you to wear fashion, and not let the fashion wear you. The goal should be "You look great in that outfit!" not "What a great outfit."

I like to dress with a degree of irony.
—Lauren Koslow

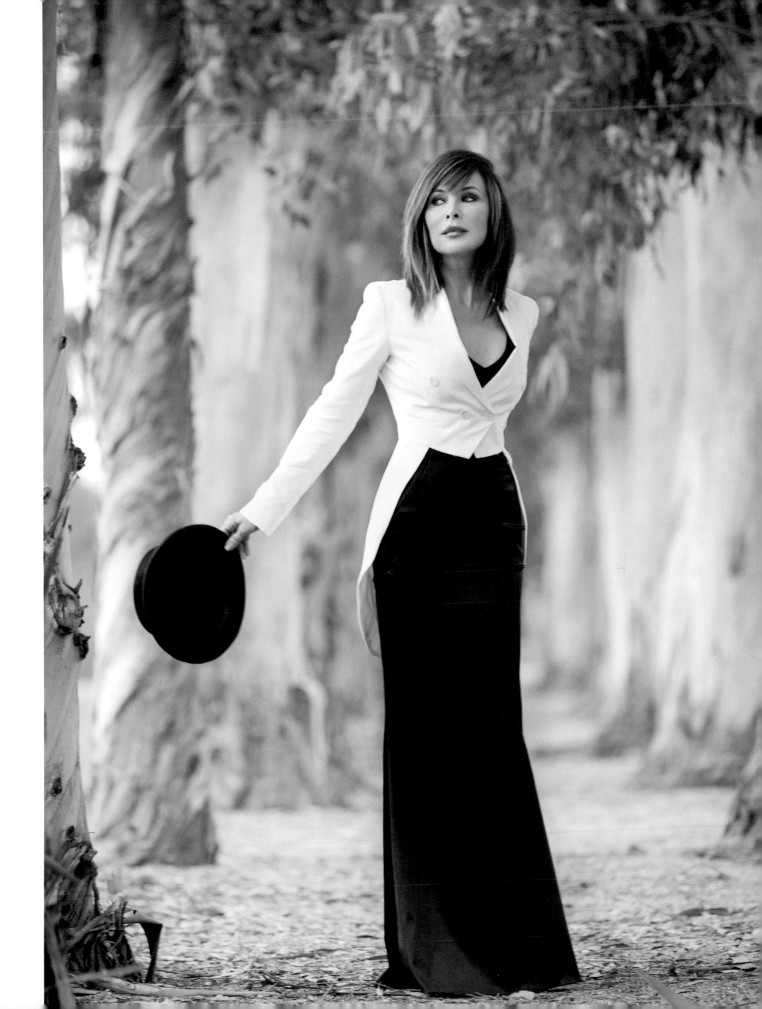

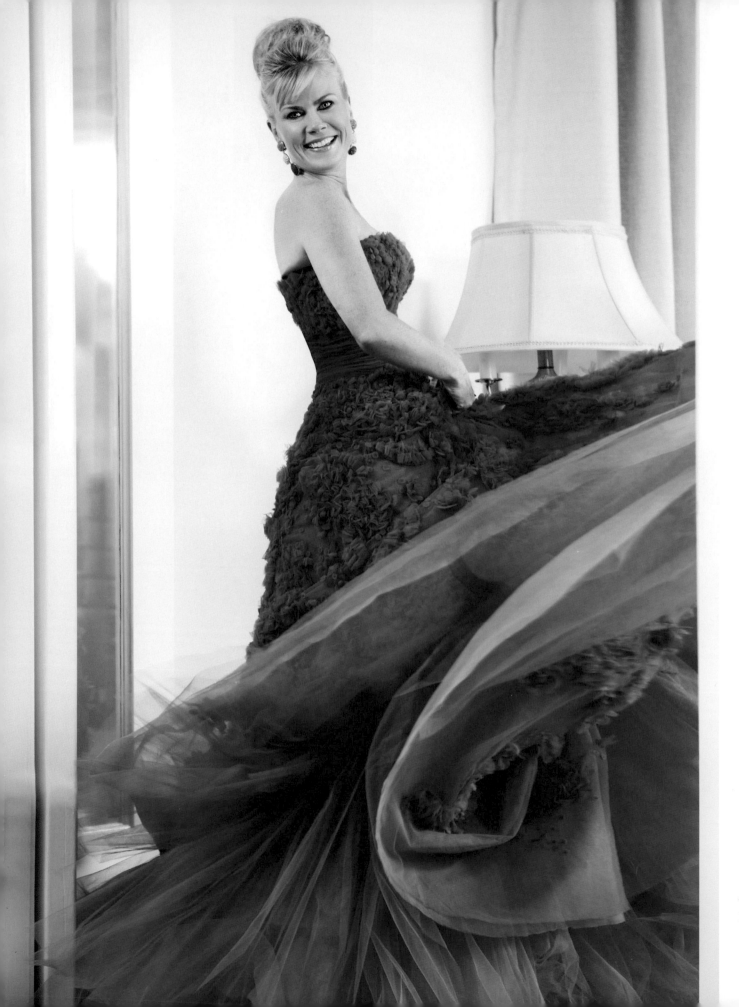

Alison
Sweeney

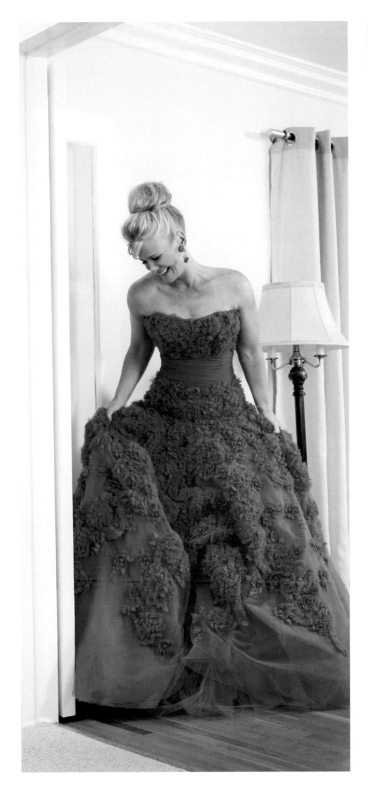

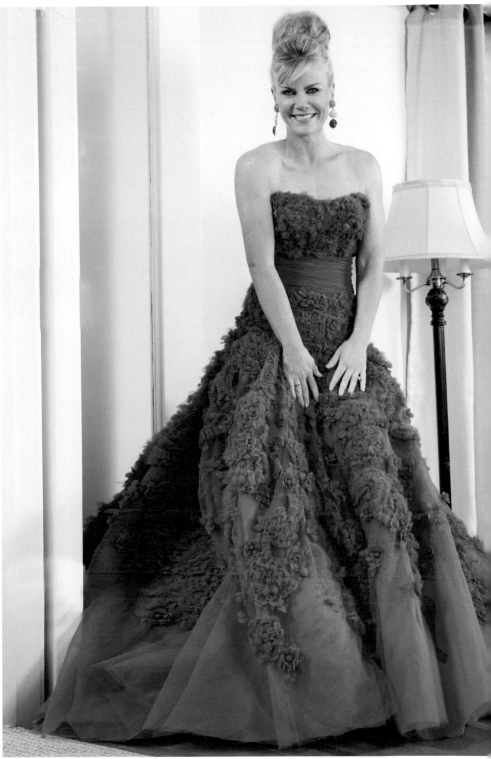

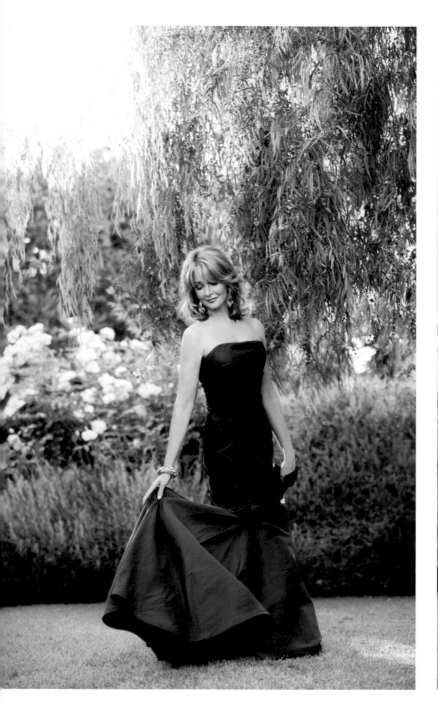
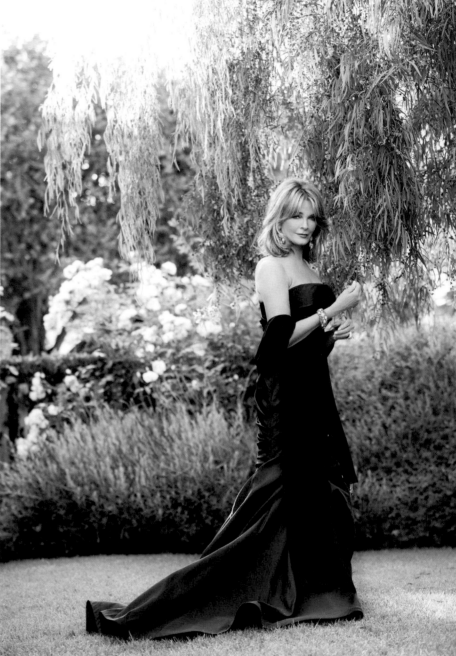

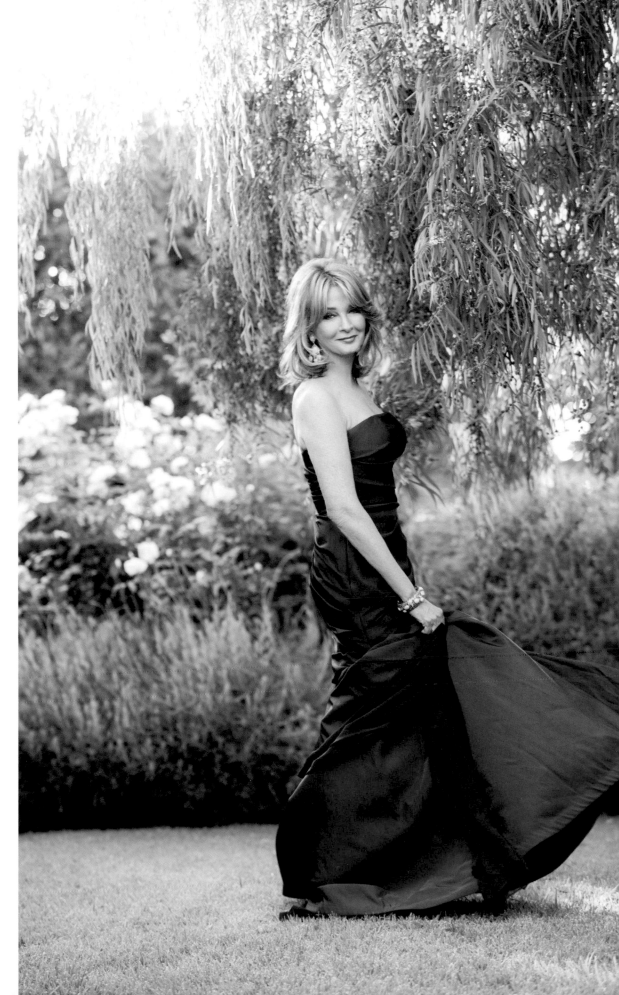

Deidre Hall

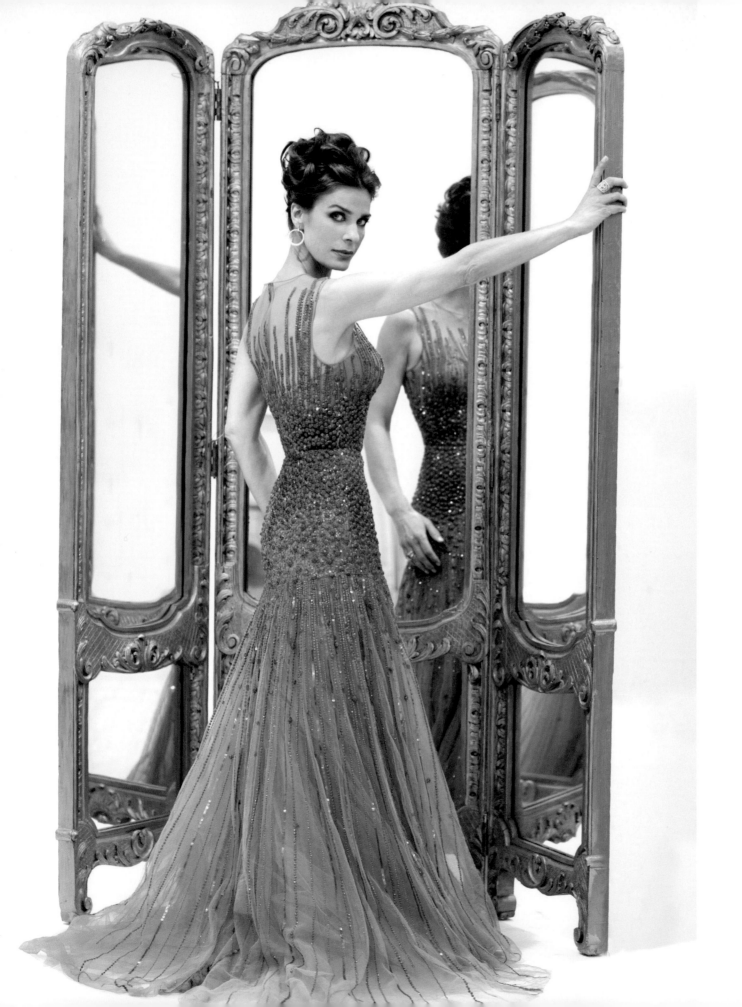

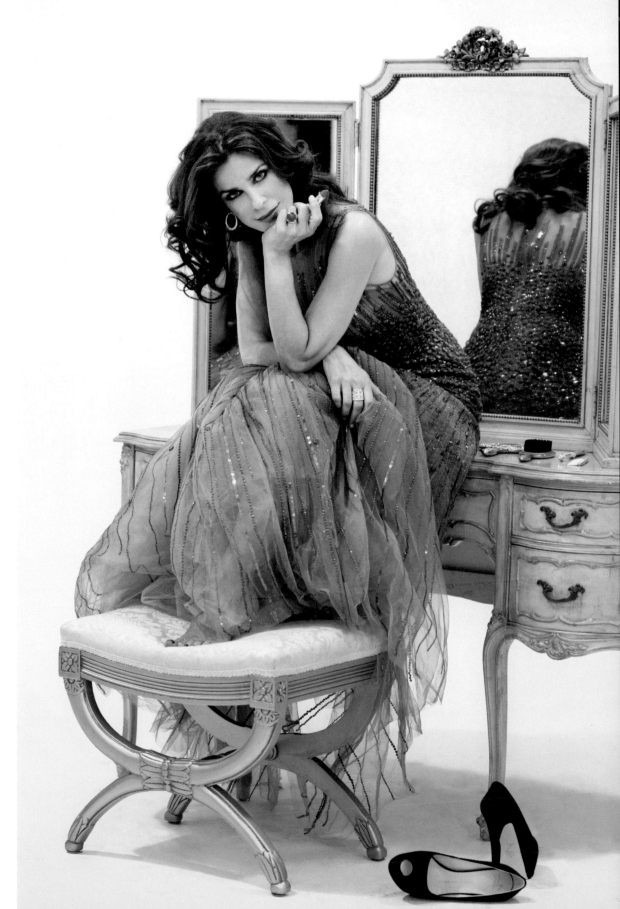

Kristian
Alfonso

inspiration, *n*

1. something that motivates

2. divine guidance

INSPIRATION

You are not a human on a spiritual journey, but rather you are a spirit on a human journey.
—*Unknown*

My positive outlook has played a significant role in my dealing with myasthenia gravis.
—*Suzanne Rogers*

I have some blind, passionate drive that keeps me going. I listen to that voice. You have to listen to your voice.
—*Molly Burnett*

If the people around you are positive then you have no choice but to be positive as well.
—*Freddie Smith*

I have become a student of positivity and spirituality. It all began when I read the book *The Power of Positive Thinking* by Norman Vincent Peale.
—*Lisa Rinna*

I have a firm belief in God. I know there is a plan...a journey.
—*Deidre Hall*

My husband is Catholic and we've been married for 20 years. He's never asked me to convert, but I've been drawn to Catholicism since I was very young and so, recently, I converted. It's one of the best choices I've ever made. After becoming more involved in church activities and helping people, I've never felt more fulfilled.

This may sound corny, but I'm glad that I have a relationship with God. And I have a great relationship with my son, too. I am pleased to say we are friends as well as being mother and son. I wanted a lot of children but my husband only wanted one. It was a sticking point in our marriage for a long time, but now I have a lot of kids to take care of through my work. They range in all ages and they all get to be my children even though it's only for a short period of time.

I have time to be with my family. Anyone who has a job where you can be with your family a lot of the time is very blessed.
—*Judi Evans*

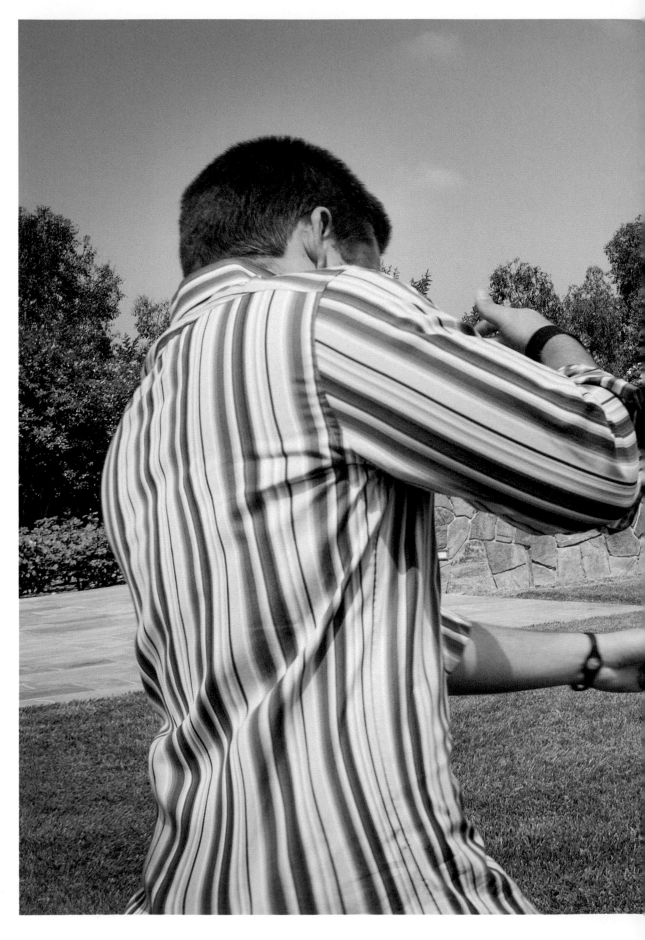

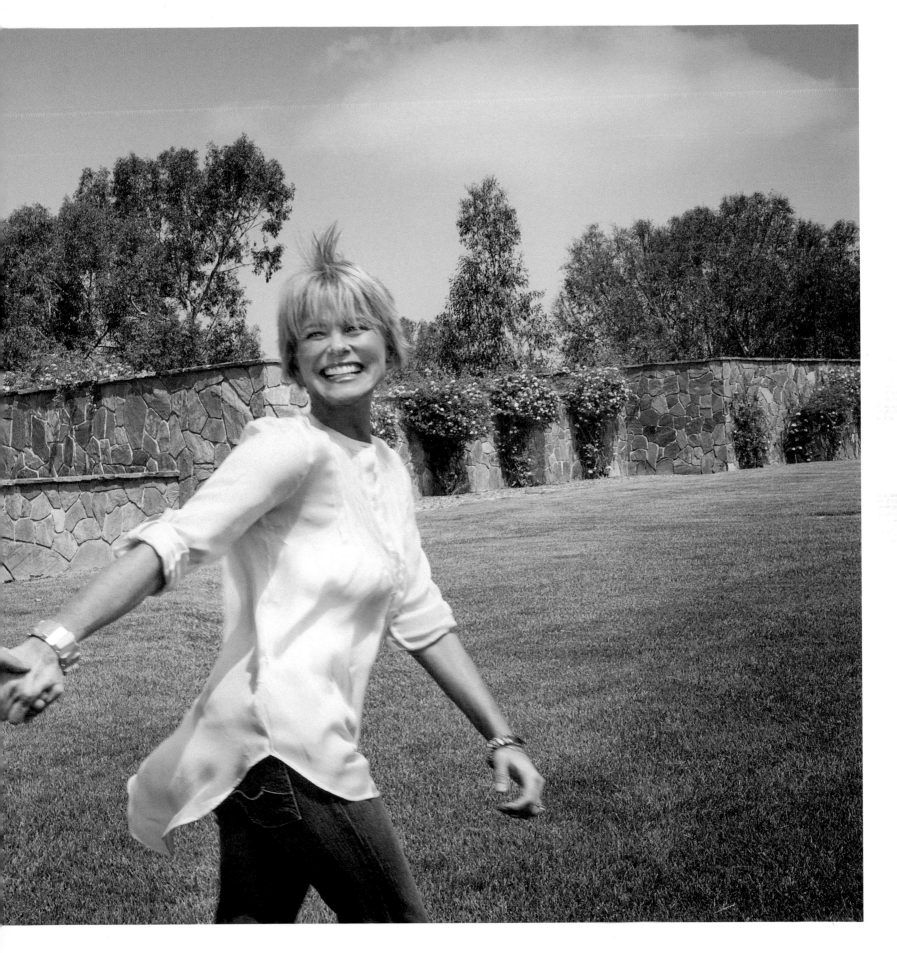

I draw inspiration from reading about other people's lives. Right now, I'm reading (President) Eisenhower's biography. I'll often read two books at the same time. One will be a mystery, thriller or western novel. I call those my "bubble gum" books. The other will be a historical work.

There is not one, single source of inspiration in my life. There are different parts to who I am. Everybody is often in different places at different times. I'm a different person at work than I am at home. There may be people who see you behave in a certain way in one environment, but they'd be very surprised to see you behaving differently in another.

People may have an issue that makes them behave angry or upset. My guess is that there's another reason that's causing their emotion. It's not about what's happening to them in the moment. It's something that has happened to them the night or the week before. People are dealing with their own issues.

It's important to respect people and not push your way of thinking onto them.
—*James Reynolds*

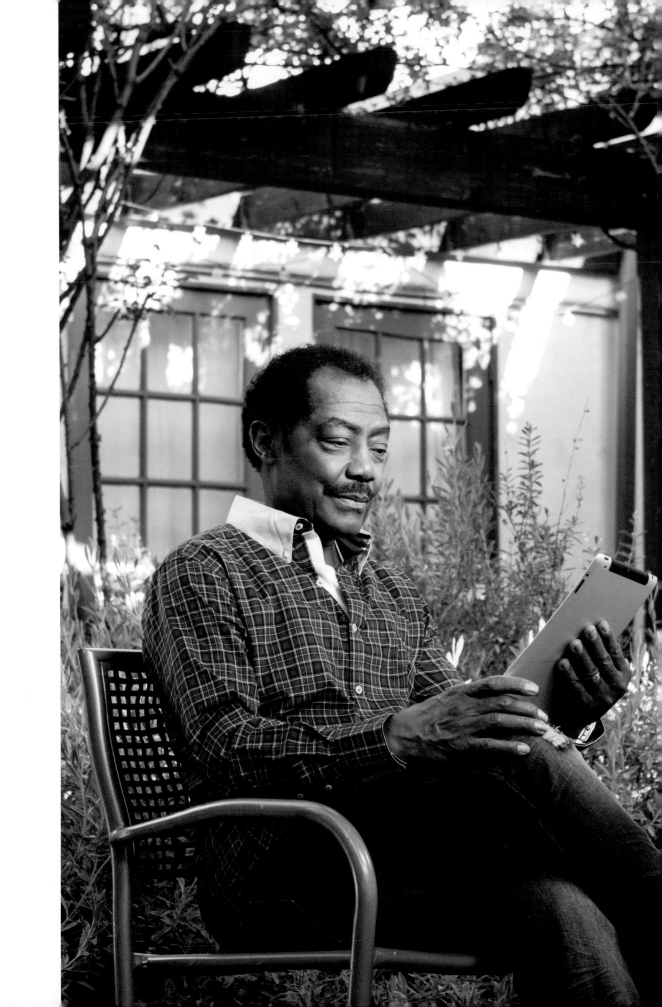

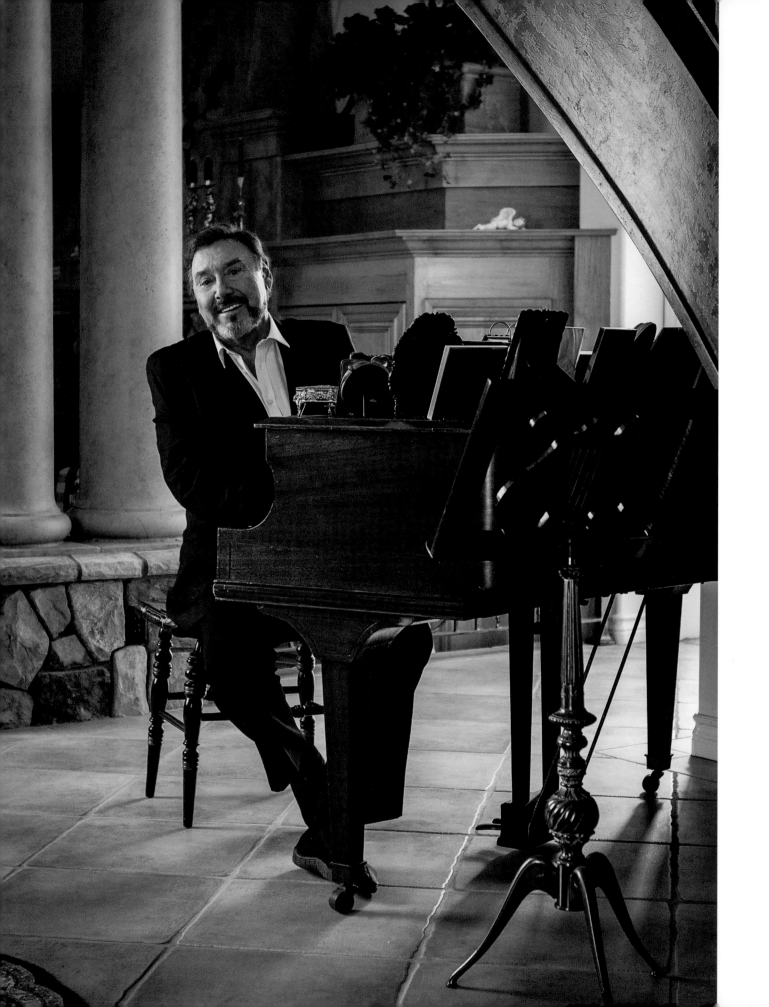

I get inspired when I see or hear great artists, whether they are writers, musicians, composers, actors, dancers, singers or anyone who creates.

I am deeply inspired by opera. Puccini and Pavarotti are my idols. And, in acting, Marlon Brando is a great inspiration. Challenges in my work inspire me. I've been blessed with many opportunities in theater, in film and in television, which, of course, includes my time as Stefano DiMera!

Above all, the closest and deepest inspiration in my life is my family. That starts with my wife, my parents, my sister, my son and includes all of my extended family. I am blessed to have them around me.
—Joseph Mascolo

I practice Buddhism. I'm a big believer in having a practice that helps you reflect on your time or your life and how you are at that moment. I do this by chanting or meditating. Finding a nice place in your house where you can be comfortable and rested to chant or just even sit quietly is a great place to start. Take five minutes just for yourself. It's extremely hard to do given how busy we all are. We feel guilty for taking time for ourselves, but we'll sit in front of the television for how many hours?

For me, it's a world peace movement. I sometimes practice in a group setting where we talk and chant. We discuss what changes we can make in our own lives and hope for a better environment with less violence. We encourage dialogue about change. This is a natural, organic outlet for myself.

By doing the PTSD (Post Traumatic Stress Disorder) story line and in talking to some military people, I learned that there's a new idea floating around called "mindfulness." It's a way of thinking and focusing that helps you become more aware of your present experience. A huge challenge exists for these people as it's difficult for them to be present with trauma-triggers found in other places. It helps you notice your thoughts and learn to take a step back from them, to let them take their natural course.

Mindfulness advocates taking some time with no radio, no cell phone and no other distractions. Do it for a minute or for five if you can. It's more challenging if you strive to do it for longer periods of time.

It's about being the change as opposed to saying, "Oh, those people over there need to change."
—Matthew Ashford

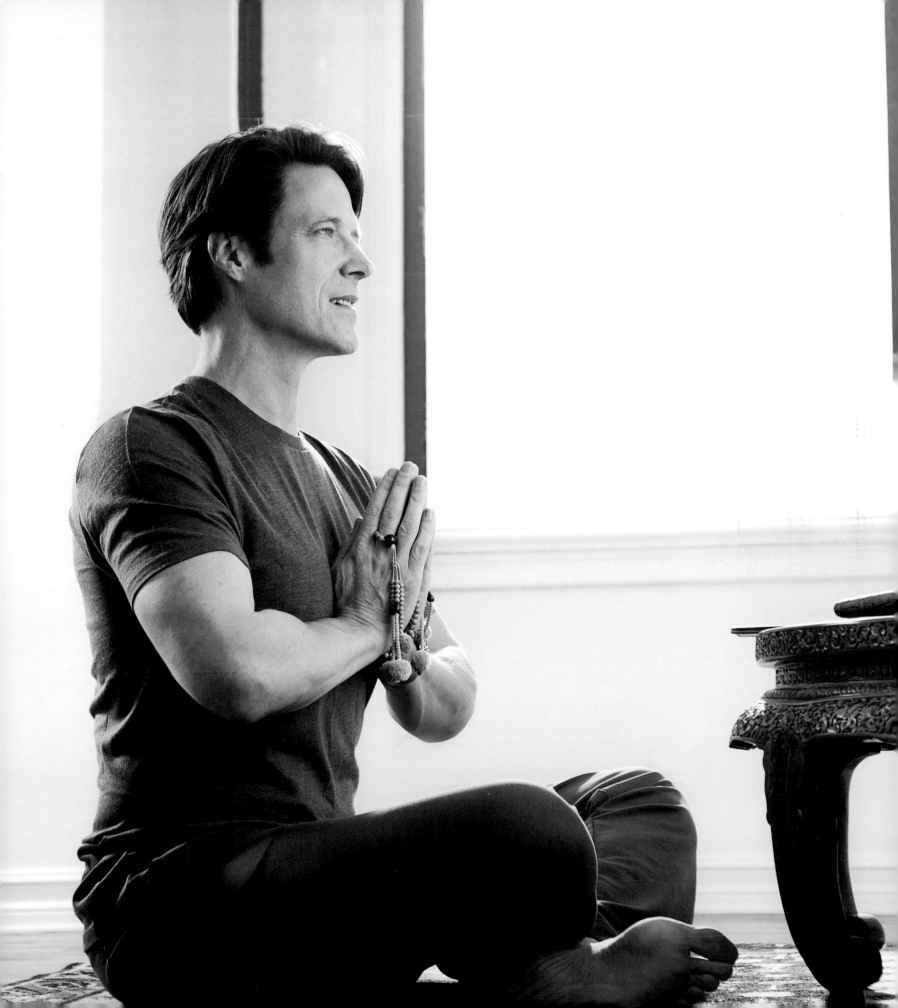

I added onto my house so my mother could come live with me. In Europe, parents come and live with their children all the time. I don't know how we, as a society, lost that. I remember saying to my parents when I was a little girl, "I'll take care of you!" Other people live with their mates or their children; my mother lives with me. Sure, sometimes we have disagreements, but that's how life is. It'd be boring if we didn't disagree every now and then!

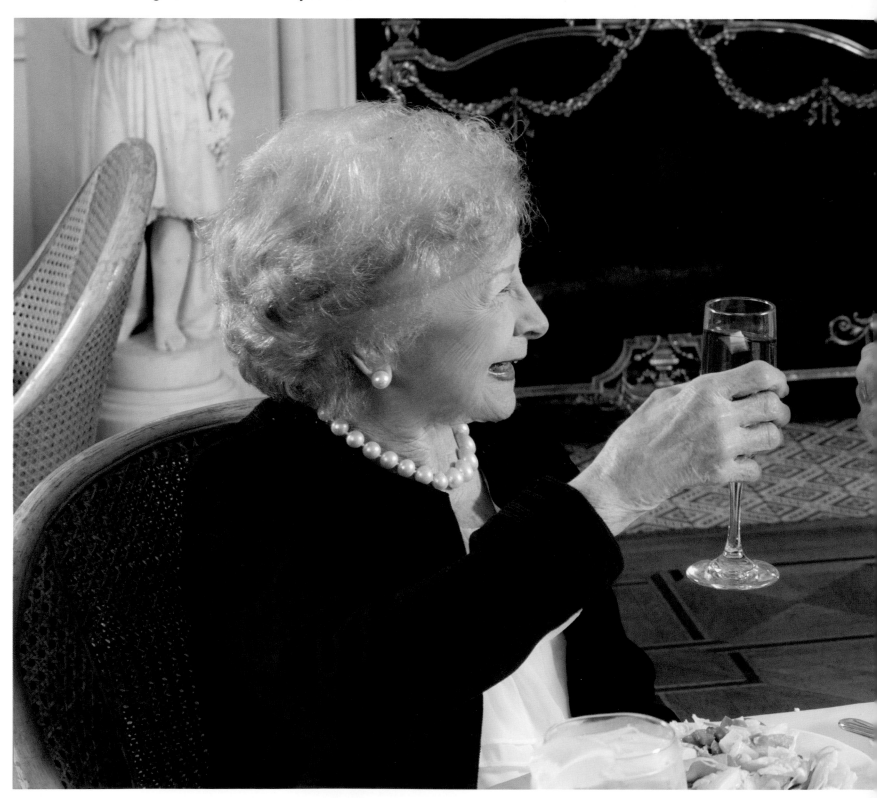

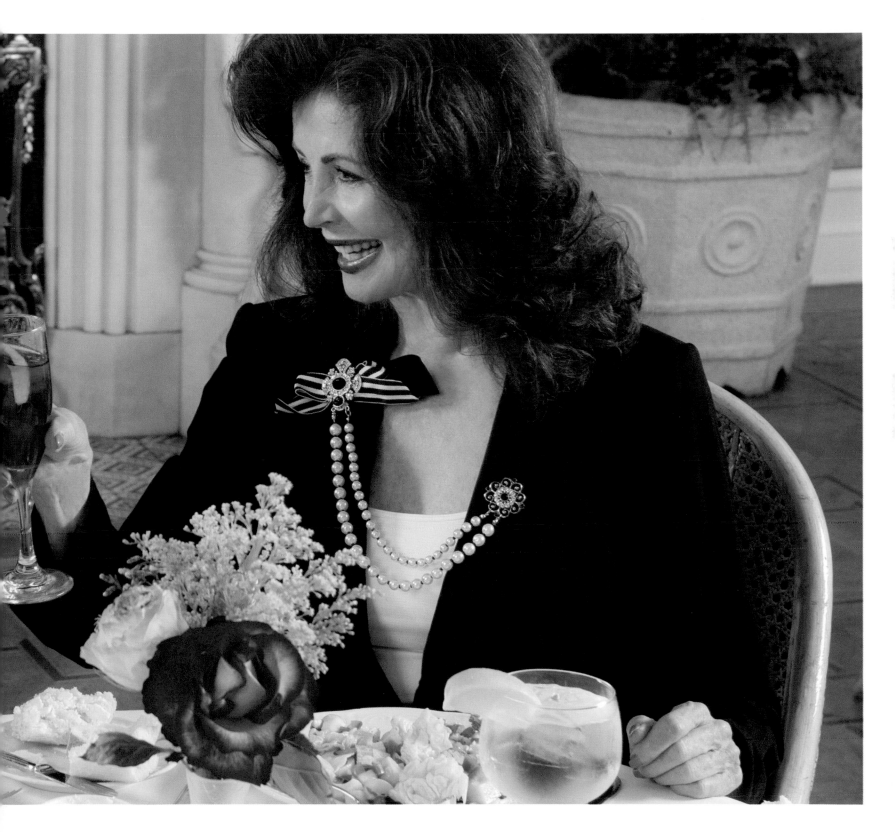

You have to get to a point where you don't care what other people think.
—*Suzanne Rogers*

People tell me I'm nice, which is great to hear, but it's not something that I particularly work on being. I think you just have to be born a certain way. I was always nice and kind growing up, I suppose. I've seen a lot of people turn (in terms of their attitude) in my line of work. The entertainment world is an intoxicating world. A lot of people are not so nice. You have to surround yourself with good people and remind yourself what's real. My parents taught me to appreciate how hard everyone in life works.

My family keeps me grounded. My girls are very young, but I'm already teaching them to be kind to others. We have a list of rules. The first one is, "Treat people the way that you want to be treated." I like living in San Francisco. There's a different attitude here than the one in Los Angeles, I find.

When I'm home, I'm reminded about what's real.
—Christie Clark

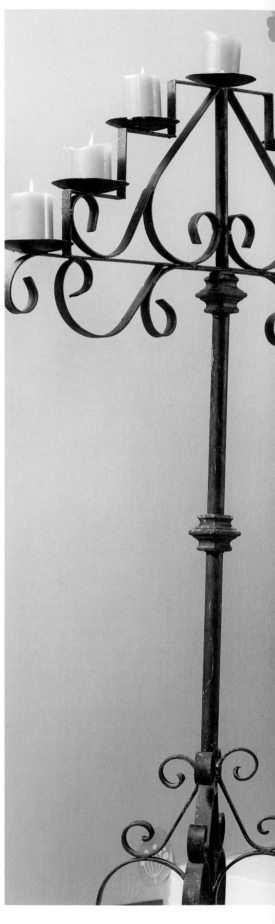

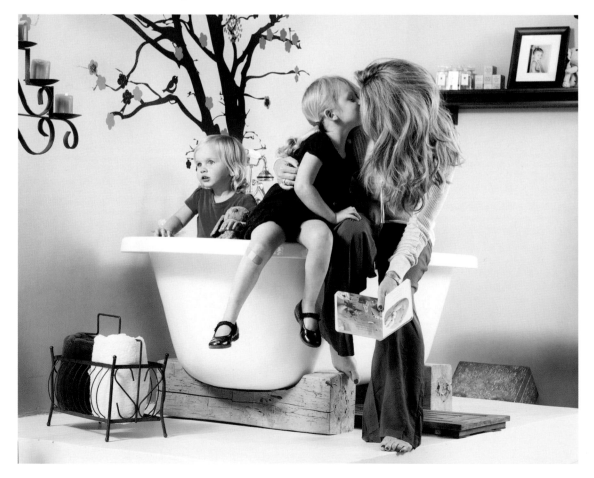

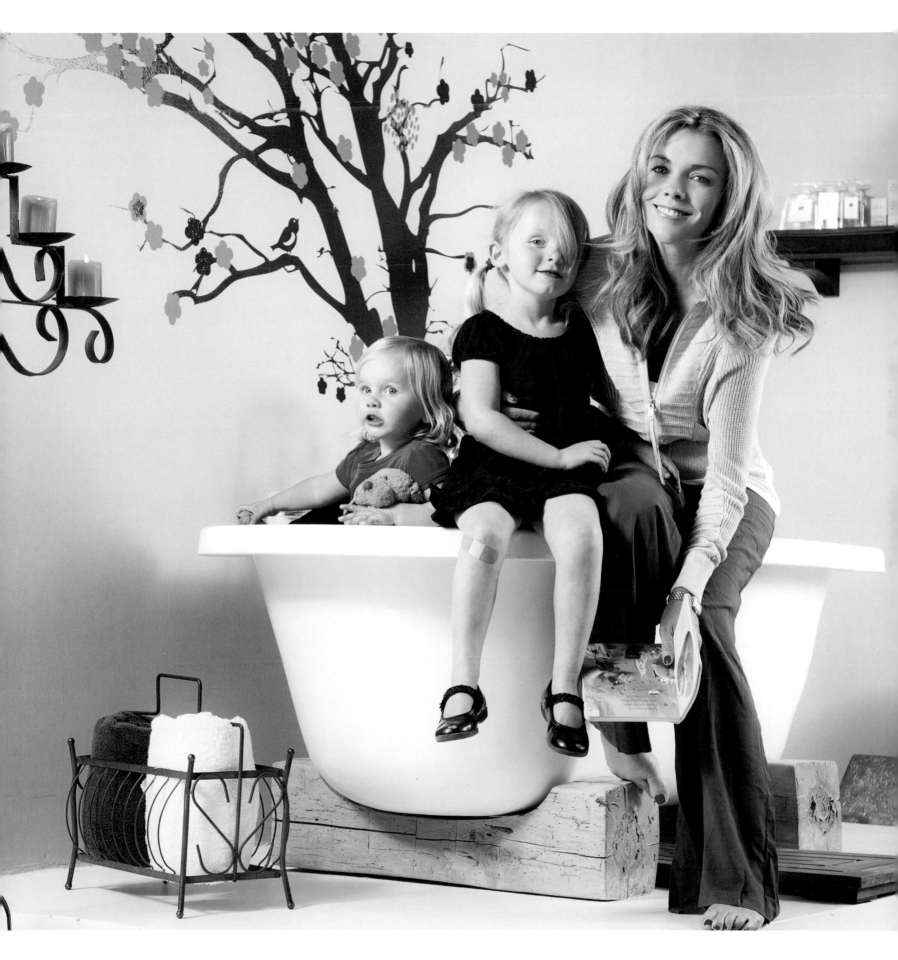

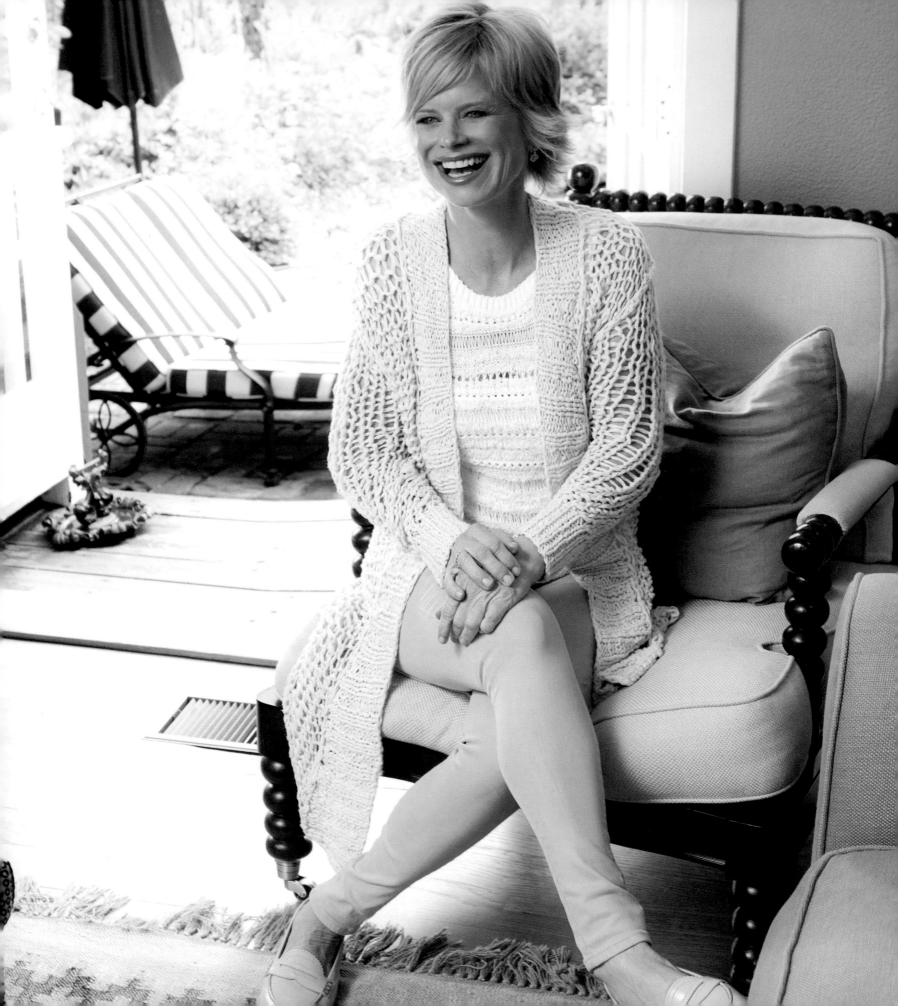

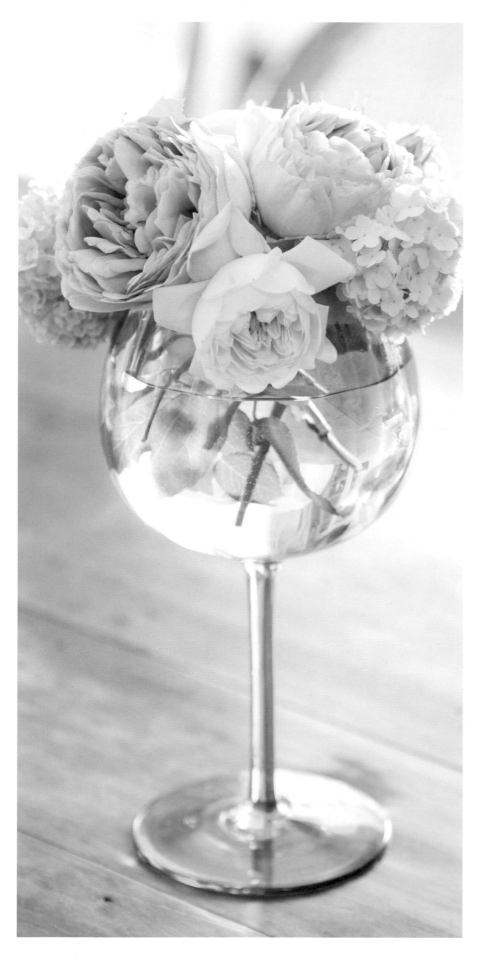

"She was flexible." I joke with my husband all the time that that's what I want inscribed on my tombstone. I say this because I think I adapt to changes well. That's helped me a lot in life. I go with the flow. I never planned to be on the soaps, but it worked out well. I met new people and grew as a person and as an actress.

My husband and my children are more important to me than anything else. I live a very domestic, happy life. We like hanging out, going to dinner and watching TV together. My son was dating a girl and he wasn't sure if she was the right one or not. I asked him if he liked just hanging out with her. I said, "Your dad and I would rather hang out with each other than anyone else. If it seems as if it is a burden then maybe she's not the right one?"

I've always felt so blessed to be on *Days*. I always feel like the luckiest person when I come to work. I don't think about what they're not giving me to do. I think about what they are giving me.

A New York soap opera offered me a contract role when my daughter was going to be a senior in high school. I thought about taking the job and she said, "Well, if you want to miss my whole senior year…" I didn't take it. It wasn't the most important thing in my life. My family is.

Life is a long, winding road, but I can't think of a single regret that I have. You can drag around what's happened to you in life or you can let it go.

I always put my family first. My family is the most important thing in my life.
—*Mary Beth Evans*

I've started taking electric guitar lessons. It's not unlike how I started surfing. I'd always wanted to surf. Then, finally, one day when I was in my thirties I said, "What am I waiting for?" And I started to do it. I got an instructor and started surfing. I'm doing the same thing now. I used to play air guitar to Aerosmith when I was in high school. Again, I thought, "What am I waiting for?" I found this great guy to teach me—David O'Rourke. I love him. He's in a band and he opens for Coldplay and Korn. He teaches when he's not touring. I've been taking classes with him for four months and I love it. I've been "shredding" with Metallica. I'm also playing a little Indigo Girls, Tracy Chapman and Foo Fighters. We're all over the place.

It's actually a fantastic thing when you get calluses on your fingers because that means you're building up enough strength in your fingers and that you're placing the correct part of your finger on the string.

Playing guitar is a form of meditation. You get into a zone and nothing else matters. When I practice guitar that's all that's on my mind. It really de-stresses me. I look forward to that time each day when I practice.
—*Eileen Davidson*

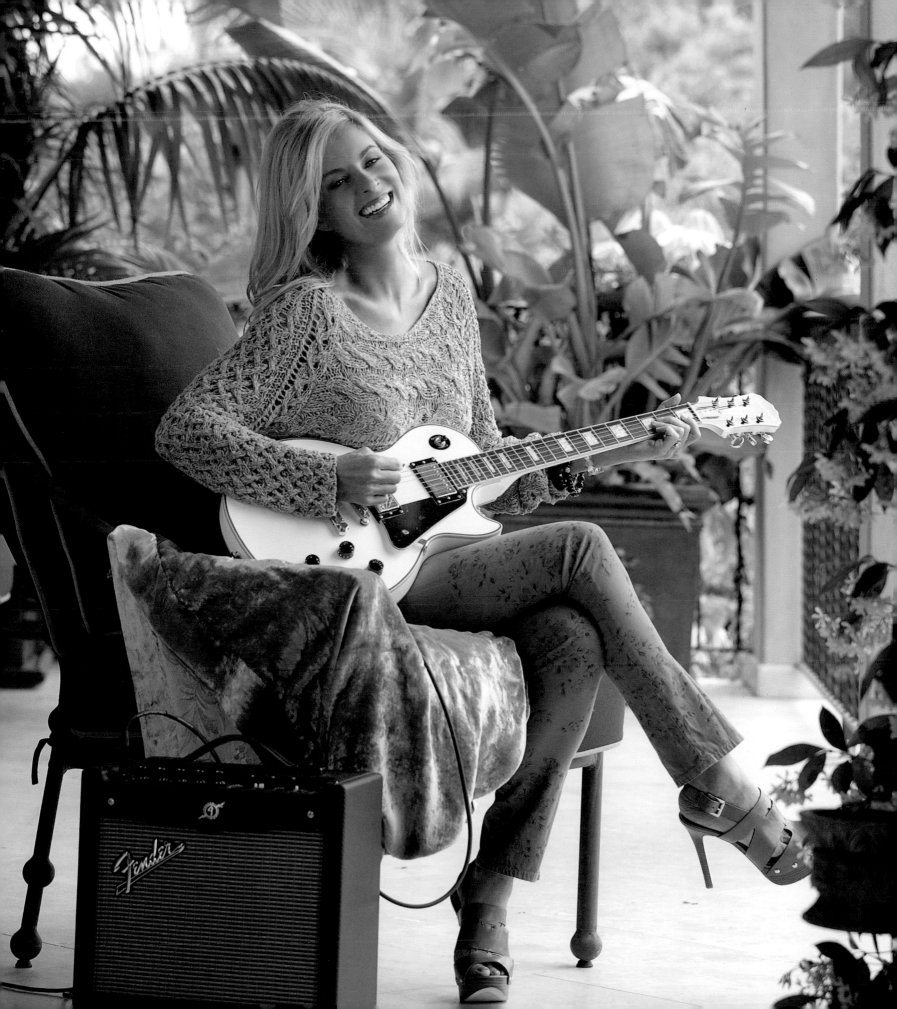

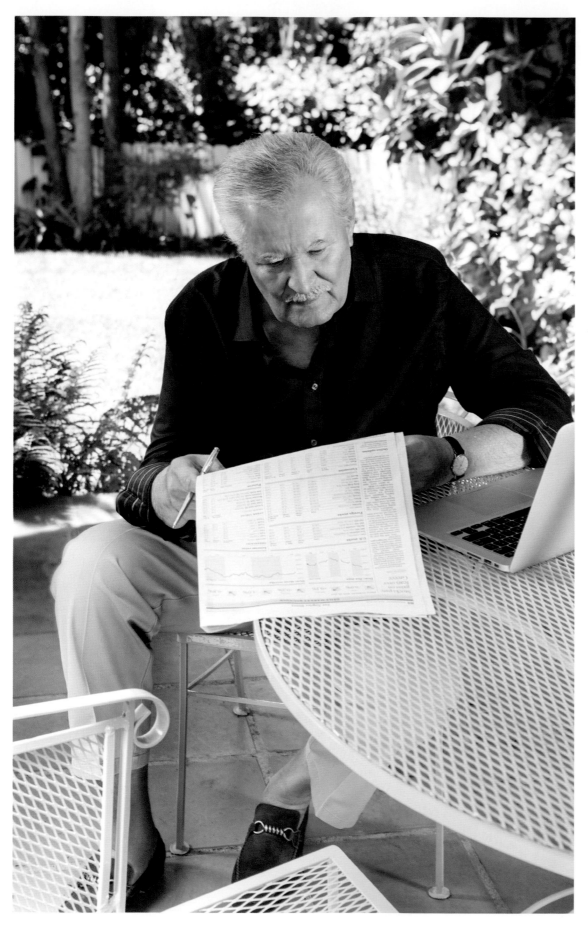

When people ask me what it's like being on *Days of our Lives*, I say, "Well, it sure beats working for a living!" People also ask me if I'm ever going to retire. I say, "From what?"

Only two percent of people who go into the profession of acting actually end up working in it. The odds of making it are horrific. When people tell me that they want to be an actor I tell them, "No. Go into medicine or law." I figure if my telling them to stay out of show business is going to work then they probably shouldn't be in it in the first place.

When you go into something, you can't think about the competition. Go and do your thing. Make a commitment. Don't go down the middle when you're giving a reading at an audition. The middle is very muddy. You have to make a definite commitment. If they don't like it, they might say to you, "Well, we had this in mind…" Then you can try it another way, but the important thing is to make a definite choice.

Do something you enjoy and you'll never work a day in your life.
—*John Aniston*

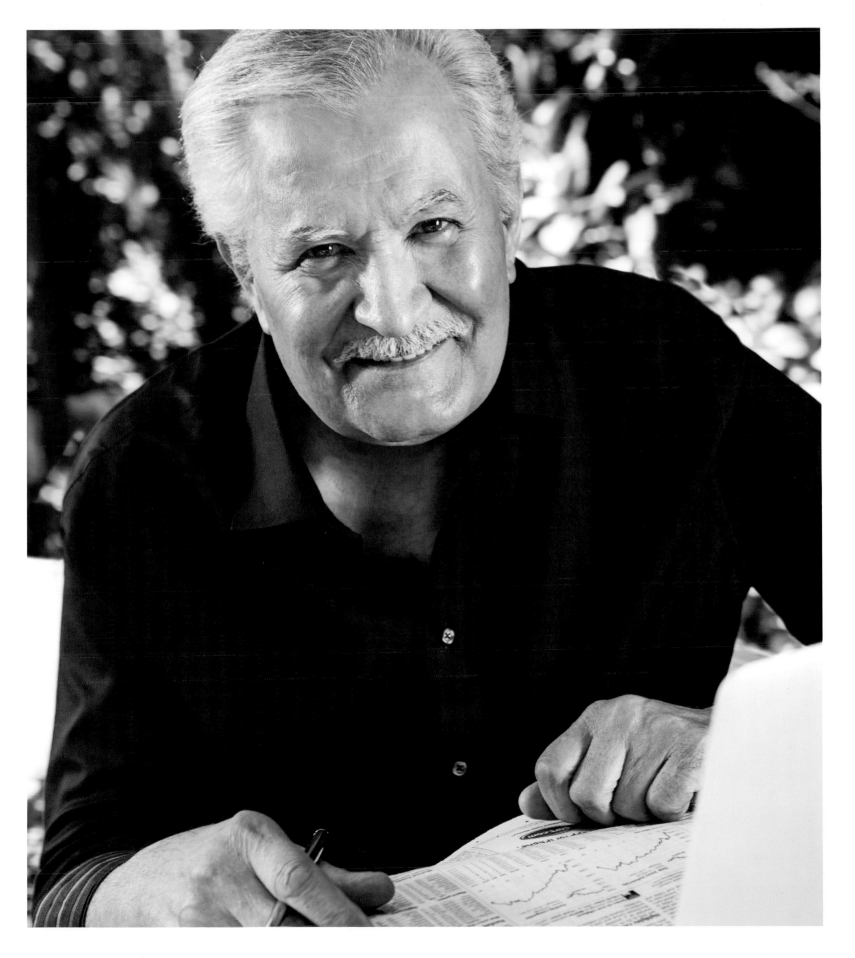

I'm active in animal rescue. We saved some show horses that were abandoned when my husband and I got our farm. They could barely walk out of their stalls, let alone be ridden. We took them in, took care of them and gave them six more months of life. We had one horse that was with us for an extra two years.

I also rescue pit bulls. The biggest misconception that people have about them, I feel, is that they're bad dogs, when actually it's bad owners who create bad dogs. Every breed of dog has a problem here and there, but this is an entire breed of dog that's been branded as being bad. Pit bulls are highly intelligent dogs. They're also very energetic, but they're often thrown into backyards without receiving any attention. Pit bulls seek human contact. That's part of their bloodline. When a pit bull bites, obviously, that's a serious issue—but to call all pit bulls naturally vicious is just not true.

I don't really think about what rescuing does for me. I do it because I want to do it. I want to make that difference. It's a good feeling knowing that I can help animals.

The way we treat animals is how we treat each other. If you mistreat an animal you're going to mistreat a human being.
—*Lauren Koslow*

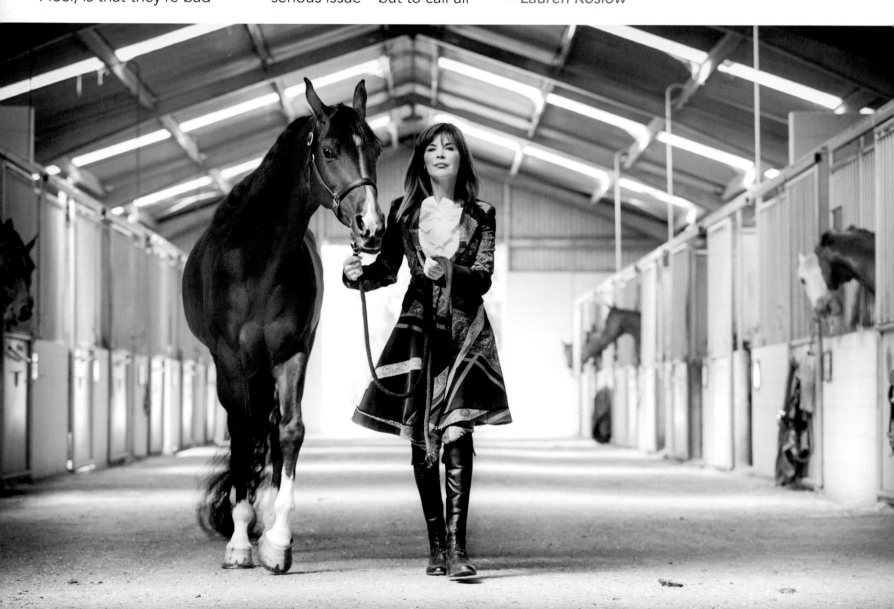

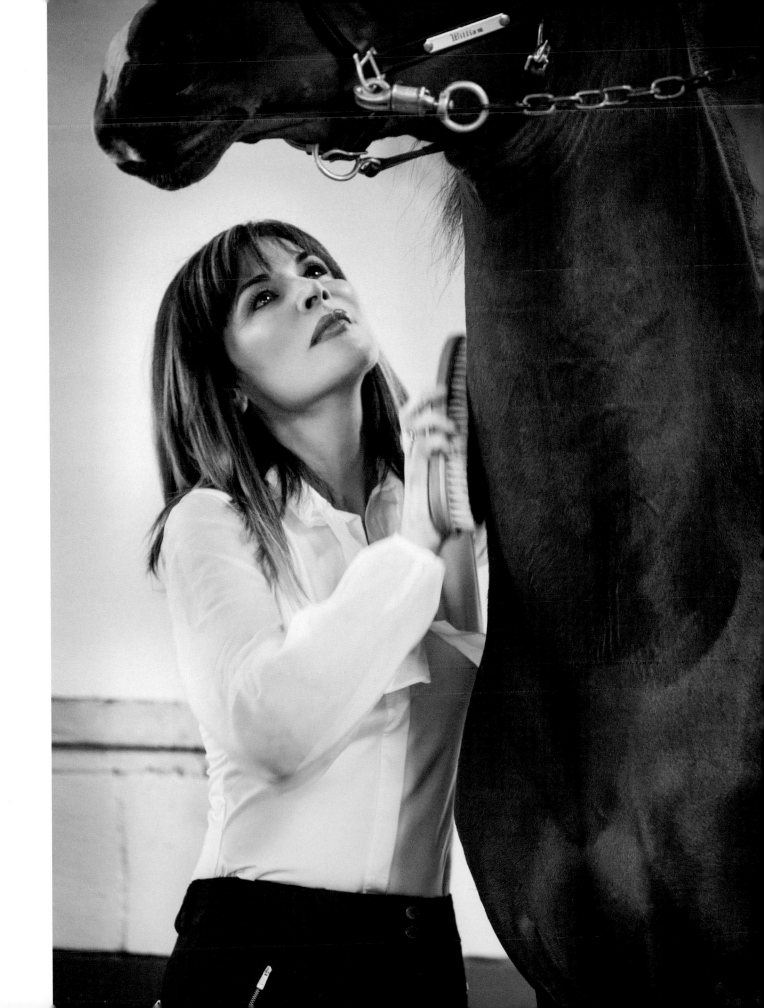

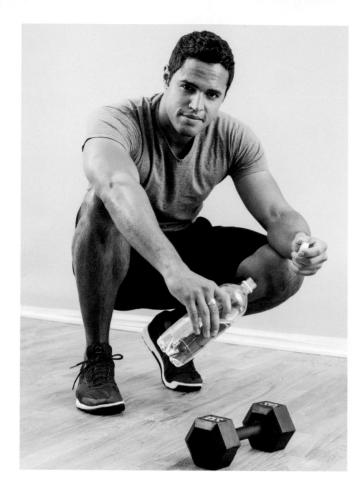

I run the gamut and work with people who are just trying to tone up and others who weigh over 475 pounds. The emphasis is on achieving real, sustainable habits—not making quick fixes.
—*Schuyler Yancey*

A friend of mine is director of operations at Live In Fitness, an extreme weight loss facility. During a time when acting had slowed down for me she said, "Why don't you check out being a counselor there? You'd be good at it!" So I did and I fell in love with it on the first day. I connected with this woman and helped her with a bike ride. I pushed her through the entire ride.

It felt so great helping someone starting to overcome something that she felt was impossible to ever do. It's like acting in Los Angeles—the impossible dream! I've never been overweight, but because succeeding as an actor is so difficult to do, I can relate to helping people achieve their goals.

How do people get off track? I think portions in this country are too big! On top of that, most people work at desks. Then they go home and take care of their kids so they don't always have time to exercise. People need to search for that one hour every day when they can go for a walk or a run.

I received my personal training certification, but it's so much more than that. As the counselor you become the client's therapist, friend and life coach, too.

Counselors work with eight people at a time. They rely on you and they can become very close to you. Establishing that trust can feel great, but there comes a time when you have to push those baby birds out of the nest so that they can do it for themselves. You build toward that final push so that they can leave.

A lot of people get nervous after they complete the program, so they stay in touch with their trainers and coaches. Not everyone has a strong support system in their lives. You have to know how to negotiate conversations about food when you get home—who's going to drag you into a deep hole and who's going to help motivate you to continue to change for the better?

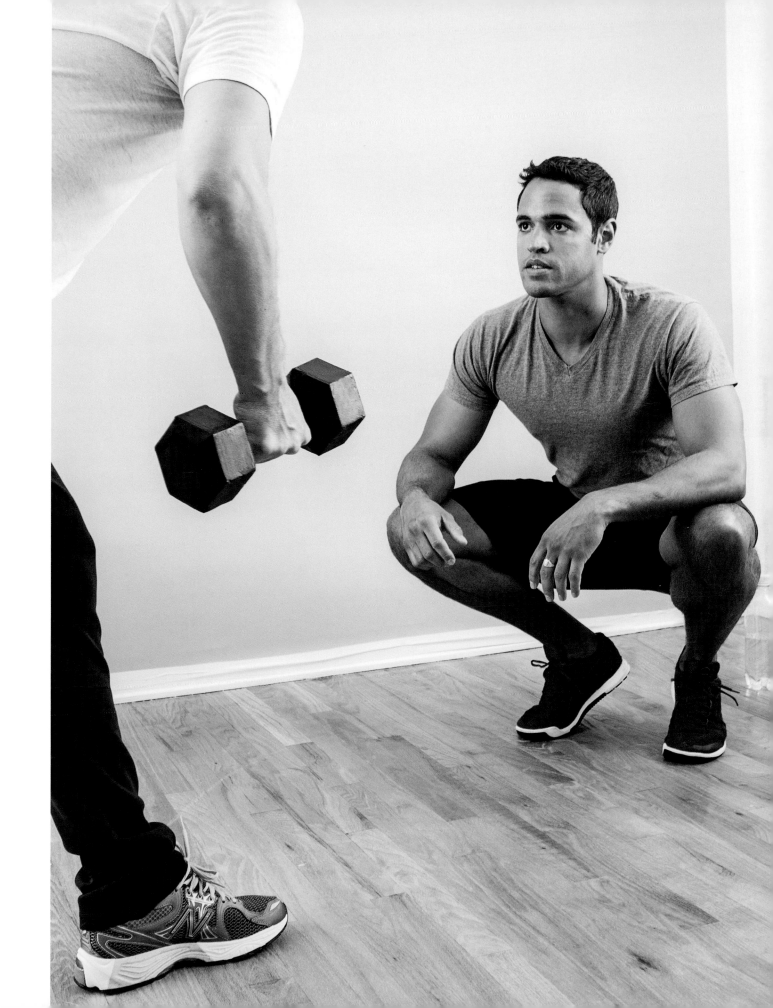

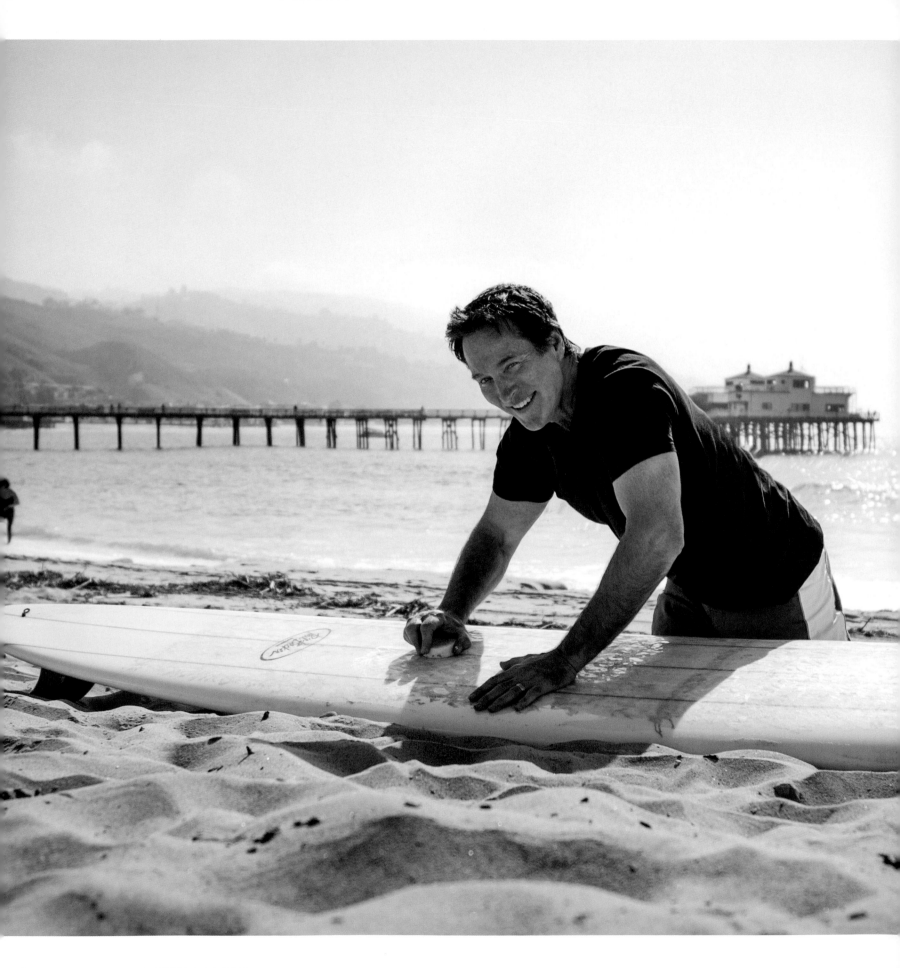

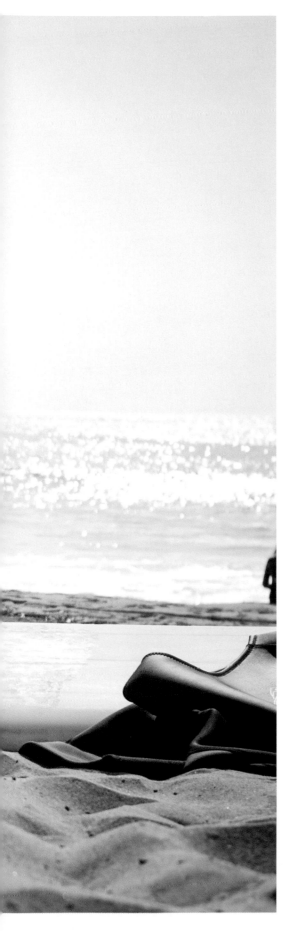

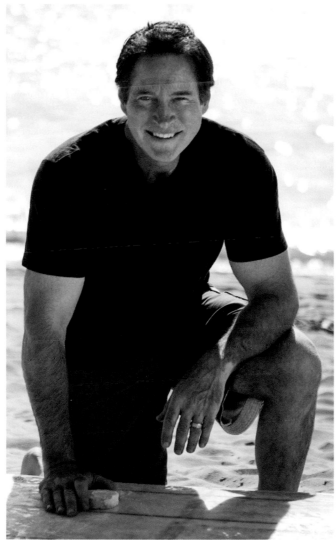

I have a fairly simple outlook on things. I don't sweat the small stuff. Life is simple.

I am inspired by the ocean.
—*Drake Hogestyn*

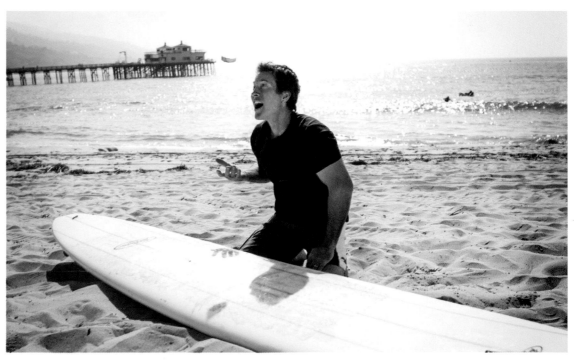

I always text this—work hard, forgive always and love really well. If you just remember those three things and love your God with all your heart, mind and soul, you're going to be fine. To see that in your kids is so encouraging. You see them put it into practice. Oh, I wish I knew that at their age! Gosh, if we could help our kids now…

I tell my kids all the time—don't search for an easy life. You don't want an easy life. It's not going to build character. You're going to make bad choices, but you don't want to make a habit of them. It can show you what you are made of.

Don't beat yourself up over mistakes. We're so busy trying to pick people apart and judge them and find their faults. I don't want to do that. I have the same faults that I'm working through every day. I look at people and say, "I have such grace for you. I don't know your life or how hard it is, so you may have said that because you're having a really bad day." If we all extend grace a little bit further than we think we can, it would be amazing how much good can be done.

I grew up back east. You're born to fight back east. I don't know. It's a tougher way. I don't know if it's because of the mind-set back east. You see it on TV shows. Not that it's a bad thing; it gave me a thick skin to move to California at a young age, but as a wife and mom that thick skin has to soften a little bit and the pride goes down a little bit. Getting older is great; wisdom comes. Getting older is the key to wisdom. It's hard to keep it balanced when you're young. Age is a good thing.

I love getting older. I love every line on my face. I love everything about getting older. I see the bad choices, the good choices…I see everything in my life and how I've grown. I'm okay with that.

Work hard, forgive always and love really well!
—*Melissa Reeves*

There's no time in show business, or even in life, to take things so personally. You can't get down on yourself and be a victim. The most important thing is to know yourself better than you know anyone else and also to have a tough skin and a good support group. That's key. My mother taught me something early on in life that is very important. She said that there will always be people who have less than you and there will be people who have more than you do. Know where you are on the scale and be grateful for where you are and what you have. People are always saying, "I wish I had this" or "I wish I had that." No. Be grateful for where you are.

I learned from my father the importance of treating people the way that I want to be treated. I was raised that way and I don't think enough people are. My father worked for an organization called Wheels Around The World. It provides wheelchairs for people in underprivileged countries. I grew up with that way of thinking. My sister and I would empty our piggy banks out and write letters to children whom we'd foster in other countries. That has resonated with me today. I'll think that I'll need a new purse, but then I quickly realize that I don't really "need" it. We're insanely lucky to live in this country. I feel so blessed.

Mother Teresa said once that people in need have enough tears, what people need are your smiles.
—Kate Mansi

During a period of time that was especially stressful, my husband talked to me about the no highs and no lows. To have the true high you have to be willing to suffer the true low. If you don't want that true low, then you have to let the true highs go, too. I understand that because I love the highs, too. In some ways you can substitute so many things there; you love the adrenaline rush, but then when that is gone…the high is gone, too. You're going to have the lows, too. That's the nature of the spotlight—it goes off. You're taking that middle path, which really is a balanced path. It means that you're willing to let things go; you're not willing to hold onto things because ultimately, you're holding on to nothing. You have to let everything go. It's really about letting it go.

It doesn't mean you still can't get excited or bummed out about something, but know that this too shall pass. When you're in the middle of some kind of horrific moment, ask yourself is it going to matter a year from now—will it be just as bad? In most cases, it probably will not be.

You have to let everything go. It's really about letting go.
—Lauren Koslow

I started playing the piano pretty late in life. I came out to Los Angeles when I was 19 years old. I didn't have any friends so I bought a keyboard when I first moved out here. I needed a hobby! I really got into playing it the last few years. I took lessons when I was a kid, too, but I've taken more since coming out here.

I really, really love classical music. Classical music is all the music I know. I really don't know any modern pop stuff. I like listening to music. It's soothing. It's a different kind of creative process when you're playing. It's a different way to challenge myself and that distracts me from the more mundane things in life.

There's a grand piano in the DiMera mansion. It's old, out of tune and there's a key that sometimes gets stuck, but I'll play it during the lunch break to unwind. It's a nice stress reliever.

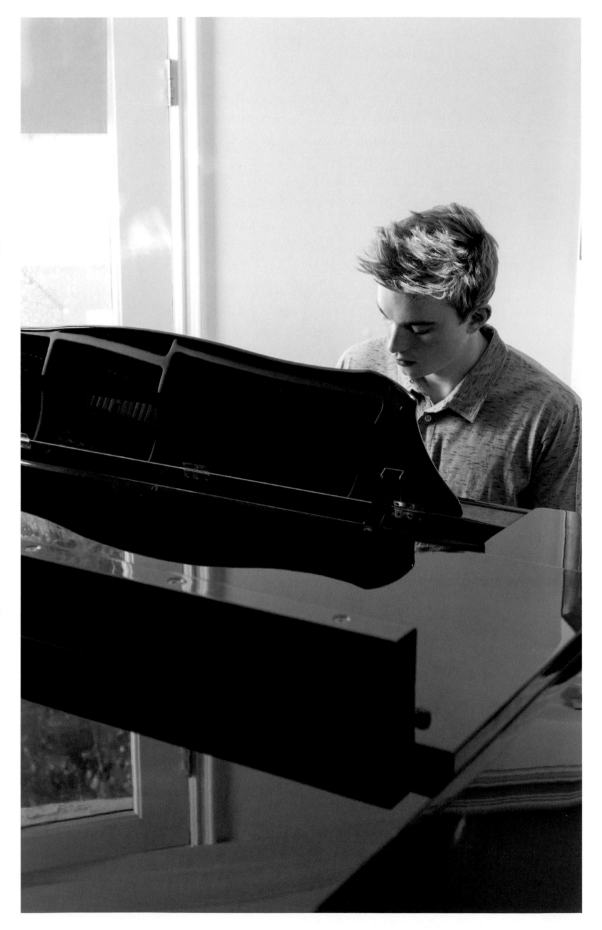

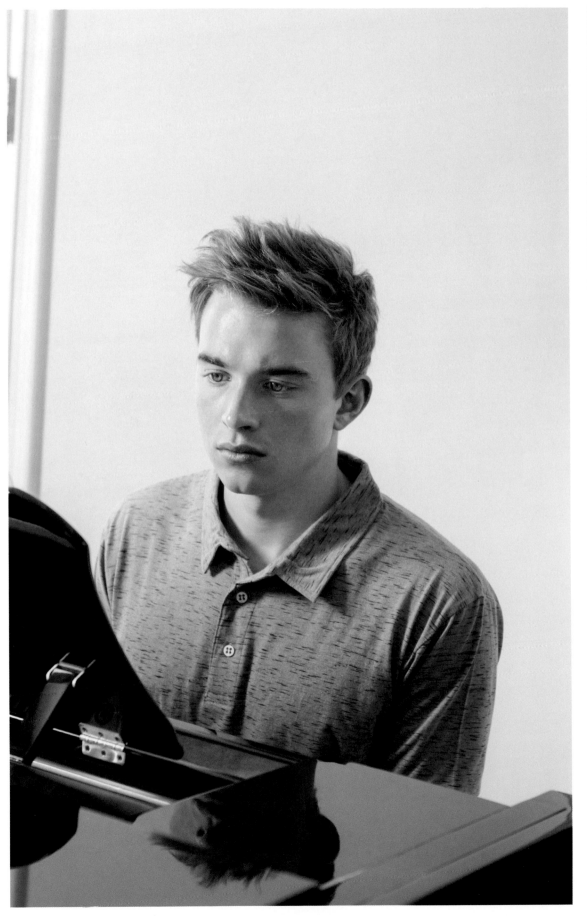
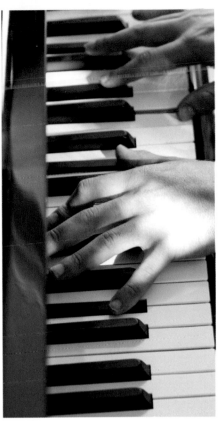

I like history, so playing music that was written so long ago makes me feel connected.
—*Chandler Massey*

I love to paint. I painted the frame around my dressing room mirror to make it look like raw wood. I've painted as a hobby my whole life.

When I was a little kid, I wrote plays and put on shows. Recently, I executive produced and played a role in a science fiction film about people who live (multiple) life spans. My character is an immortal who needs to solve the mystery of his mortal brother's death.

I've always gravitated towards creating something out of nothing.
—*Shawn Christian*

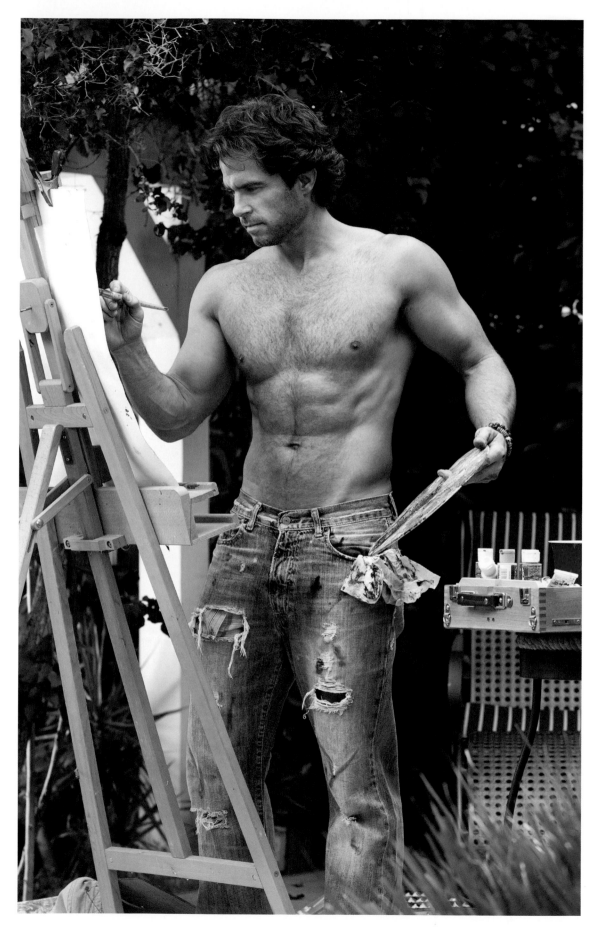

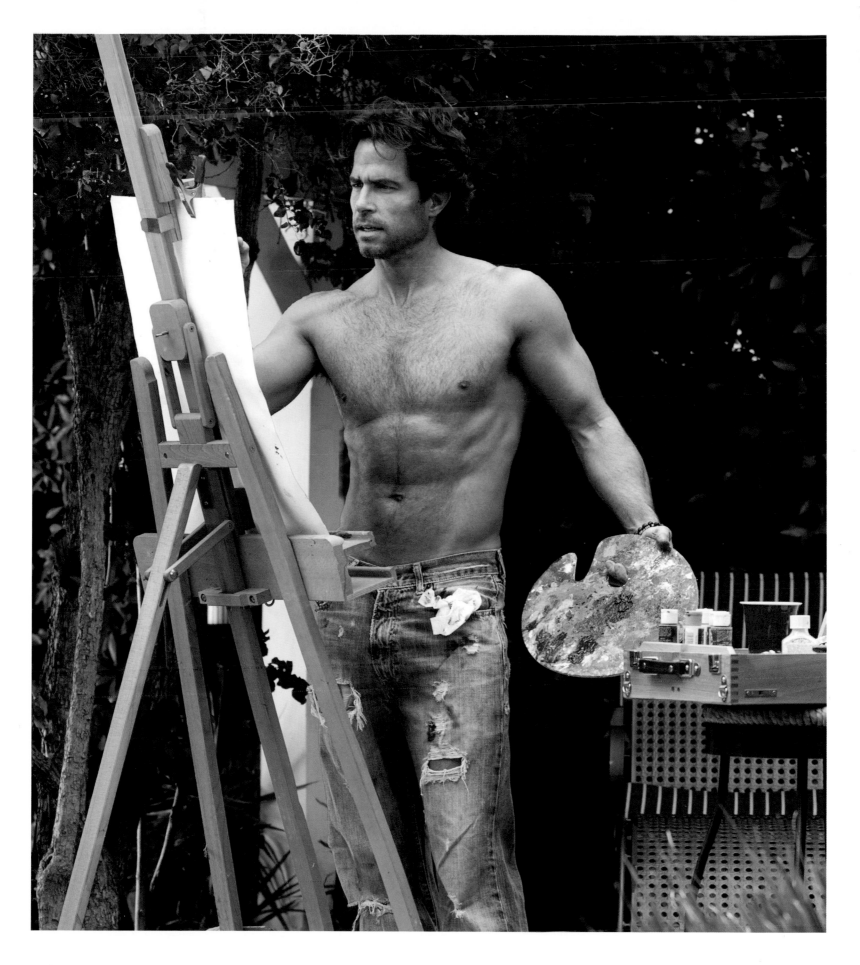

I was fortunate enough to come from a mother who is one of the most positive people on the planet. I've had some help. It's not really that hard for me because I was trained in it: my mother sees everything as happy and great; even if it's not, her attitude is it's going to get better and everything's fine and don't you worry!

When you're brought up by a cheerleader, you can't help but have it in you. I search for that and I strive for it on a daily basis. I think I've taken it to another deeper, more spiritual level because I've had to—I'm in a business that requires me to go even further to find the positivity because there is so much rejection. I've become a student of positivity and spirituality. It all began with the book *The Power of Positive Thinking* by Norman Vincent Peale. That book changed my life; it's so much about how everything is in our own control. We create everything that happens to us. I truly believe that. I believe that what you put out there tends to come back. It's about taking responsibility for your life. And if you can be happy and filled with love, your life will bring you just that. That's my mantra. That's my motto. I think everything I put out there, whether it's negative or positive, will come back to me.

Realizing what's important in life doesn't come to everybody at the same time. You get it when you get it. It's a process. Once you take responsibility for it I swear I think your life changes so quickly. You don't blame people. You're less of a victim. If there's something in your life that's not what you want, you may have to say, "No, I created that. I own it. If I want it to change then I need to change it."

I think being positive and how you treat people and being kind says a lot. It's helped me lead a happy, happy life. Do unto others as you would have them do unto you. It's so much basic stuff that we've all grown up knowing and learning. It's about getting out of your own way and finding joy and if you're not in joy then find it. Take risks and chances. Never rest on your laurels—especially if you're not happy.

When you're brought up by a cheerleader you can't help but have it in you.
—*Lisa Rinna*

My mother passed away last year. She had a lung disease. The only cure was a transplant. It happened so fast. She was an Army brat and moved all over the world with her dad and her mother; she was in places where they used asbestos before they knew of its danger. Her passing has brought my father, brother and me closer together. I'm so lucky. My mom and dad fought like hell, but they loved each other. That helped us get through. My brother is my best friend. My dad is also my best friend. We are all really close. My brother and I used to fight a lot. It was terrible. After I moved away to college we got closer; there's 20 months between us. Five years ago we started getting close and he became my best friend.

I'm a very spiritual person. I believe there's something else out there.
—*Molly Burnett*

I like artists because they're looking for beauty. They're creative; also people with humor. Listen. Try to be helpful. People don't listen to one another very much.

A therapist said that listening can be the greatest gift you can give anybody. Openly, quietly, really listening to what they're talking about; it's healing and it's so simple.

Just keep going. It doesn't matter what. When things don't go your way then you keep going, if there's something in the way, when you're discouraged.

I was nominated for an Emmy once and they moved it to the non-televised ceremony. I won prime time guest actress; I found out the last seven years before mine they got no recognition. I won it for *The Trials of Rosie O'Neill* with Sharon Gless. I played a homeless mentally disturbed woman; she was a quiet woman. Sharon, who played Rosie O'Neill, discovered her and decided to help her. She helped her find a place that was good for her. She couldn't sign the document; she was afraid she'd be put away in some horrible place. She does something, she's so panicked and she goes to the other side.

I would hang with people you connect to, with values that you have.
—*Peggy McCay*

Every town is mercurial and has change. That's what I love about L.A.—there's diversity and change. You can live slow or fast. I love L.A. because there's so much change. I grew up in a small town in the Midwest. It was a nice place, but I much prefer a big city. I had a wonderful time growing up there, but I love L.A. I love diversity. Small towns can be somewhat stagnant and a little provincial. There's not a lot of diversity. Some people are fine with that. They're a little "too" fine with it. Some people don't expand their thought processes.

I love that I have all kinds of friends, of all nationalities and persuasions. That's something I probably wouldn't have if I hadn't come to L.A.
—*Josh Taylor*

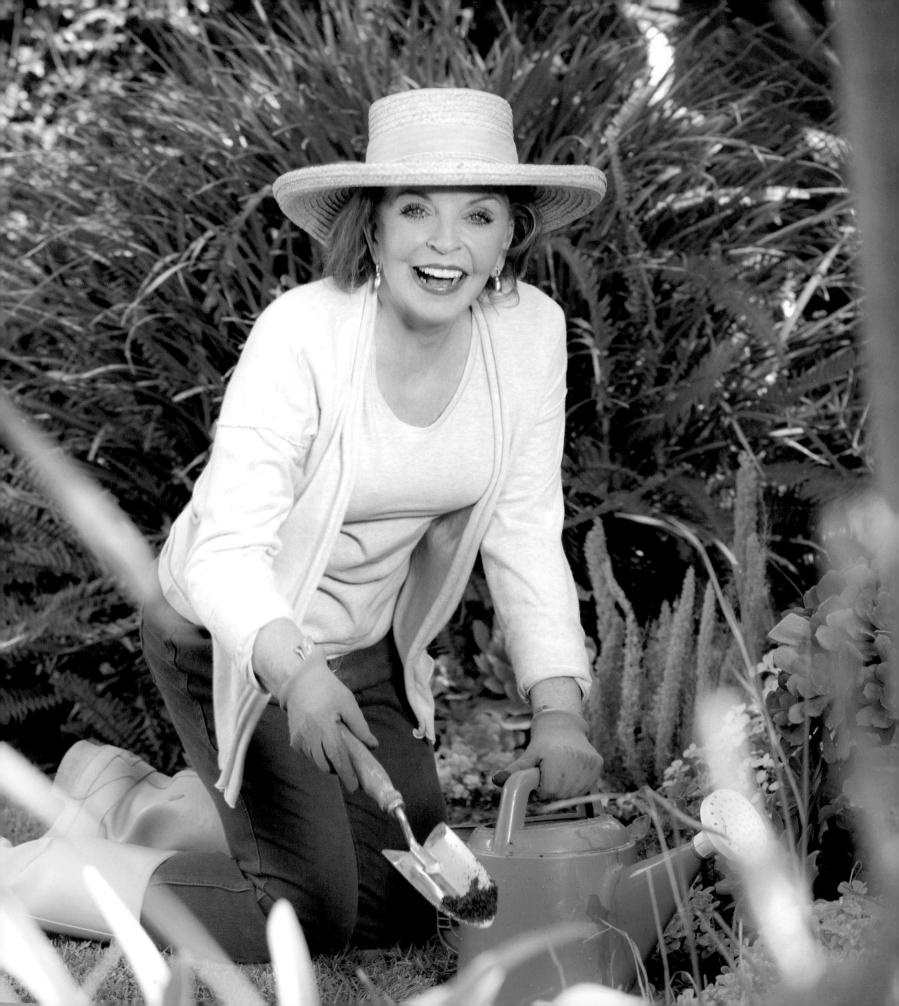

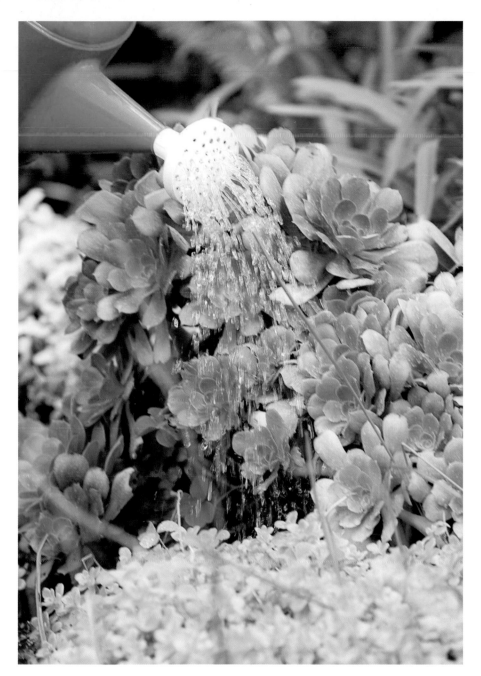

Gardening involves stretching, lifting, kneeling, stooping and carrying. I'll make a thousand trips back and forth and around because we have an extensive garden. It's a big deal for me.

In my darkest moments, I find peace and serenity in my garden.

Working outside in my garden throughout the years is very therapeutic. It gets me plenty of Vitamin D...and a great payoff of flowers in the spring!
—*Susan Seaforth Hayes*

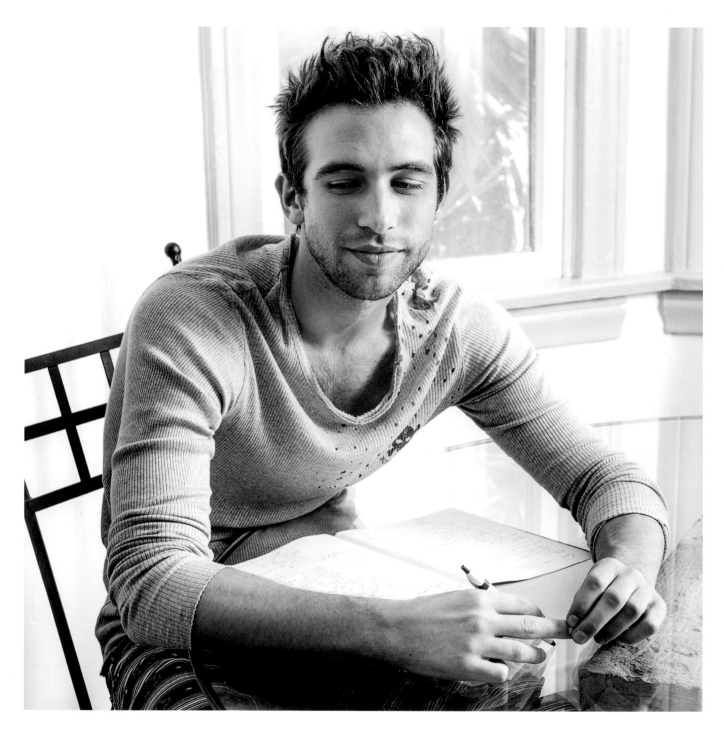

I recently started writing screenplays. One's in development and one has been optioned and has a director attached. We're going forward with it. Writing is something I've done on and off for many years. I studied a lot of playwriting in college.

Two of my favorite playwrights are Kenneth Lonergan, who wrote *This Is Our Youth*, and Arthur Miller. I saw a production of his play *All My Sons* in college, which was inspiring.

I'm not just posing here in the shower for the photograph. I actually do some of my best thinking in here. There isn't much time during the day that I'm by myself outside of my car and the shower. Those are places that I have a lot of my "Aha!" moments.

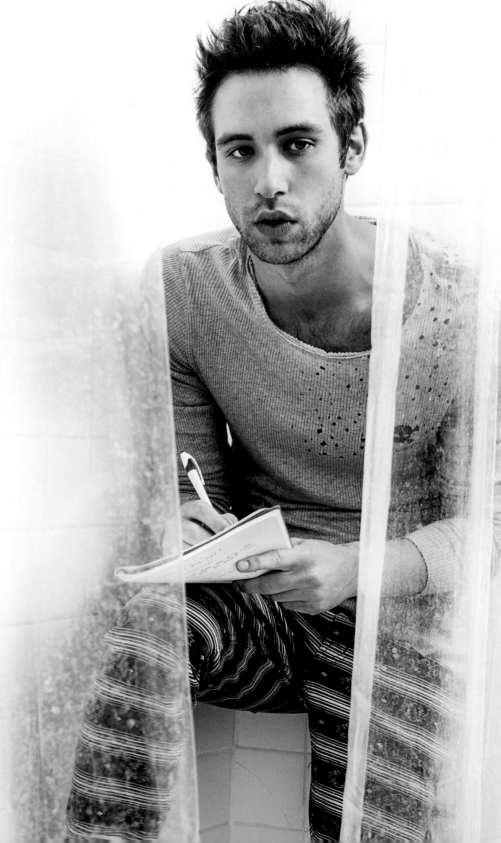

I've actually rushed out of the shower on occasion, interrupting my shower, so I can go straight to my computer to make sure my thoughts aren't lost.
—Blake Berris

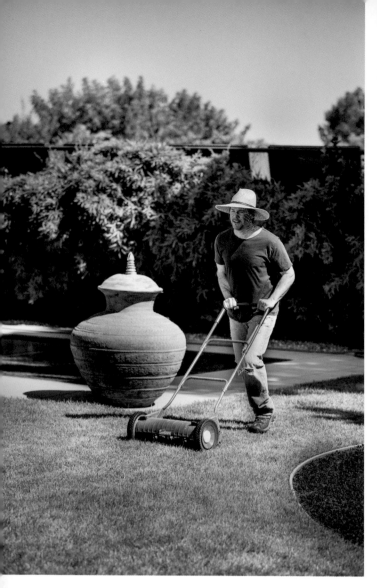

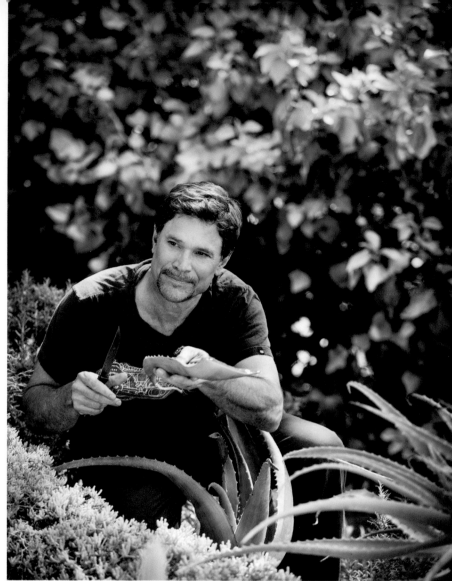

When we're in hard economic
times, we naturally conserve.
When we're not, we don't, but
why not do it all the time?
—*Peter Reckell*

My house is green from the ground up. We built it from scratch. People have always asked me how I got interested in all this. When I was a child, there were six of us and my dad didn't make much money. We had a cow because we needed milk. We'd trade milk with the people down the street who had chickens for eggs. We weren't being "green"—we were trying to survive.

We have solar energy in our home. (My wife) Kelly is a musician and she has a sound studio that absorbs a lot of the energy. If it weren't for that, the panels would take care of almost the whole home. We hardly ever use air conditioning. My lawn mower isn't electric.

People conserve energy during a recession. Once we come out of a recession SUV sales go up again. It's kind of crazy, but that's how people are. We are inspired by a need.

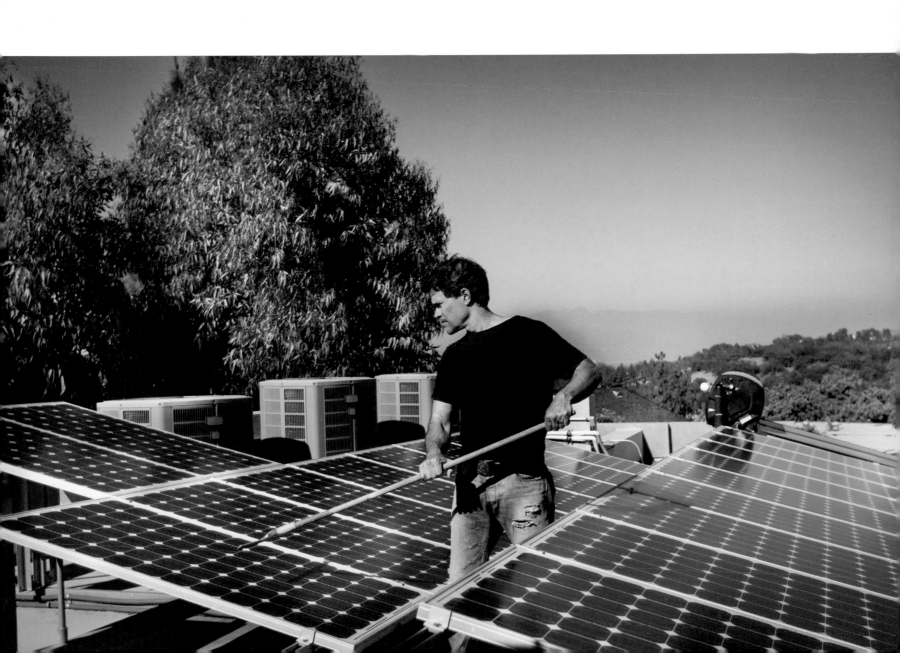

I have to say I'm incredibly happy and lucky to have a terrific job. I live in a house that I absolutely adore with my two dogs. On a given day, I can walk out my front door, go down the driveway and take a hike for 20 miles through the mountains if I want. Happiness is one of the most powerful forces in the universe, the most powerful being love.

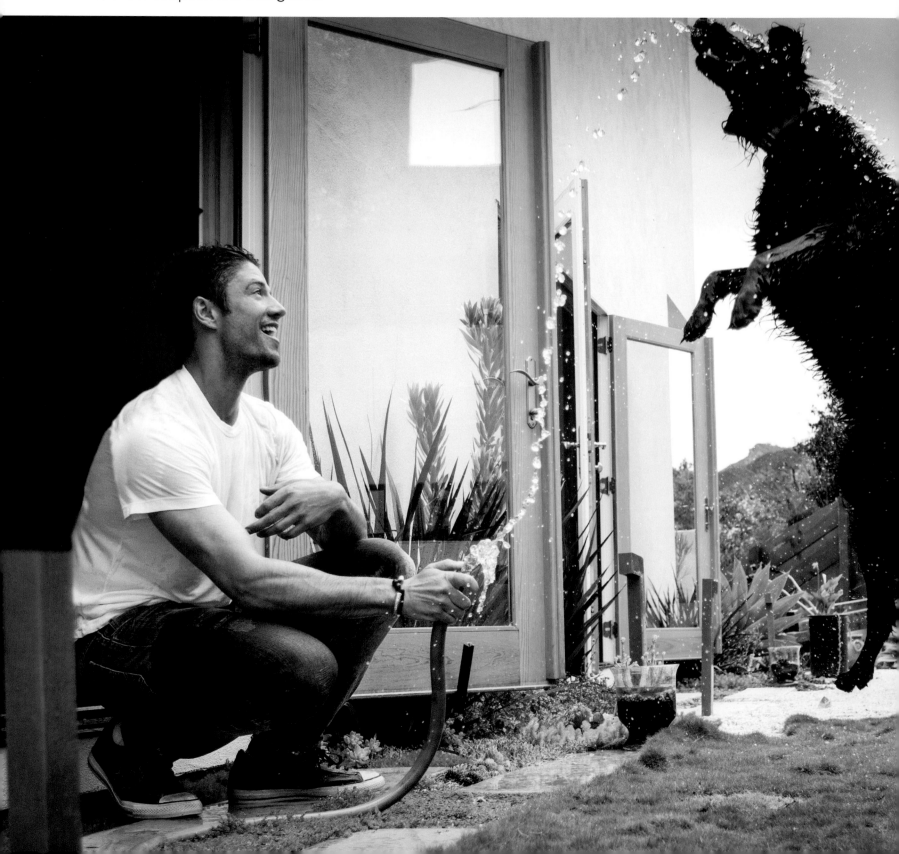

I am the opposite from my character in that I prefer no drama in my life. My home and my dogs bring me tranquility.
—James Scott

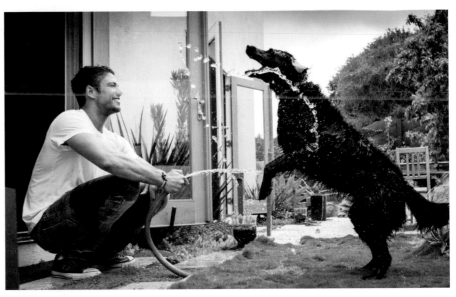

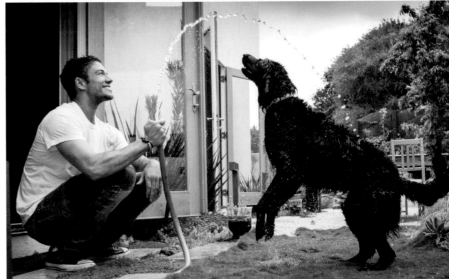

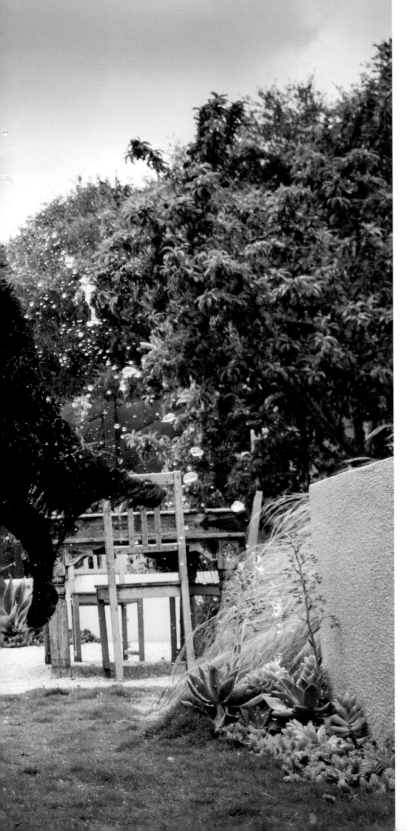

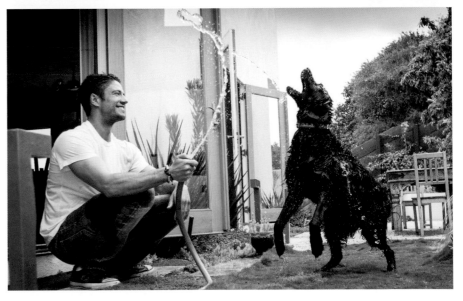

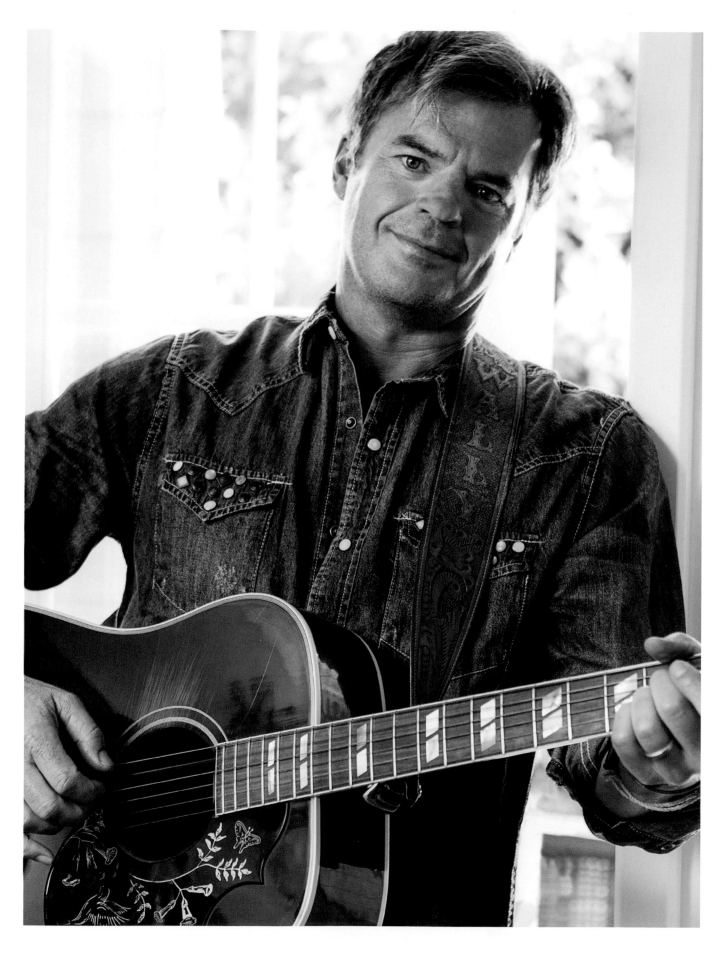

My music has always been very important to me. I definitely keep up with it. The Kurth Taylor band still performs concerts. We're still active.

If I have time, I'll try to learn how to play a song that I heard on the radio. If I can't figure it out by listening to it that way, I'll go on iTunes and download it. I'll try to figure it out myself. I'll research the chords and say, "Oh, that's how it is."

I'm much better at saying "no" than I was when I was younger. I guess that's what my son has taught me. I never had that huge thing where I felt I "had" to be a movie star. I love soap operas and being a "blue collar" actor. A television executive once asked me how I was doing and I said, "I'm the happiest actor in daytime. I'm doing two things I love—acting and singing. This is as good as it gets."

As I've gotten older I've realized that you don't have to do everything. You can do what you want to do.
—*Wally Kurth*

I have a firm belief in God. I know that there's a plan, a journey. I think it's ordained. With a higher power in our lives, I'm comfortable with whatever is put in front of me. I feel as though there's a plan. You might have a day when you say to yourself, "I'm going to go to Bloomingdales and I'm going to get those shoes," only as the day progresses you learn that you're just not meant to be there that day. I was not meant to have my own children. I was not meant to conceive because I did everything there was—every test, two years of surgeries, medicines and shots. I gave myself shots. I was not meant to have my children be put in my arms until after I met Robin. We bonded. We promised each other that we would have these children and we would keep them safe. She kept them safe until she could put them into my arms. There's no mystery in that to me. It's just the journey.

I see the things my kids are experiencing and I have a motherly desire to adjust and protect their world, to shield them from pain and disappointment. I know that's dumb. You have to prepare them.
—*Deidre Hall*

I get pretty simple. My wife has heard me say it a thousand times: life is simple. It shouldn't be this difficult. When you see people going through all these problems, I try to reduce it to the simplest level and not let all the little stuff that consumes people and gets them all worked up. I think I read in OMNI magazine when I was in college that 99 percent of your worries never materialize. That really made an impact. You can say "don't sweat the small stuff" or whatever but I just think that life shouldn't be that difficult.

As far as the mantra goes: Life is short. We're here for a short amount of time. I lost my dad a few years ago. He was a real tough, smart guy. He didn't sweat the small stuff. He always embraced challenges. My daughter, Whitney, came to me with a problem one time and I said it's a pebble in the road. We'll find a way to kick it out of the way and move forward. She looked at me funny. I said you're going to face this stuff all the time. There's always five ways to solve a problem. Let's just take a look at it. That's what it is.
—*Drake Hogestyn*

I practiced transcendental meditation for a number of years; I have a mantra that I use for that. They give it to you and you're not supposed to share it with anyone and I never have.

I find Los Angeles to be one of the most angry and aggressive cities; it's filled with people who have incredibly low self-esteem and therefore they feel that everyone is trying to take a piece of them away with them. In the last few years, one of the changes that I've made that has had a profound effect on my mental well-being living in this environment is that I've made the choice not to be angry. It doesn't change anything. Being angry is a waste of time. The Buddhist philosophy comes down to…attaining a sense of happiness and peace with one's self. My ability to do that is not just because of a certain amount of work and focus; I have made it a major focus of my life. I'm 33; I was 27…you think you know but you know nothing in your 20s; that's when you're supposed to fail. You haven't had a successful relationship yet; you haven't worked out really how to be an adult yet or how to balance your career or make informed educated choices; you have no idea about building or planning a future. If you're married you shouldn't be, in my opinion, because you haven't started to become who you are. Contemporary psychologists have the same opinions I have; they suggest that women's brains and personalities don't finish evolving until they're in their late 20s/early 30s. For men, it doesn't happen until their mid-30s. You hear people in relationships say: "I met this guy and then he became somebody different." Well, yes, he did because he hadn't finished becoming who he was going to become. In your 20s you can't expect that you've figured these things out; although everyone in their 20s thinks they have. I did.
—*James Scott*

I'm more of a "go with the flow" type of guy. I look at life with very different eyes. I'm kind of a loner. I think people make things more difficult than they have to be. Playing a gay character and seeing what they're going through makes me ask why? Why can't people just leave it alone? No one is hurting anyone.

Make your own decisions and live your own life—life is way too short.

It's easy to pull from Sonny because he's a very positive, energetic type of person and so am I. I should write a book on how I see life. People make things far more difficult than they should.
—*Freddie Smith*

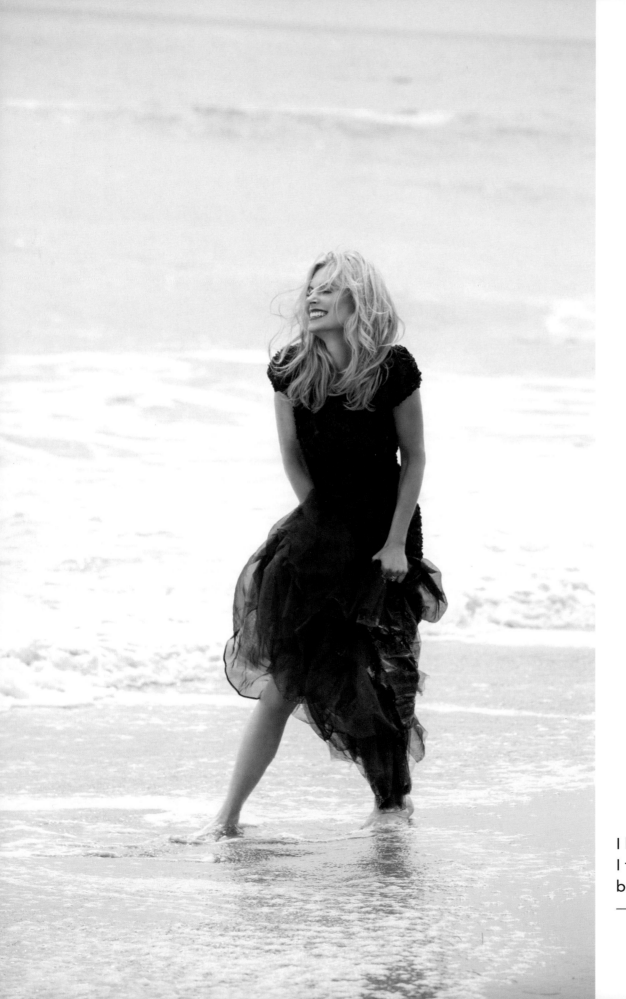

I live near the ocean because I find that walking along the beach is so invigorating.
—*Eileen Davidson*

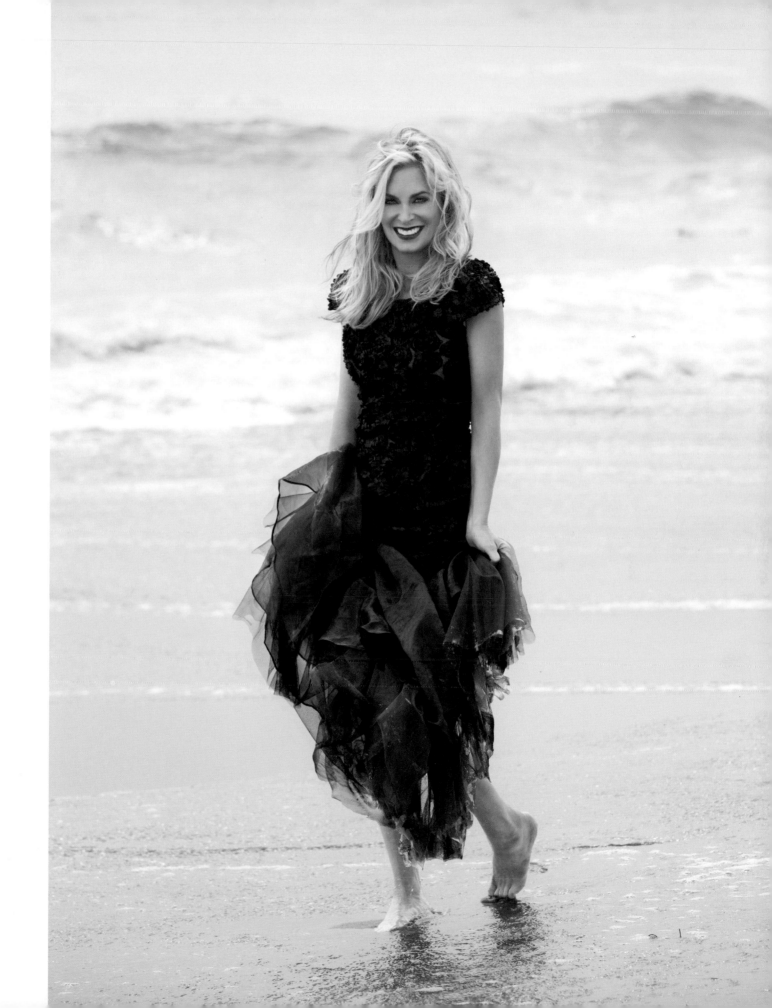

Bill: Religion is part of my life. I like to include it not only as part of my life but part of our life together. I've been singing in the church choir since I was 14. Attending church together helps us remain grounded and it builds strength for the future.

Susan: I'm enough of an "Old Testament" girl to say that you should bring your cleanest and your best to the temple of God—or you can wait a little farther in the back. I have seen people come to church in ripped jeans. They put their feet up on the pews and throw back a latte during the service. I find that's just a tad too relaxed. We'd like a little more respect and reverence. God is everywhere. Let's worship together.

We don't have a message to sell, but we believe in the power of love.
—*Bill and Susan Hayes*

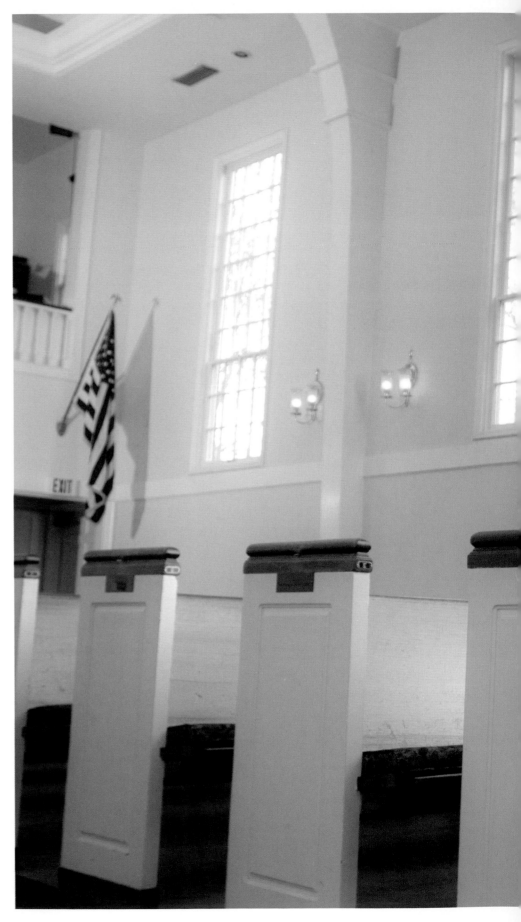

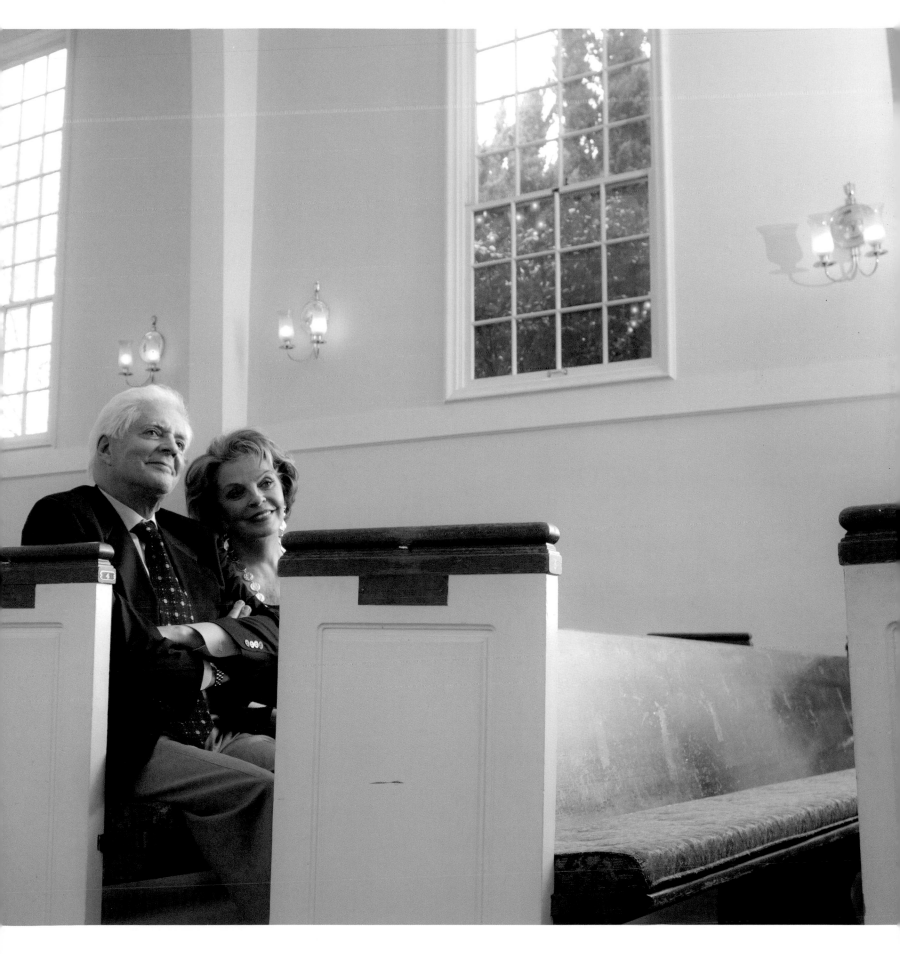

BALANCE

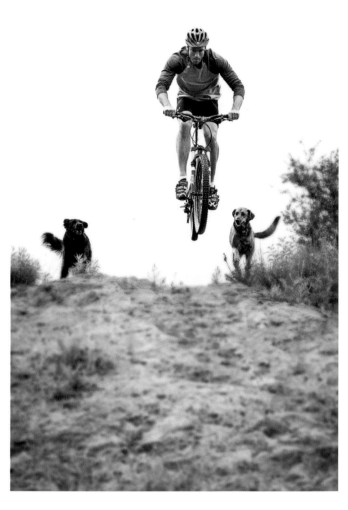

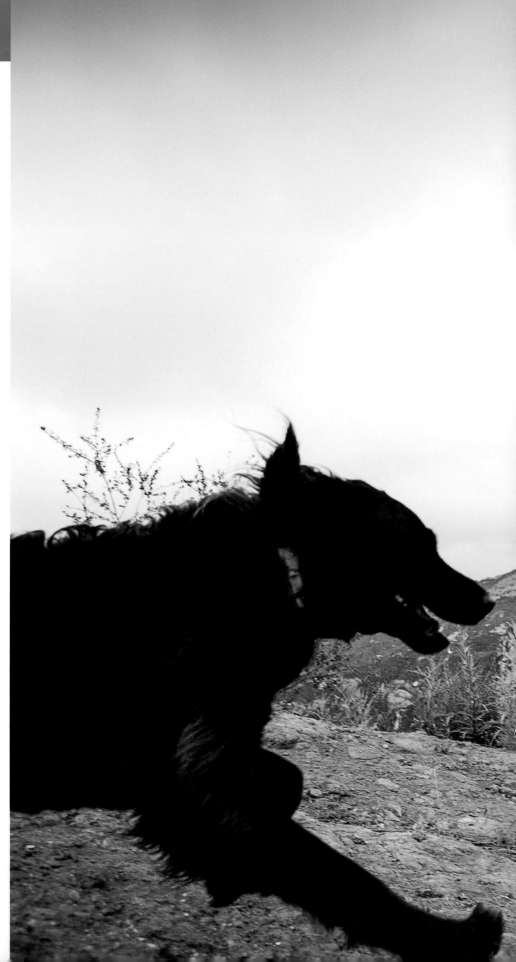

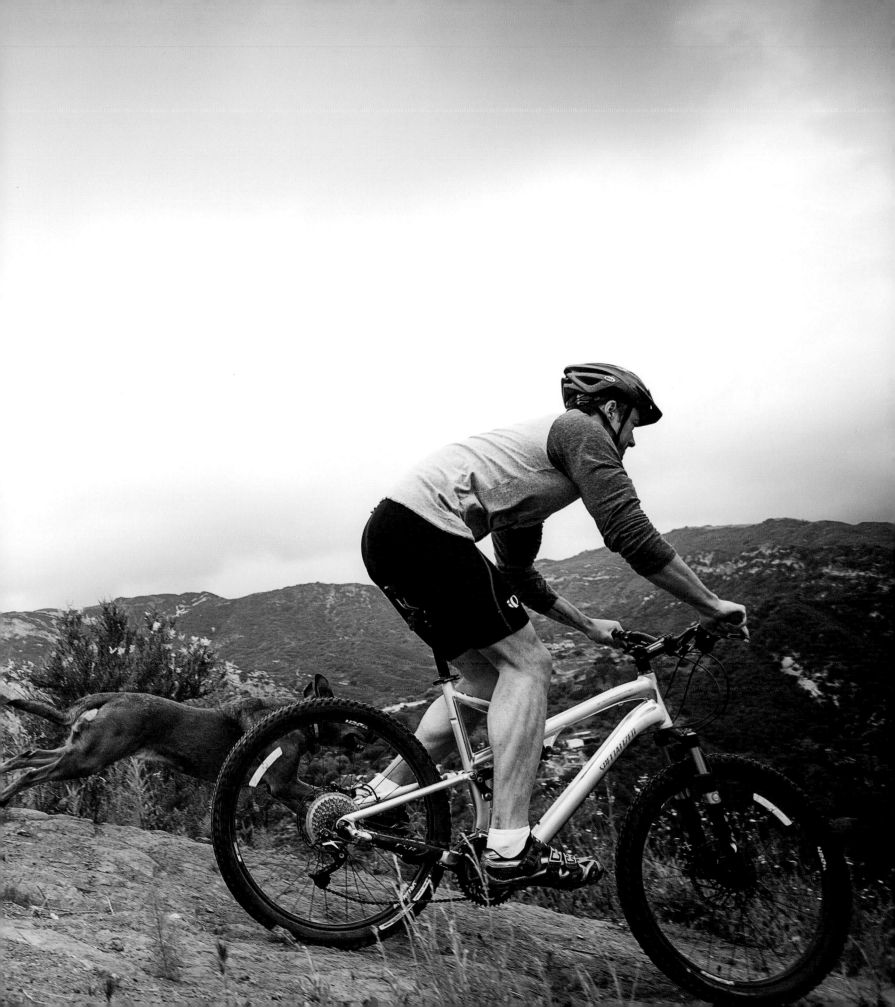

balance, *n, v*

1. mental or emotional steadiness

2. harmonious

BALANCE

Life is like riding a bicycle. To keep your balance you must keep moving.
—*Albert Einstein*

Balance is about having compassion for people in the world and opening yourself up and having the capacity to really embrace and love strangers as much as you do your family.
—*James Scott*

Facing your fear and doing something. It is good for you to shake things up. It keeps you young and alive and excited about things. That feeling of not always being safe creates balance.
—*Eileen Davidson*

You know on an airplane they say if there is an emergency to put your oxygen mask on first and then your child's? You have to take care of yourself first. I wake up in the morning and I have to choose to be happy. This is balance.
—*Arianne Zucker*

I love photography. I love taking pictures. A picture lasts forever. Something about photography and capturing a moment that stops is wonderful to me. Do something you love.
—*Melissa Reeves*

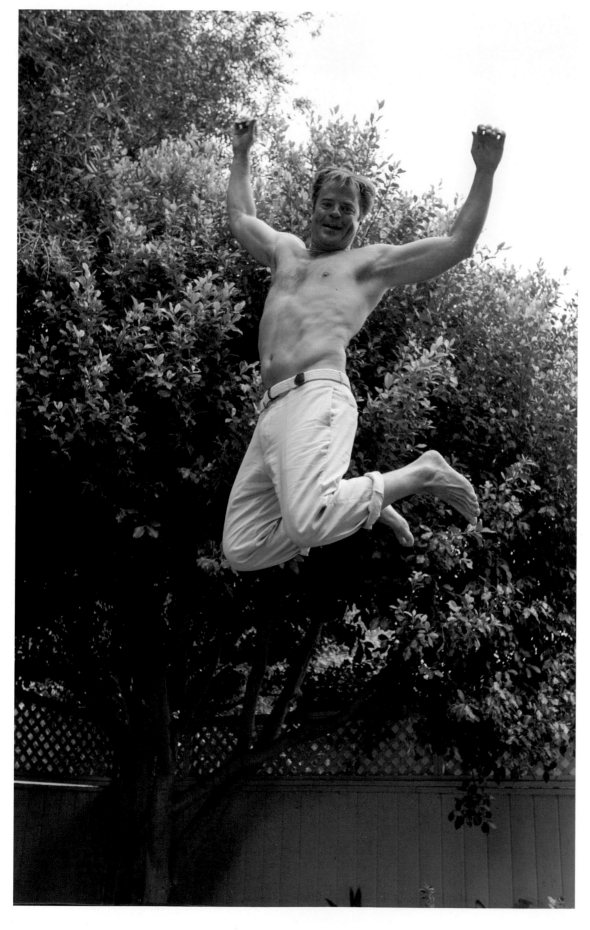

We have a huge trampoline in the back yard, which my son, Brogan, just loves to jump on. I go out and bounce on it early in the morning with him sometimes. I spend time with Brogan each day in the afternoon, too, after I pick him up from school. I'm "Mr. Mom" and I love it! I have my other children, my daughters, too. This time we have now is a blessing to both of us. That's how I look at it. Jane Elliot, who played Angelica on *Days*, once told me, "Don't freak out if you're not working. This is a chance to do the things that you're supposed to do in your personal life."

I'm "Mr. Mom" and I love it!
—*Wally Kurth*

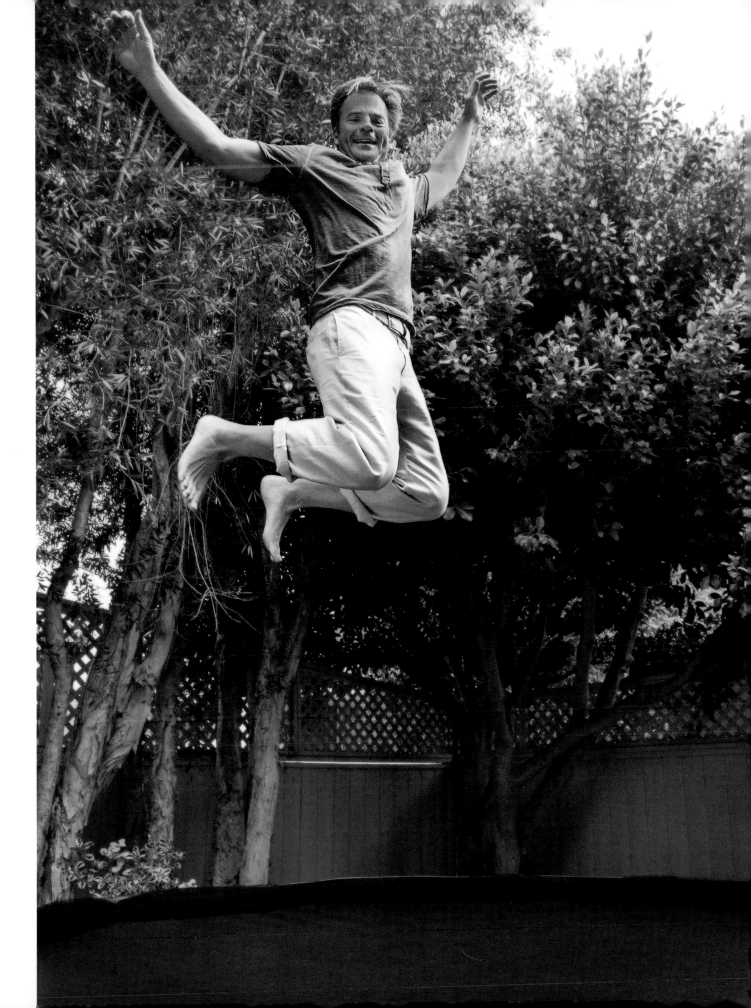

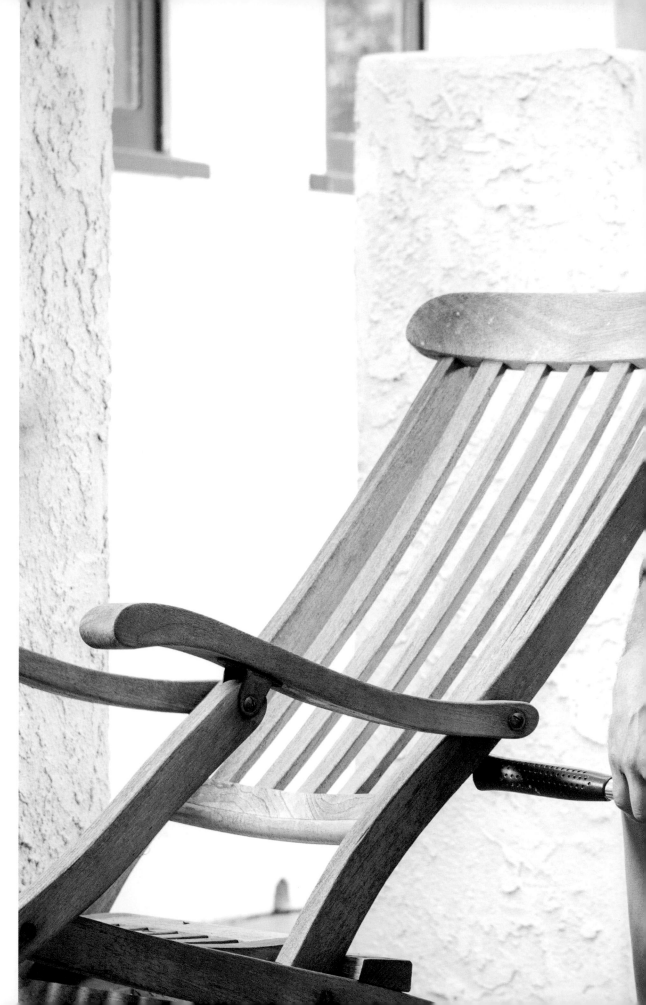

I love to build things. While I was away from the show I built teepees. There's actually a demand for them. People would see one that I'd made and then they'd want a teepee, too. I also make tomahawks and I've worked in construction.

But it's hard not to put "being a dad" at the top of the list if you're asking about what I do when I'm not acting. When you're responsible for other people and there's a possibility that something could happen to you, you ask yourself, "How am I going to take care of them?" "How am I going to keep my house safe?"

You don't just think about yourself anymore.

I love being physical and being outside in the sun. I love making something out of scratch that will last. I love the planning that goes into the buying of materials.
—Bryan Dattilo

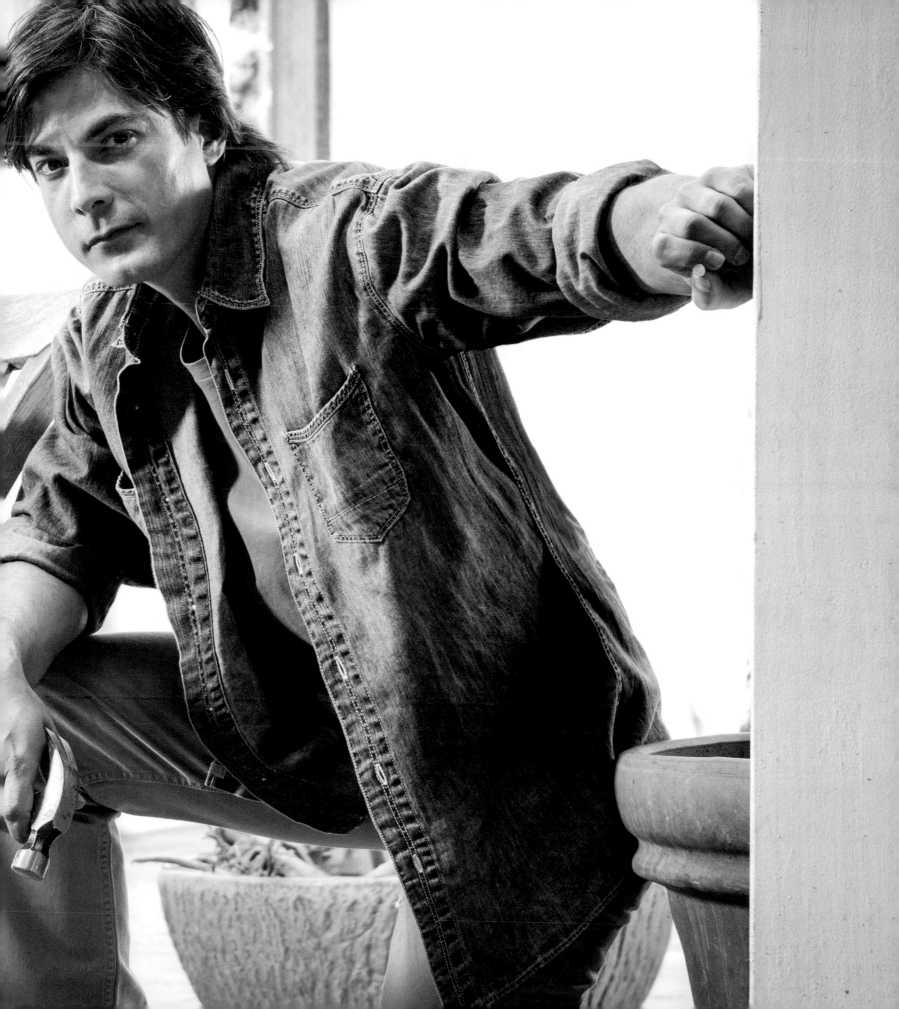

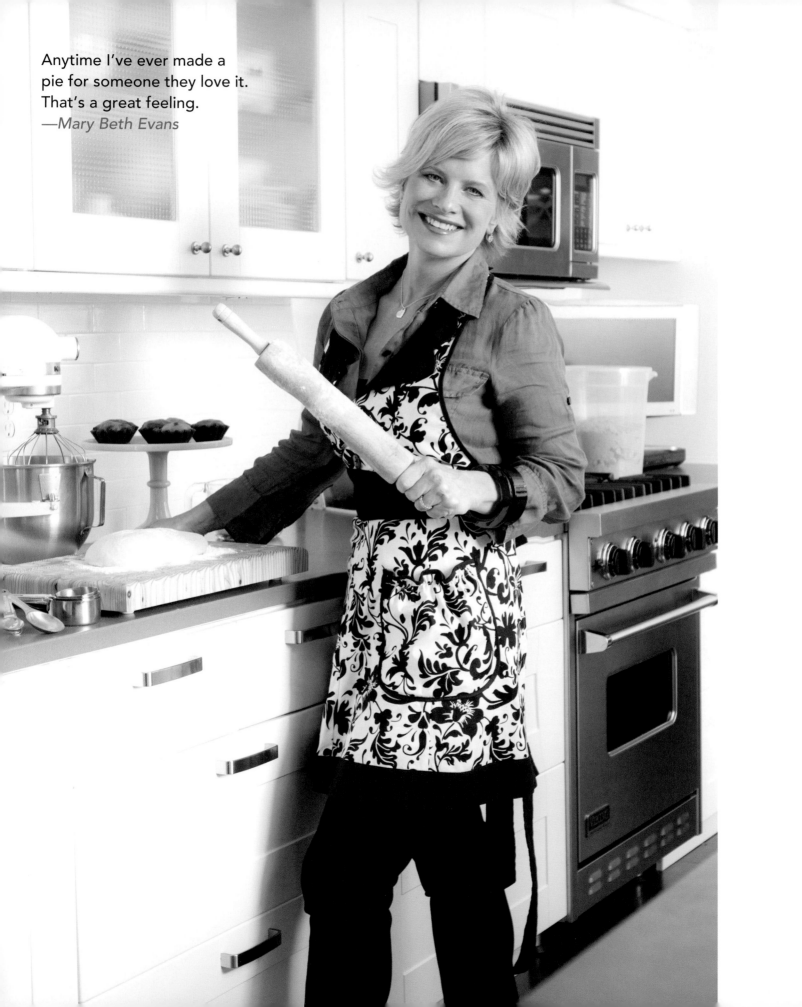

Anytime I've ever made a
pie for someone they love it.
That's a great feeling.
—Mary Beth Evans

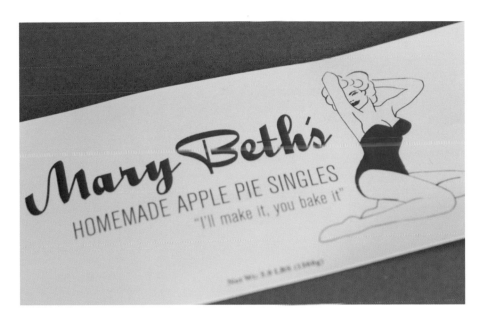

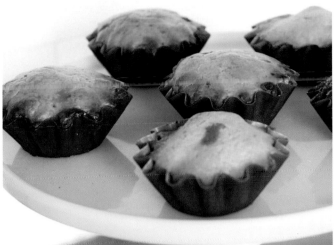

I've been making pies since my kids were little. I have a recipe that's been passed down from my husband's mother. I'd ask my kids, "How many pies do you need this year for gifts for your teachers?" One day, my husband read an article in the Wall Street Journal about mail-order pies. He said I should try that. I went ahead and gave it a shot. It must have been when there was a lull in the show for me.

Friends helped me with a logo and a mailing list to reach out to people. I got 100 orders right off the bat. My kids and everyone helped me make them. The business only grew after I took out an ad in a soap magazine and The Today Show did a whole segment on what I do.

Sometimes I think about not making them anymore, but then I think—why? It'd be so sad to stop. I should get a distributor someday, but the problem is all my pies are handmade and they would be hard to mass produce. We're still trucking along!

www.marybethsapplepie.com

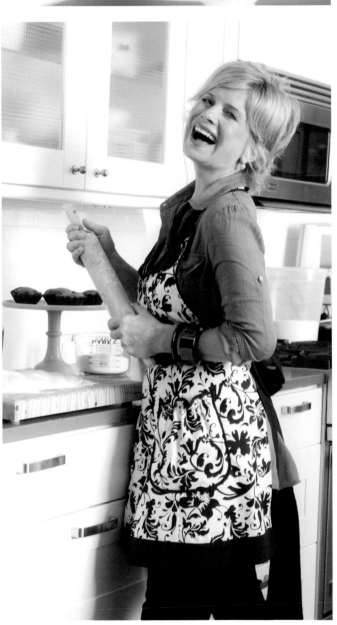

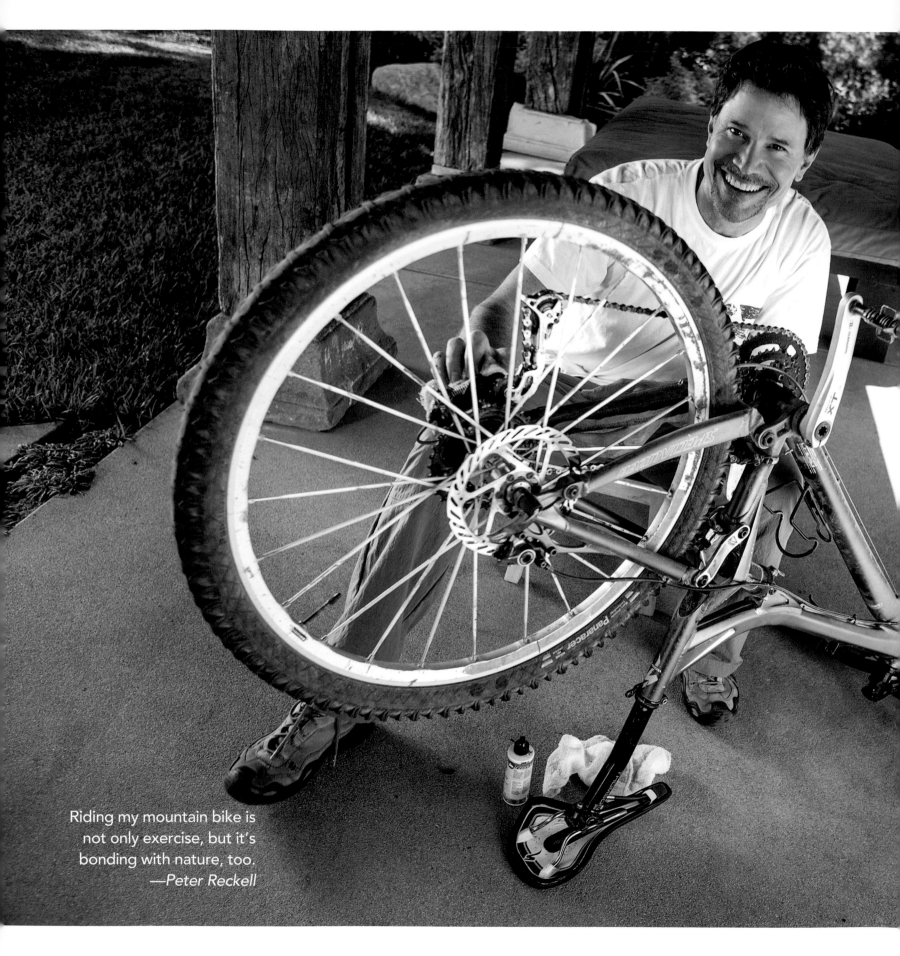

Riding my mountain bike is
not only exercise, but it's
bonding with nature, too.
—Peter Reckell

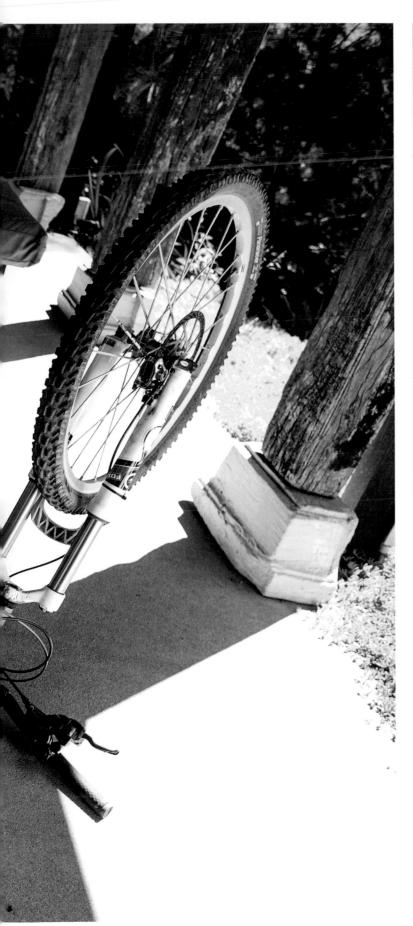

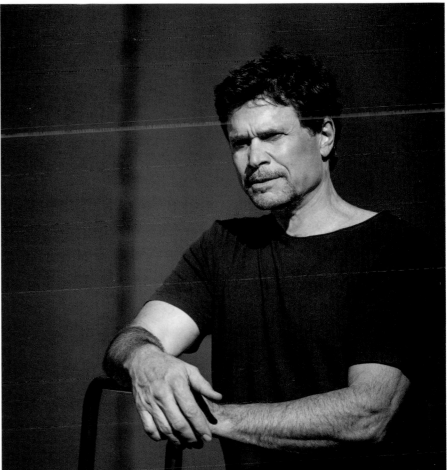

Going out on my mountain bike into the wilderness is meditation for me. It helps me sort out my thoughts and the energy of the earth and nature is cleansing. If I get irritable sometimes (my wife) Kelly will say to me, "Maybe you should go for a ride?" I'll come back refreshed.

You see the bigger picture. I call it self-medicating. When I was in high school I just started running. It wasn't a conscious thought. I'd just put on my sneakers and say, "See you later, Mom!"

I had a biology teacher in tenth grade who came up to me and said he was also the cross-country coach and that I had to go out for the team and run for him. I never did because for me it was just therapy and being by myself. Competition would have made it a whole other animal.

I'd love to put on my snow shoes in the winter and feel the power of a storm.

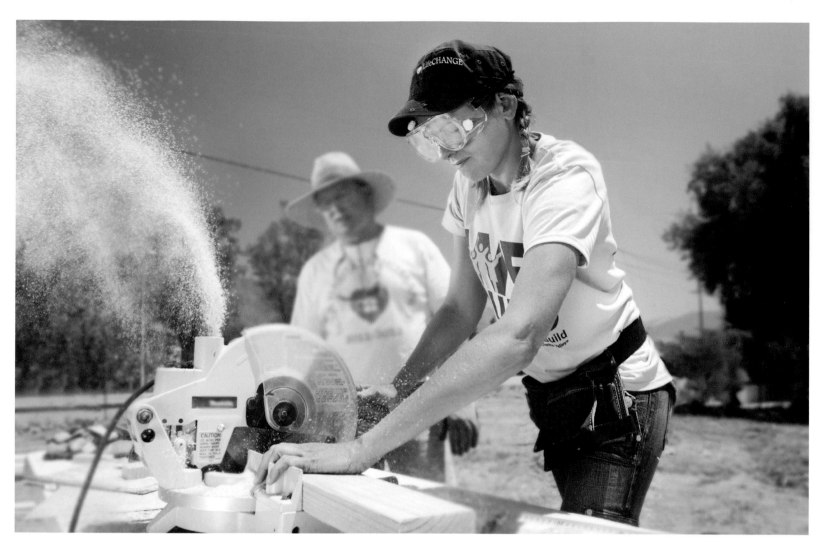

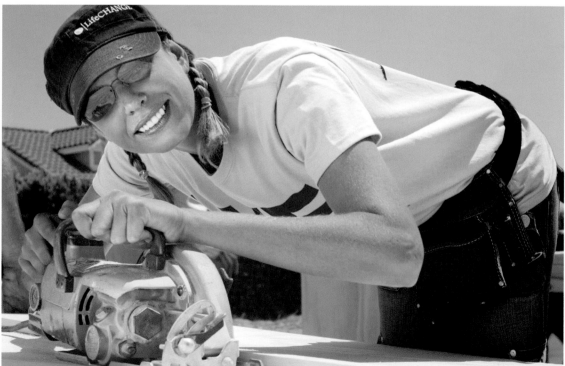

My philanthropic endeavors
are huge. I hope LifeCHANGE
is a lifelong project.
—Arianne Zucker

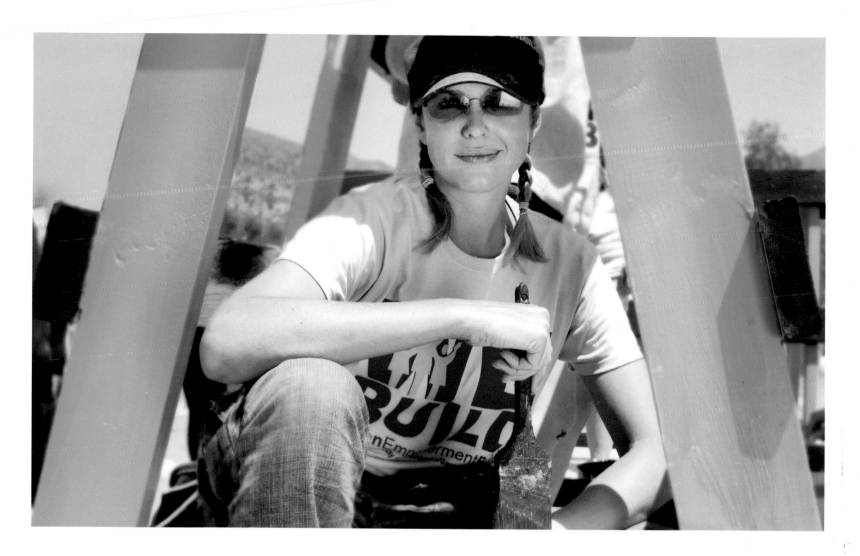

I've worked with a lot of charities over the years including Habitat for Humanity. I've started my own organization called LifeCHANGE, which helps young adults to achieve their full potential and help others to do the same.

LifeCHANGE helps kids who are between the ages of 18 and 24. I chose that age range because when I was at that time in my life I had no direction and truly needed to find myself. I went to school at night during my senior year of high school so I could work three jobs during the day.

At 22, I started some pre-veterinary courses and was studying theater, too. Around that time I got the audition for Days of our Lives and got the job. I thought, "Great! Now, I can pay for college." Then, I realized I couldn't go because I was too busy working. My mom gave me great advice around this time. She said, "School's not going anywhere. You're only young once." So, now, here I am. I've been on the show for a long time now.

I've always been inspired by families who do something instead of just going on vacation. Some families actually take a vacation and do a "build" where they help construct a home for other people. They can still go to Fiji, but they can do something important there, too.

www.officiallifechange.com

I garden and landscape at my home. I bought my first house when I was 24. My wife and I have always been building and flipping homes, renovating them. That's always been a side business. If I weren't acting, I'd be doing something in that field, but I went to school to write and direct.

It's really nice to know as an actor that there are other financial streams in your life so you don't feel "Oh, I have to get this job or I'm done" when you walk into an audition. Nothing smells worse than a desperate actor.

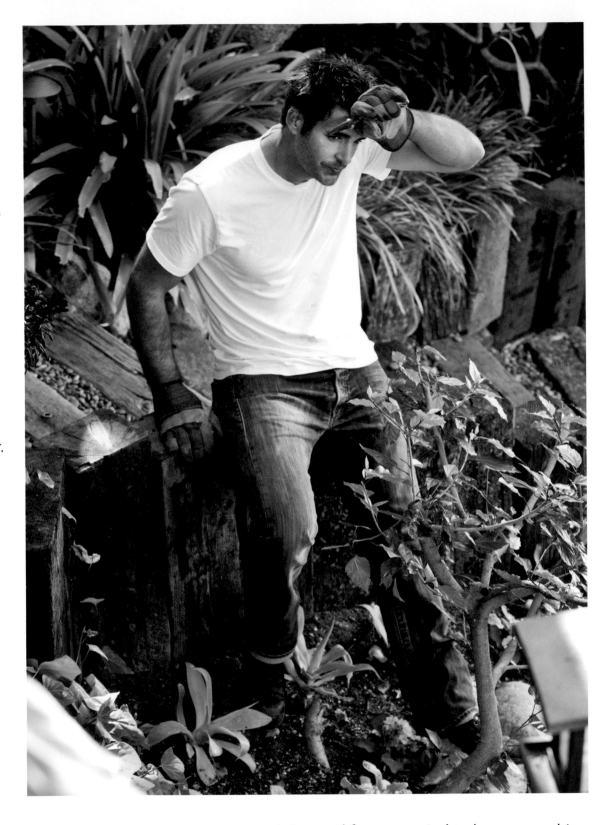

It is good for your mind to have something else to do in addition to whatever you have as your main job or career.
—Galen Gering

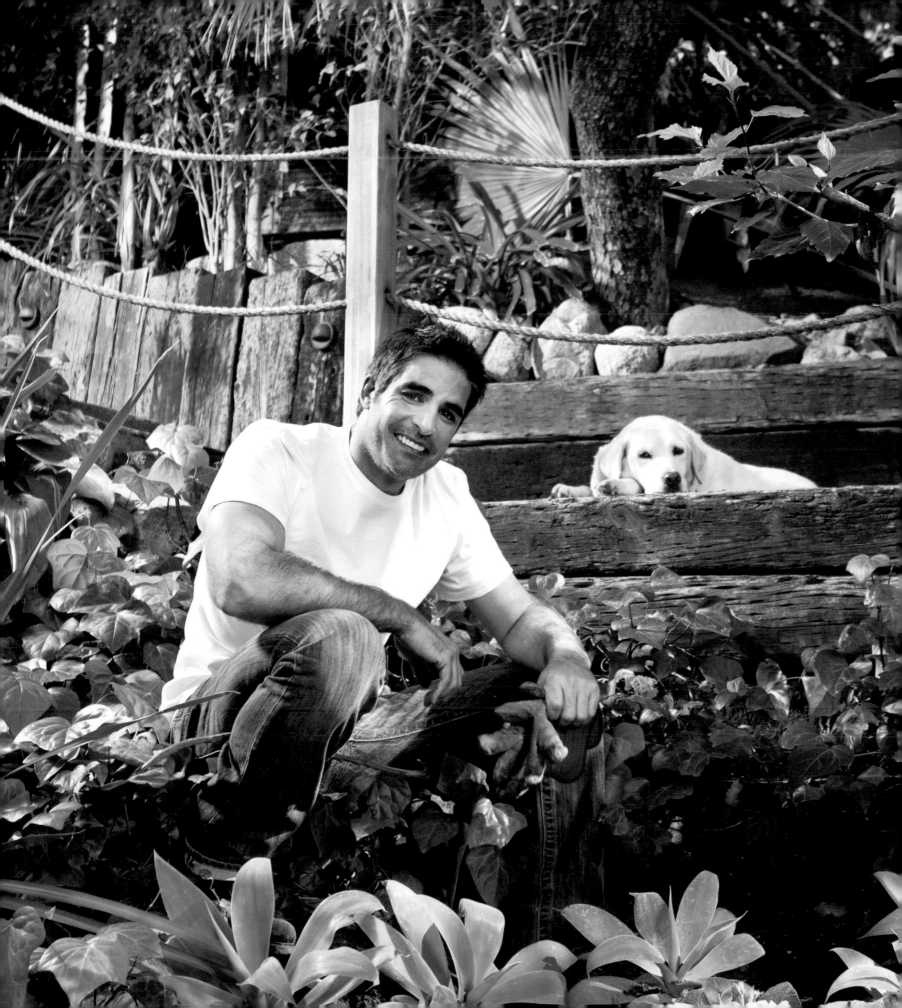

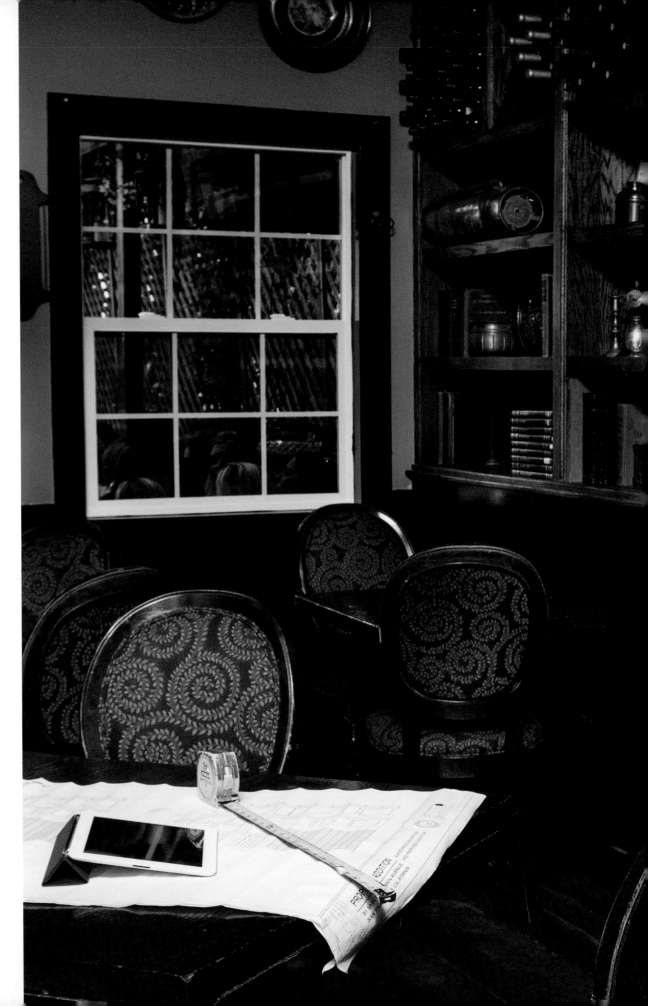

I've always liked decorating and designing my houses. My cousin, Nate, started opening restaurants about seven years ago and he and his business partners asked me to do the design. I did another one two years later for a place called "The Tipsy Pig" in San Francisco. The name comes from pigs actually getting tipsy on farms after apples end up fermenting after they fall from trees and the pigs eat them. My father-in-law came up with the name and it's golden. We go there quite a lot. It's like a Cheers thing.

I love to decorate. I'll collaborate with an architect and devise ways to make things better. For "The Tipsy Pig," I worked on what went up on the walls, the lighting and the paint color. I envisioned wood floors and I used a lot of eco-friendly products, too. I went to flea markets and got some vintage books. It was so much fun spending other people's money!

We didn't want the type of restaurant where the seats would be uncomfortable. We want people to feel like they could come here to eat and stay awhile so we made the seats and the booths as comfortable as possible.

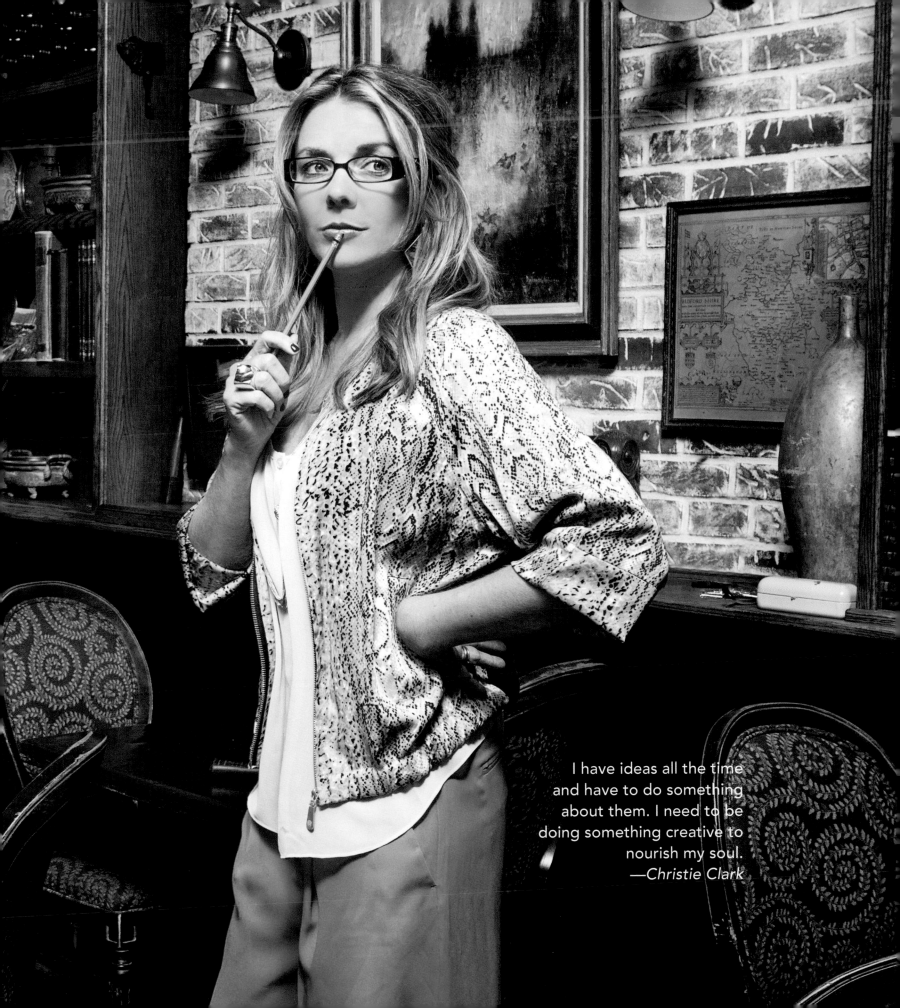

I have ideas all the time and have to do something about them. I need to be doing something creative to nourish my soul.
—Christie Clark

I used to be a semi-pro skateboarder. I did that my whole life while growing up in Hollister, California. I moved to Colorado for my freshman year in high school and in both places all my friends loved to skateboard. It's how I lived my life.

My buddies and I would grab our skateboards and our cameras and shoot each other going down the stairs. That was a normal day for us. One time, I went down 16 stairs and hit the bottom and smacked my head on the concrete. It was a surreal moment. I remember being in the emergency room and they were cutting my shirt off. My mom made me promise to wear my helmet from then on. I'd always bring it with me but I wouldn't always wear it. Sorry, Mom!

I stopped skateboarding after I was cast on *Days of our Lives*. I miss doing it. Now, I go snowboarding. I learned about the importance of money from skateboarding. I'd go through a skateboard a week back in the day and that'd be $60 right there.

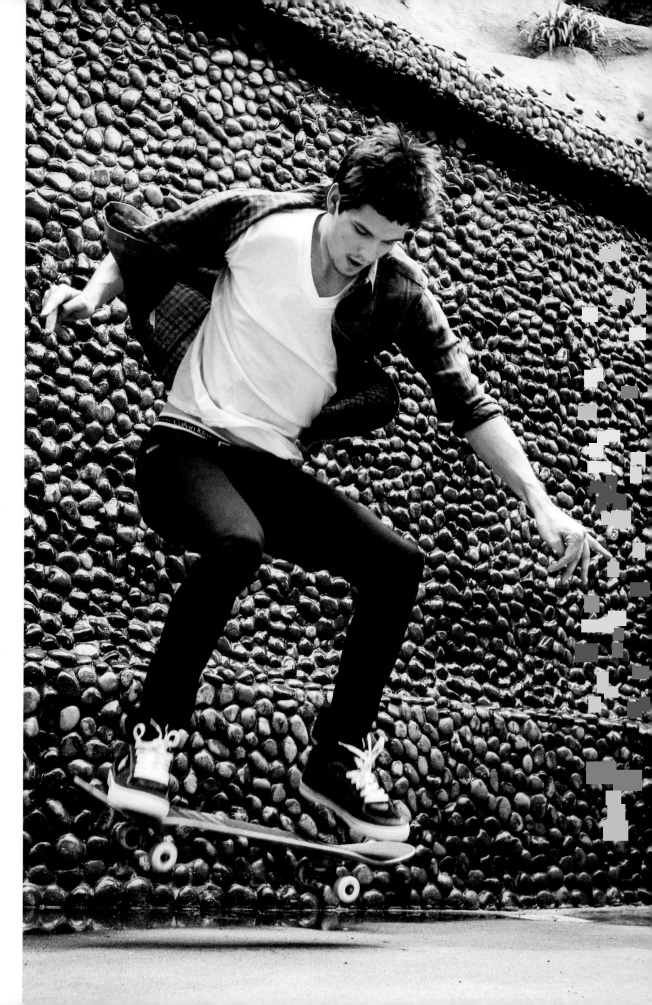

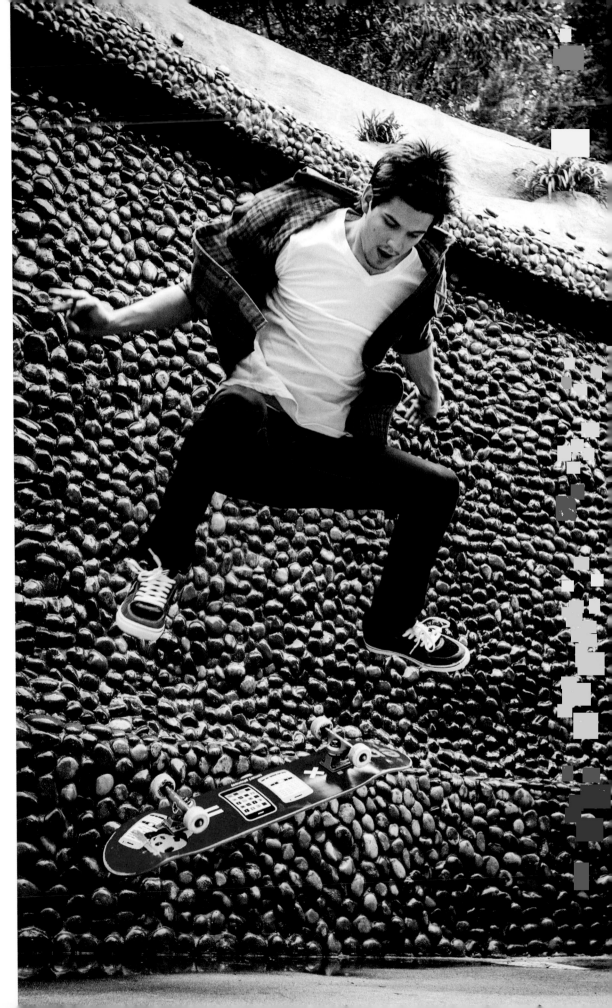

Skateboarding is a mind game...and you have to find a way to overcome your fears.
—*Casey Jon Deidrick*

I grew up in the restaurant business and later owned one in New York when I was on *Love of Life* in the mid- to late '70s. I was talking to one of the crew members one day and he was telling me that he and a bunch of other guys were thinking of opening a restaurant by 11th Avenue and 57th Street in New York City. I thought about it and asked if he'd like to go in on it with me. I said that I'd get it open and then he could run it. Four months later, we opened the place and called it "The Fives."

Later, we decided to put in a cabaret. It worked on the nights that I booked it. We had one girl come in to audition and she was sensational. We asked her how long she'd been in New York and she said a week. She didn't know anyone in the city. Who would come to see her? The ideal bookings were 18-year-old kids from Long Island, who came from big families, preferably Italian. A kid's father would hire a bus to bring the whole family into the city to see them perform. It wouldn't matter if they were good!

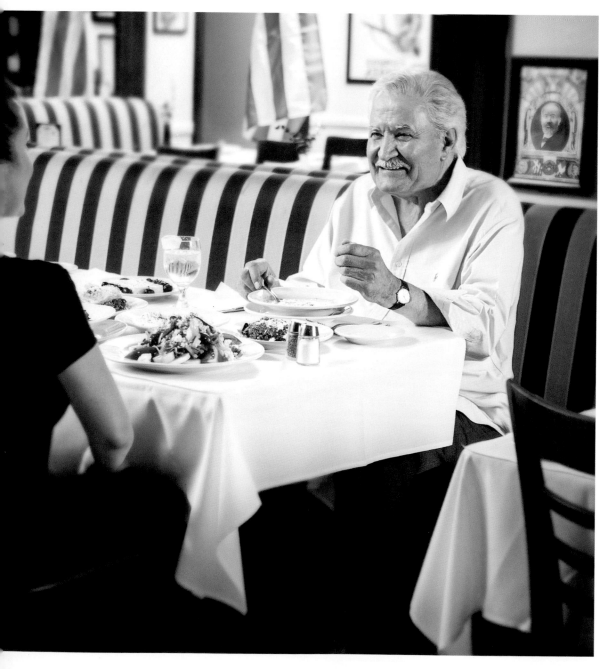

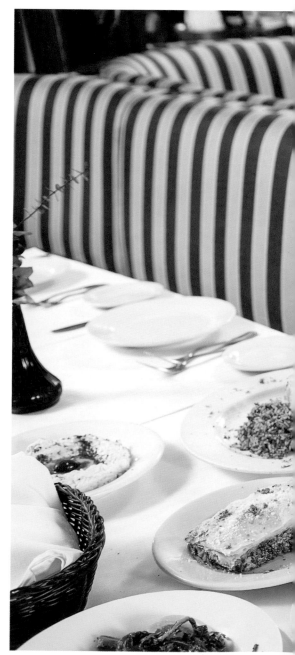

It was a fun time. The top three floors of a nearby building were for the DEA (Drug Enforcement Administration), so there were a lot of agents and police officers there. On any given night I had 15 guns sitting at the bar. I kept waiting for some poor bastard to come in and try to rob the place! It never happened, fortunately.

The nice thing about owning a restaurant in New York City is that I got a couple of parking spots with it so I was able to drive to work every day!
—John Aniston

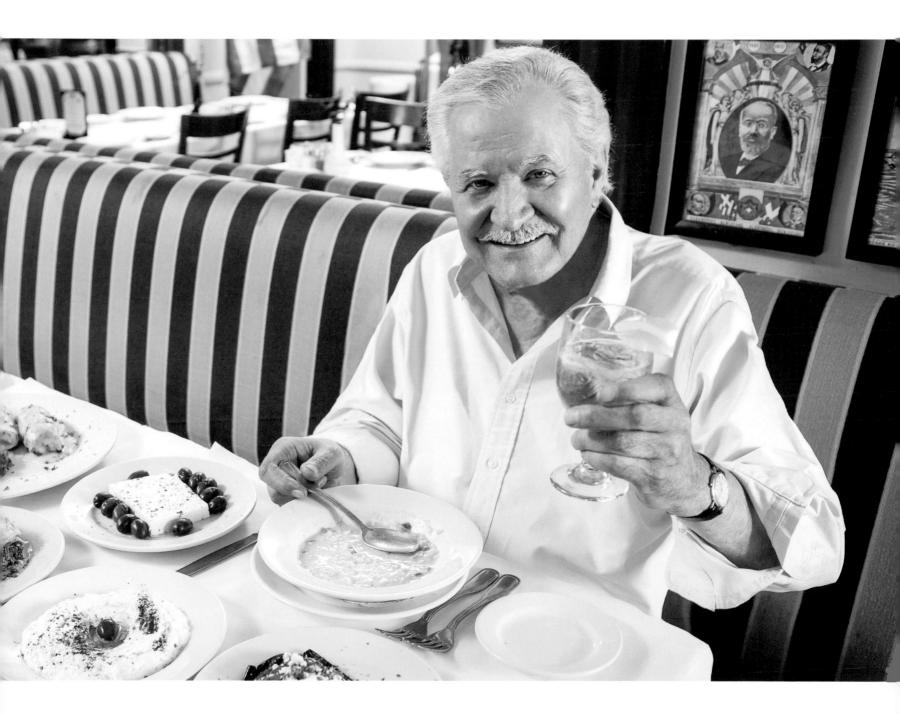

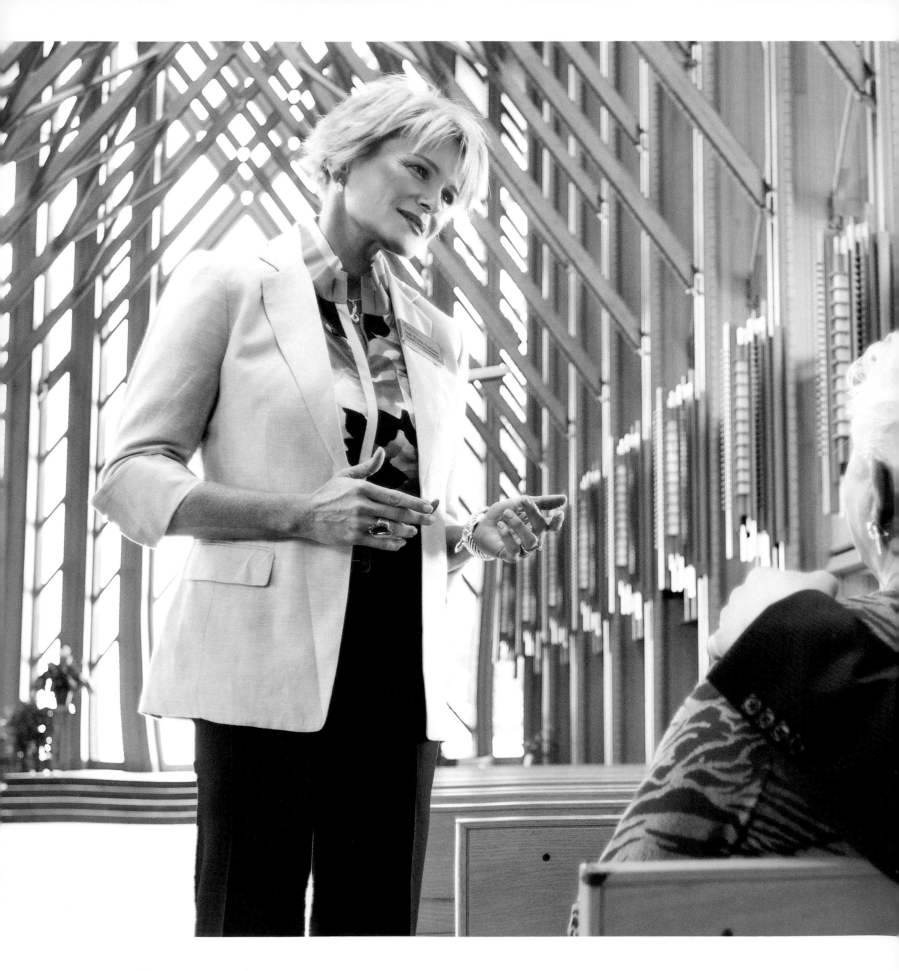

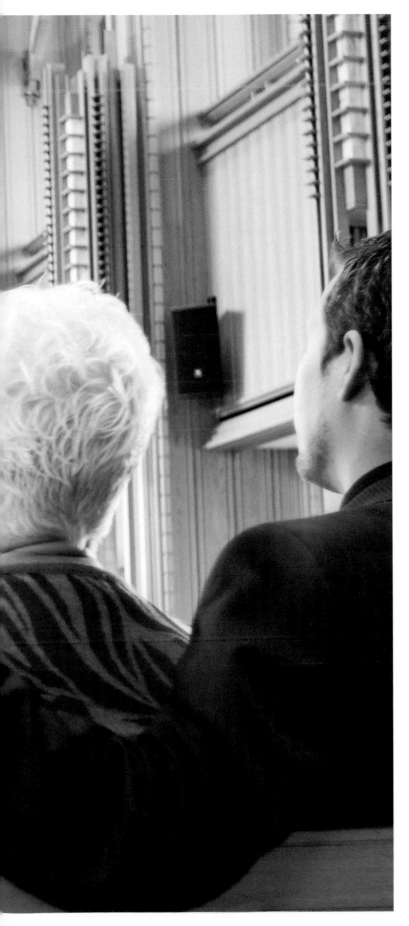

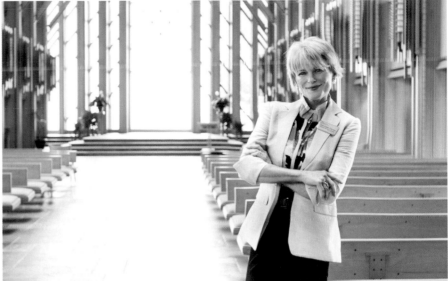

I work as a family service counselor at Rose Hills Memorial Park and Mortuaries. I help grieving families. It brings so much to my life—more than I ever thought possible. I wanted to do something that would help people. I know the show helps a lot of people, but it's hard to directly see the positive effect. A girlfriend of mine had a friend who worked at Rose Hills and she said I should apply. They asked for a resume. I wrote a paragraph. I don't even remember what it said, but one of the vice presidents of the company called me and said he had to interview me because I sounded funny.

I try to help people through this time, give them an ear and be there for them. It's worth more than any dollar amount there is. I love to go to my job there. I love being able to help somebody. It warms my heart knowing that I may have helped make a horrible experience for someone a little less horrible. You really feel for the grieving families. I never detach, but there's a part of me that has to hold back. There was an instance in which I cried for what felt like days when I had some time off because I just had to let the emotions out. I try to help people through a difficult time and be there for them. I can't tell you how emotionally and spiritually rewarding that is for me.

The thought of being a little ray of sunshine in someone's darkest day really appeals to me.
—*Judi Evans*

I like machines. They're fascinating. You take care of them because they take care of you. It's a guy thing.

I've had my Corvette since 1983. I got it for a song and a dance when I finished being on *Seven Brides for Seven Brothers*. It's a rolling sculpture and so easy to work on. When something goes wrong, it's usually only one of three things. I get it right the second time if I don't the first, but I usually zero in on what's wrong right away

Being in a garage with the ball game on the radio and smelling the oil is a guy thing. It works for me. I find it to be very peaceful.
—*Drake Hogestyn*

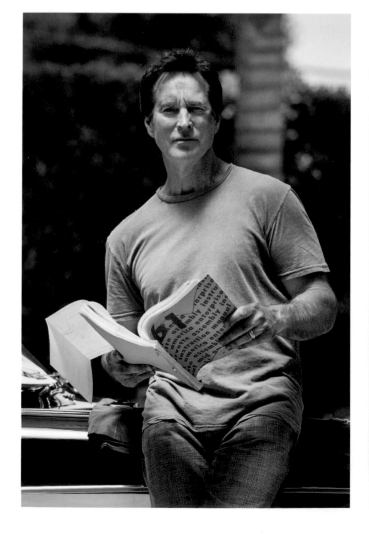

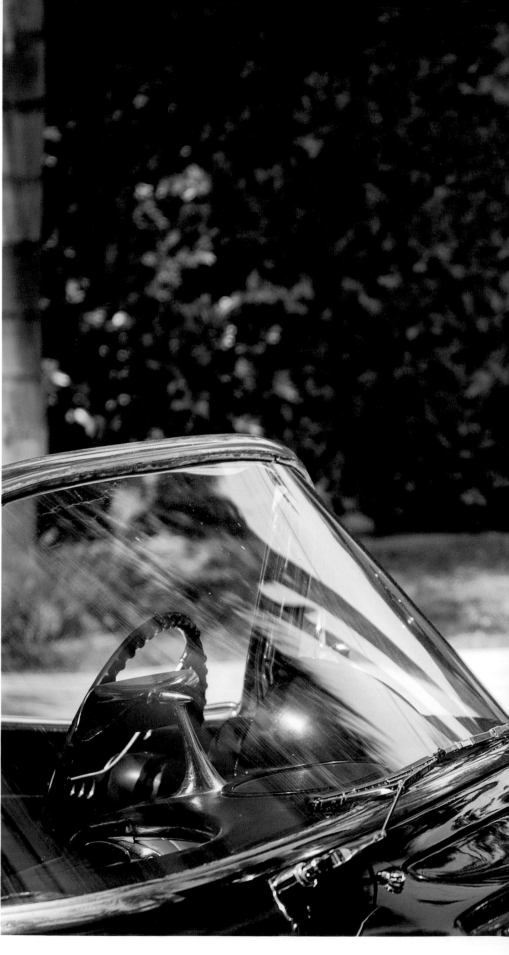

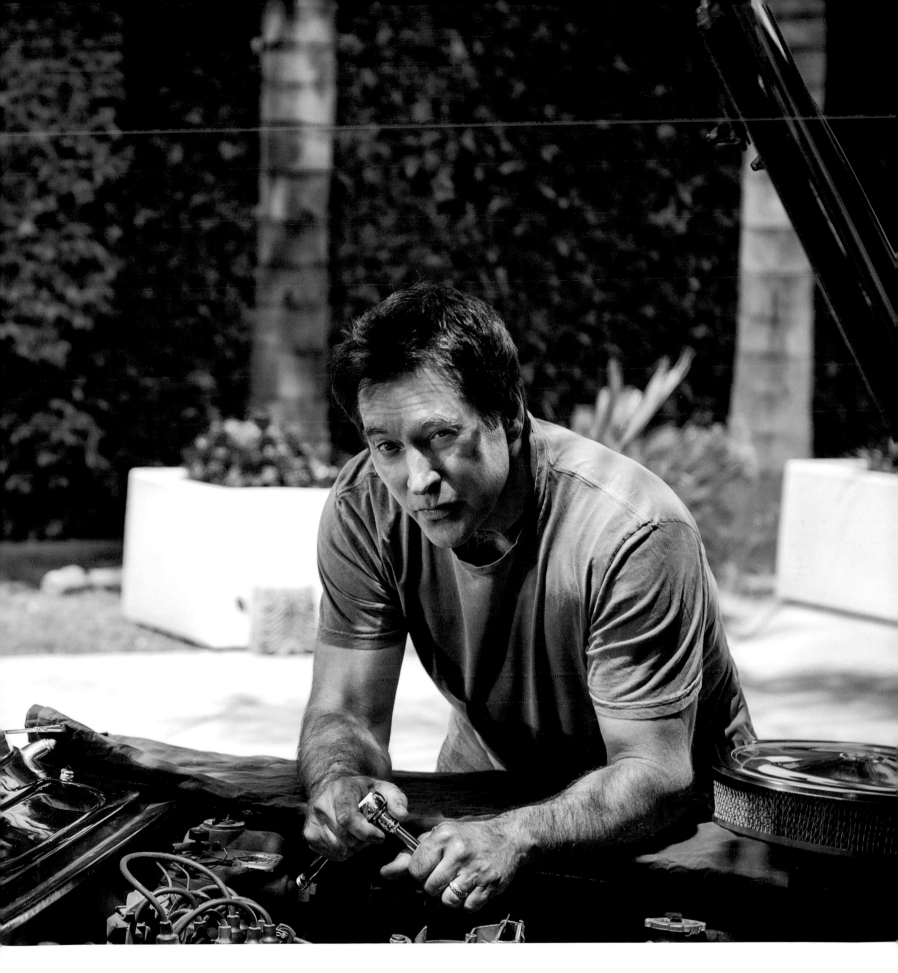

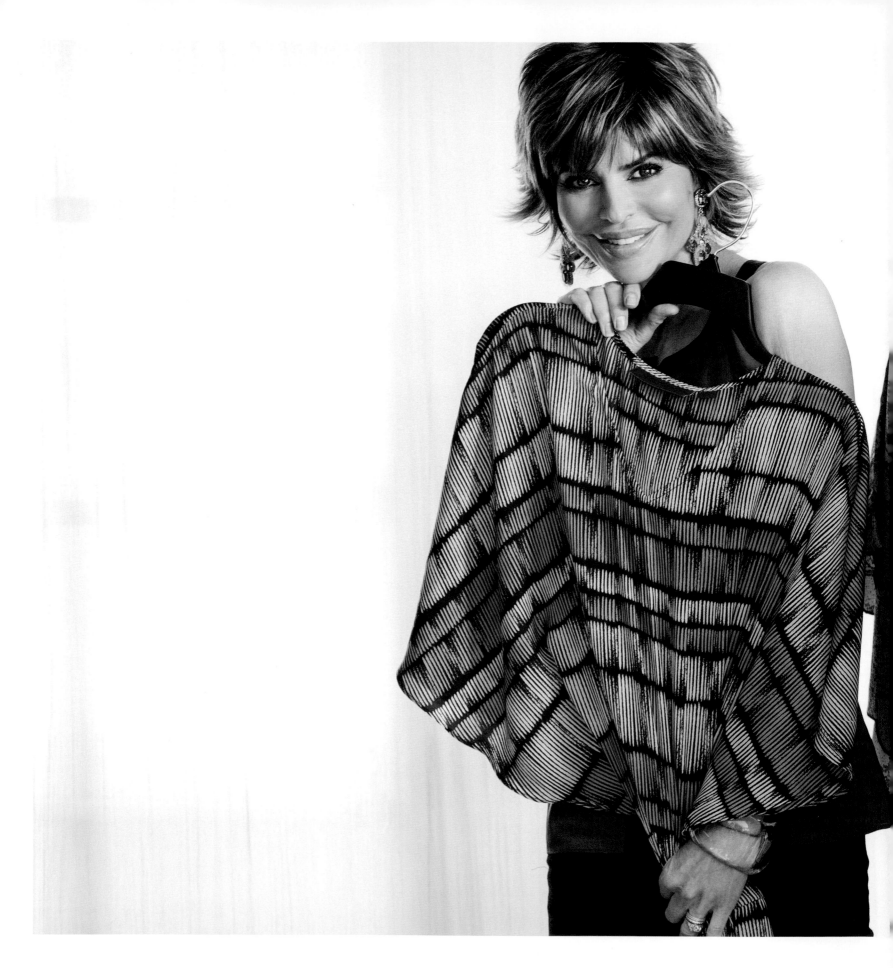

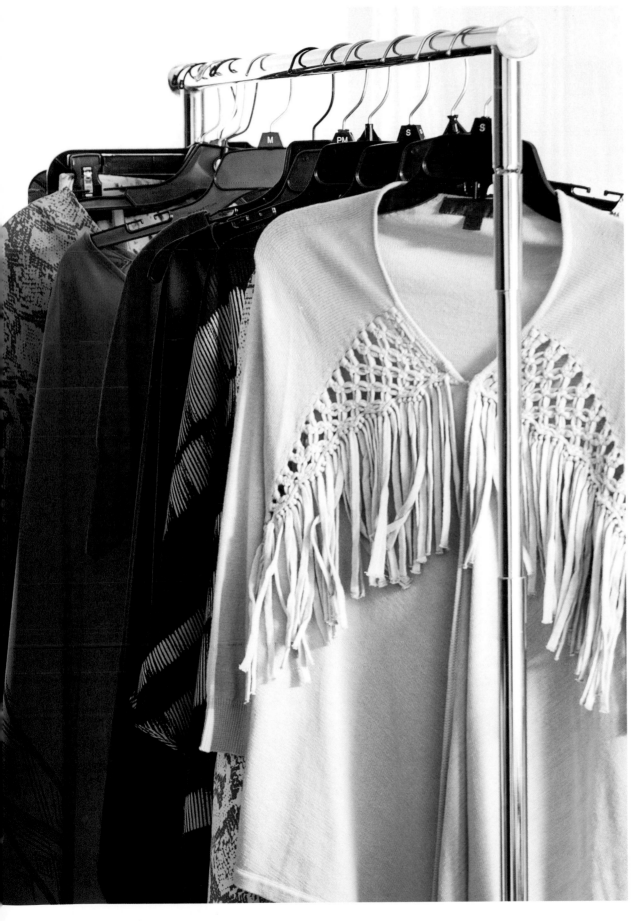

My line is called "Belle Gray by Lisa Rinna." It's named after my daughter's middle names—Delilah Belle and Amelia Gray. I used to have a store by that name, but now we're taking it on a much more global and expansive way. Now it's about the masses and getting it out there to all sizes of women, not just a small percentage of the population. We're hoping to expand the line into lifestyle, too, from handbags, accessories, beauty, hair, skin care and a home section, too. That's my goal.

www.lisarinna.com

I truly like the idea that I am combining what my hobby is with being an entrepreneur.
—Lisa Rinna

I like working on worthwhile causes that don't get enough attention. For me, that's animals. I am deeply and genuinely moved by their plight. I've always cared about animals, but it really started for me in 1988 when I was doing a movie called *Winnie* with Meredith Baxter. We were filming on a college campus in Los Angeles that had a biomedical research building and there were dogs in some pens. I went over to say hi to them when we were on a break. But I noticed that when the dogs barked they coughed as if their throats were hurting them. I asked a man, who was smoking a cigarette, what was wrong with their voices. He said, "Well, we have to cut their vocal cords so you don't hear their screaming." I said, "Screaming?!" He said, "Yes, we use the dogs for medical research."

When I got home I called a friend who loved animals and asked her for the name of the most radical animal group in town. She said it's Last Chance for Animals. I joined the next day.

I said to myself that this kind of animal cruelty has to end. I thought medical research was more humane. The public didn't know. People would say, "Oh, that can't be!" I've testified in Sacramento (about) how the eyes of kittens would be shut (in medical testing.) Why? To see how babies act in the dark! Ridiculous! That was it. It's never stopped for me.

I will appear on behalf of anyone who's trying to do the right thing for animals. I even have my own sanctuary for dying and handicapped animals that are in the pound. I want animals to be treated with respect, compassion and acknowledged for why they are here. They are a part of this earth. They have certain needs. The main thing is to educate the public. I have two rescue dogs right now. They're very sweet.

There's something inspiring about animals. They're pure and beautiful and I can't stand to see them treated badly.
—*Peggy McCay*

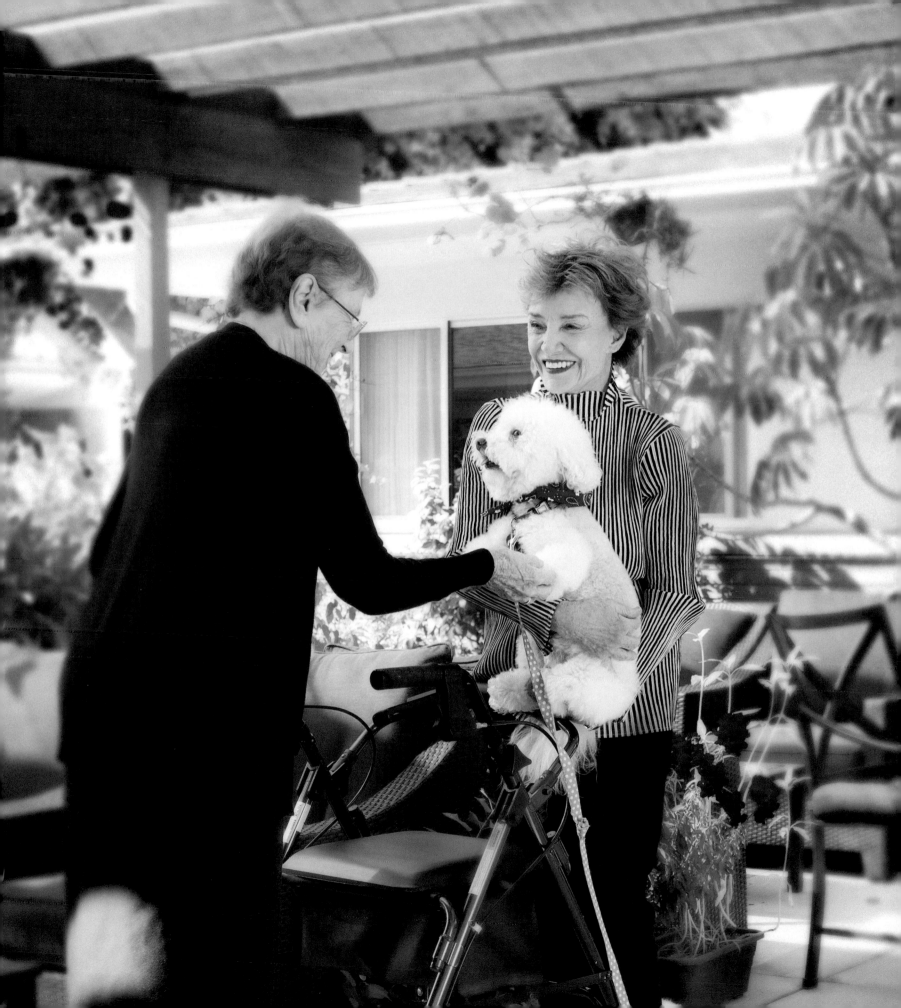

The theater is certainly one of my interests. My wife Lissa and I own and operate the Fremont Centre Theatre in Pasadena. We're now in our 15th year. I direct a few plays there a year. I also act as the spokesperson for hospitalized veterans. That keeps me very busy, traveling around the country and visiting veterans. There are a number of other things I do that keep me busy and moving, but I'm very close to the theater. I've run about five different theaters in my life. I produced and directed the first play in which I ever appeared. I've been doing this for quite some time.

Running the theater is a challenge in every possible way. We have a 99-seat plan and we're constantly challenged. The biggest challenge is keeping the doors open and presenting high-quality theater.

www.fremontcentretheatre.com

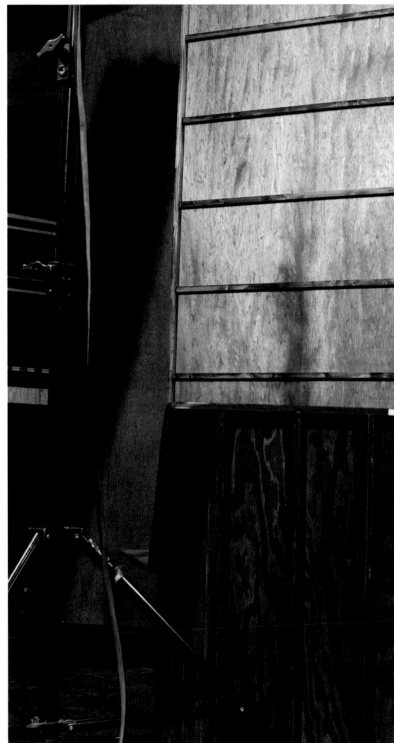

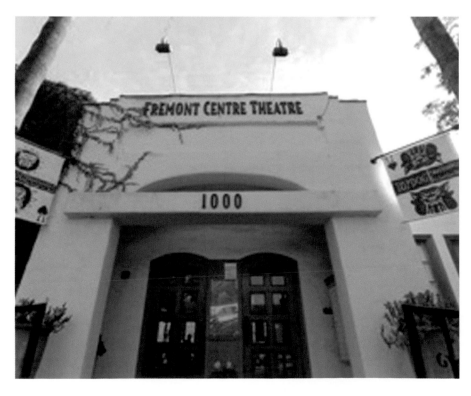

This isn't something we do for profit. We do it because we're committed to the arts and to theater.
—*James Reynolds*

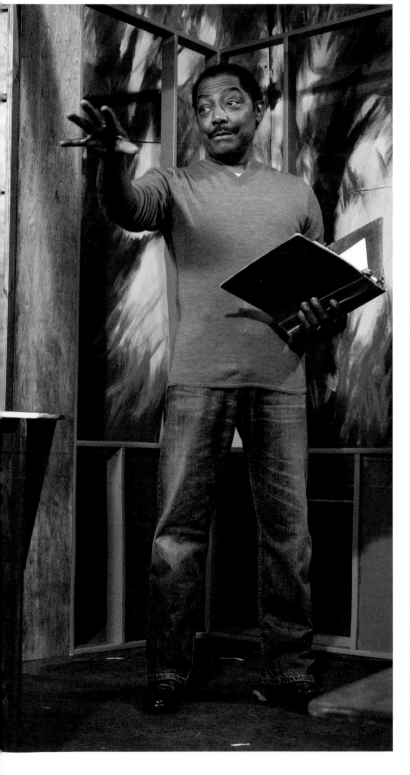

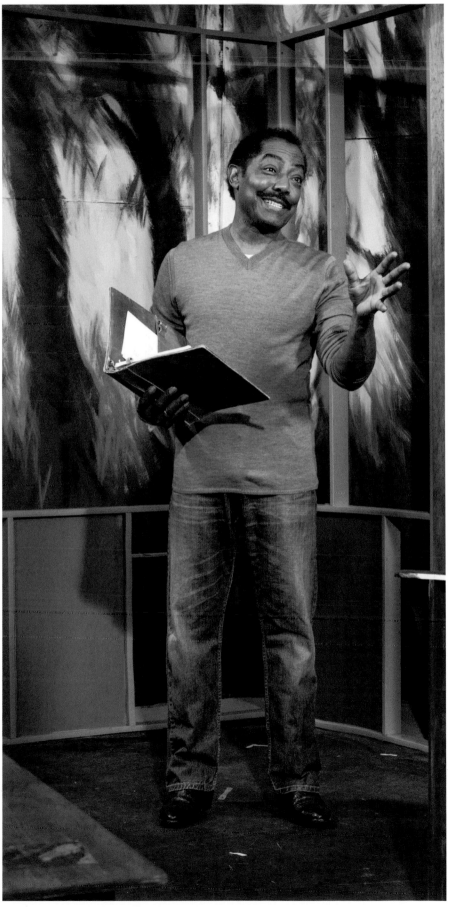

It's working out. That's a big lifestyle; just hanging. I hang out with friends and I do different things. We go paint-balling or we'll go to the park and play Wiffleball or basketball. When people say, "How are you doing?" I say, "Good. I'm working or hanging out." Work can consume you all day—preparation, auditions. It's not hard labor but it's mentally exhausting. I'll go to the beach and play volleyball with my friends to unwind. That is fun for me. I love hanging out when I'm not stressing about work.
—*Freddie Smith*

I just signed up to start volunteering at the Children's Hospital. I love working with little kids. I used to work as a nanny and provide childcare before I was acting full time. I just love kids. I decided to do it after I was watching the National Football League draft and I saw this player who'd become friends with this little girl who has leukemia. They became good friends through a charity. I just want to go outside of my own world and the stress of this industry. This is such a selfish, self-absorbing industry. It's why I like to read the newspaper and be involved with things that aren't about your own vanity.
—*Molly Burnett*

These are things that satisfy me. I like machines. I was weed-whacking here a couple of days ago; then the weed-whacker was done. It was ten years old. I got a lot of use out of it. It was old. I took it into the shop and I broke it apart. I think it was $8.95 for some new fuel lines and the primer ball; the filter and carburetor gasket for 12 bucks. Now it runs better than new. Those little victories are really nice.

If you really want to drop out, I'll take my board and go out there and look for a wave. You don't have to be a surfer—you can get out there and paddle around and it's a great upper-body workout. My board isn't a paddle board per se; it's a 10-foot, 2-inch board; you can stand up on it and paddle. Just to be out there on the ocean and see a dolphin or whale and to see the sea life…it's quiet out there and it's the best. I'm blessed to live where I live. It's the best. It's beautiful, removed, quiet and peaceful; it's all of the above. It's important that you find that in your life. I don't care where I've lived…I know I've needed to live in a place where I can look around, stop and appreciate at any moment anything. I got a big kick out of the partial eclipse. I told my girls about it.

You need to live in an environment and be able to look around and appreciate it. You can call it "stop to smell the roses," but I find a lot of joy and solace being right out in the middle of it all and looking around.

—Drake Hogestyn

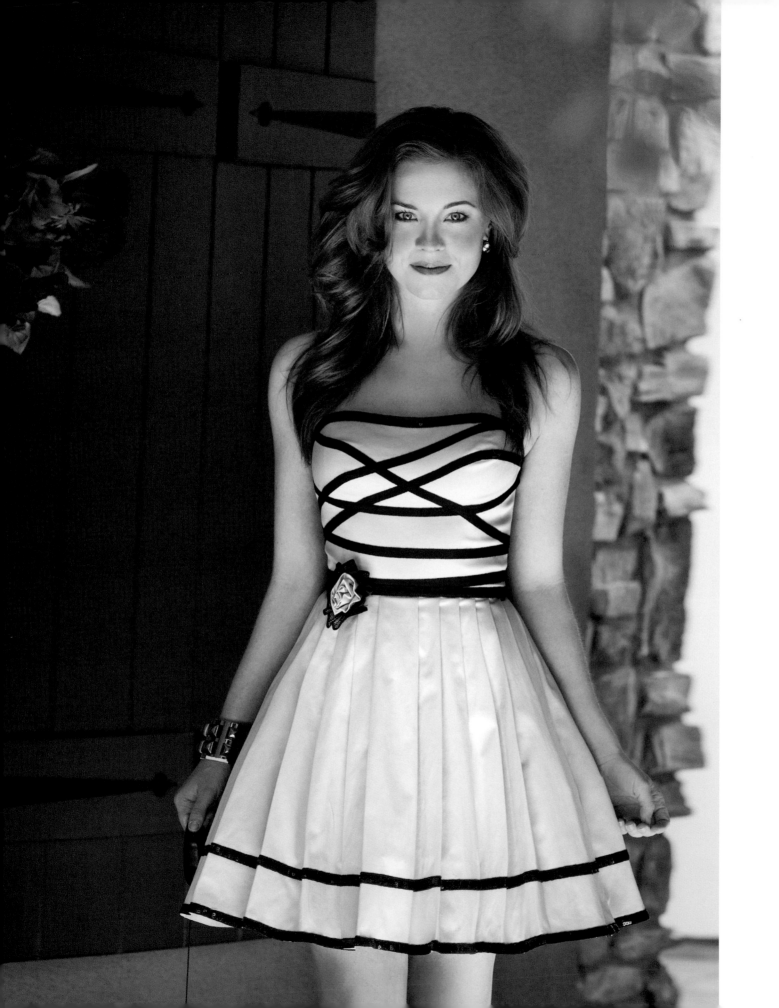

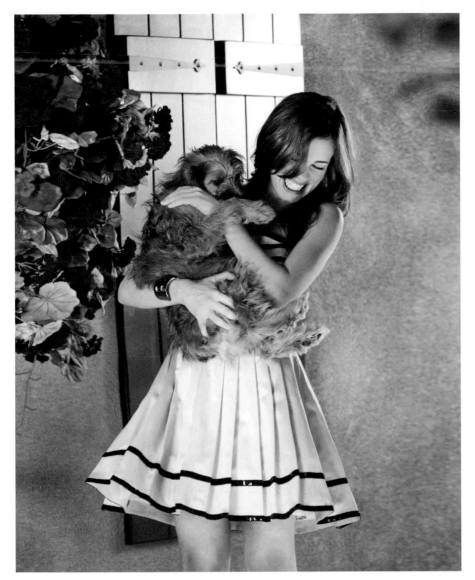

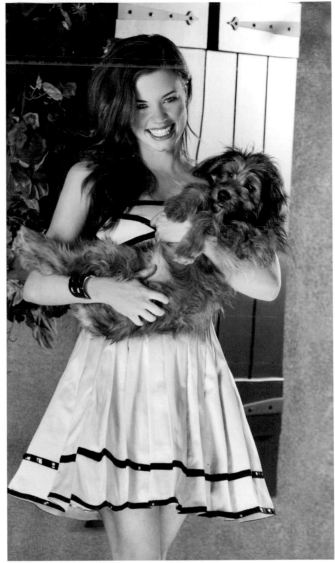

I have a new puppy. I play with her all the time. Her name is Eloise. I have no idea what she is, but she looks like a little brown bear. I got her when she was eight weeks old and she's been with me ever since! We go on hikes together. And she's fast! She beats up on (Casey's dog) Nanuk all the time, but they're best friends!

It makes me feel good when I take care of someone. I used to volunteer at nursing homes. I try to volunteer once a week. I love going to charity events or going to a hospital where you meet a fan. I love giving back. It sounds cheesy, but it's not.

The people who are the most important and are in the most need of receiving joy and attention are the ones who don't always get it—the elderly and little kids.
—*Molly Burnett*

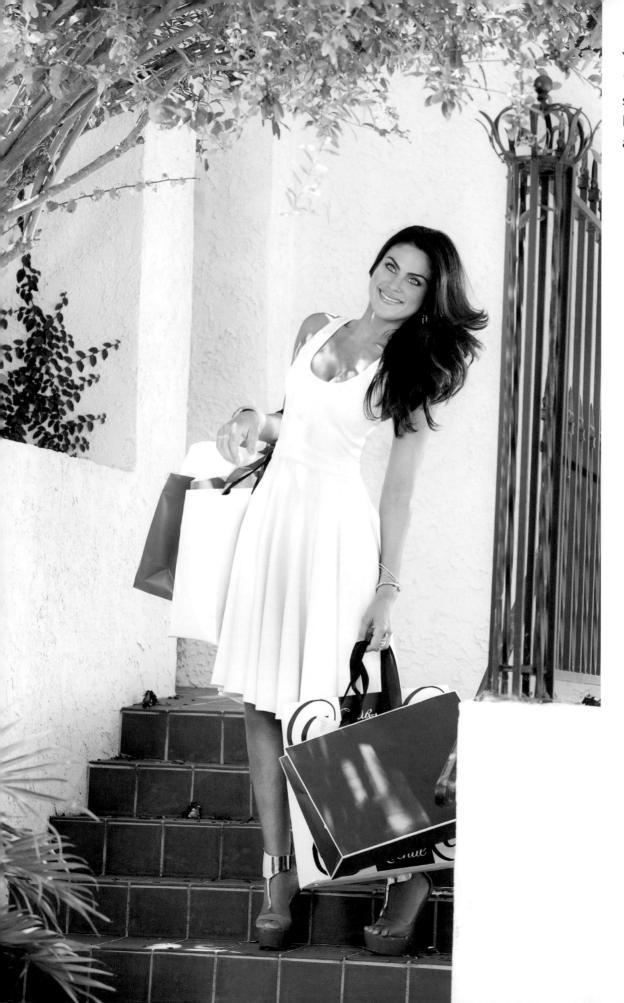

You could say I'm a fan of "retail therapy!" I do love to go shopping, but by no means do I think that shopping can solve all the world's problems!

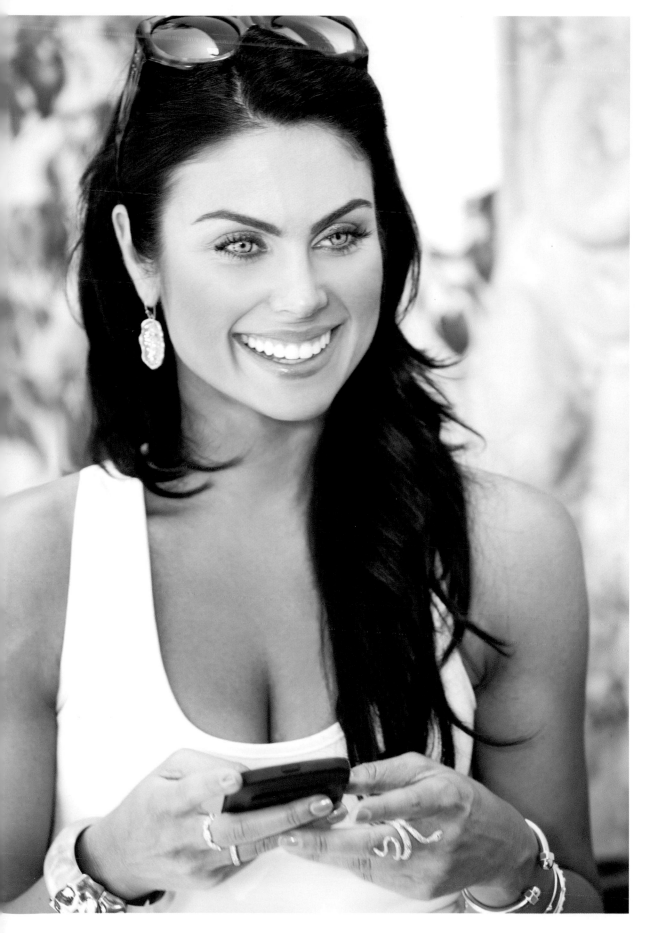

Twitter is amazing because it's a great way to stay connected and communicate directly with fans around the world. It's also a great tool to promote charities and causes by "rallying the troops."

I love staying in touch with my friends when I'm out shopping in case I see something that one of them might like. I'll shoot them a quick text to see if they'd like me to pick it up for them or if I want their advice on something I'm on the fence about buying.

—Nadia Bjorlin

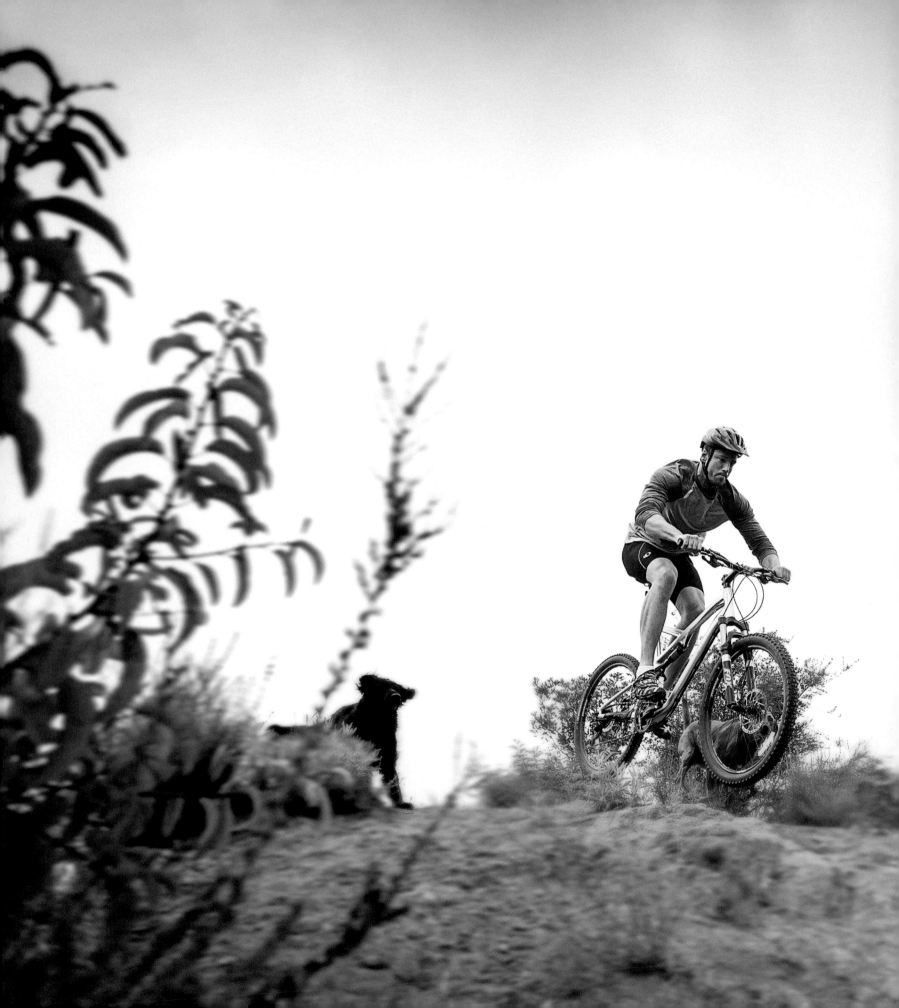

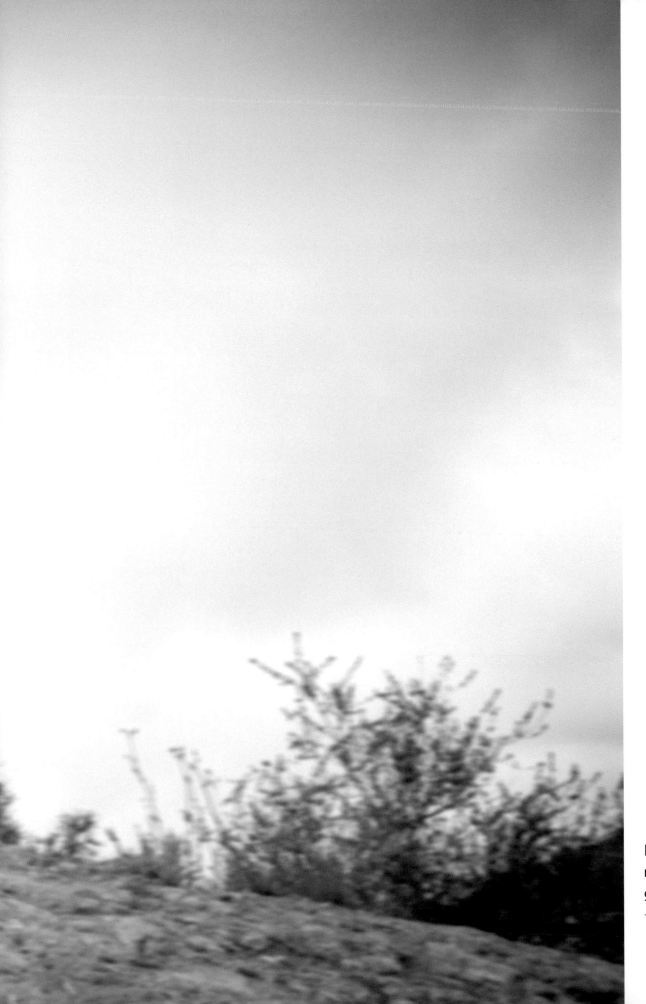

I go mountain biking with
my dogs so they can
get exercise while I do.
—*James Scott*

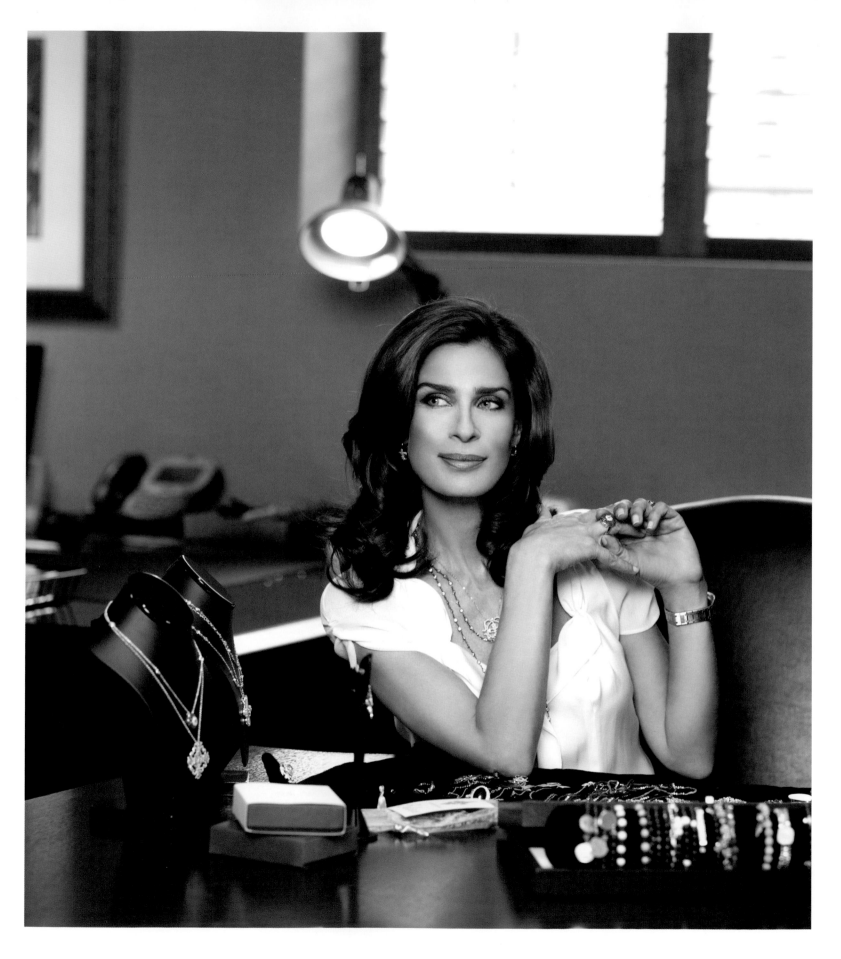

Over the years, people have written the show wanting to find out where they could get some jewelry that I'd worn as Hope, but they couldn't because they were either pieces I'd made or that I'd picked up during my travels. So I started my own jewelry line, Hope Faith Miracles. Originally, I'd make pieces for myself and one for my mother. We had very similar tastes. She'd buy something for herself and a second one for me, thinking, "Oh, Kristian's going to love this!" I would do the same for her. My mother introduced me to the fleur-de-lis (symbol, the basis for my jewelry line.) "Fleur-de-lis" is French for "flower of the lily." It's such a beautiful symbol and it has so many variations.

I get such joy from seeing people enjoy my jewelry.
—*Kristian Alfonso*

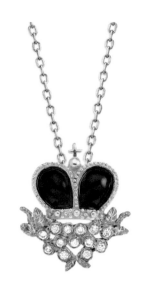

Blue Enamel Necklace

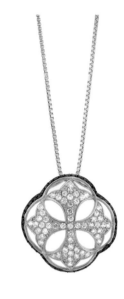

Maltese Cross Pendant

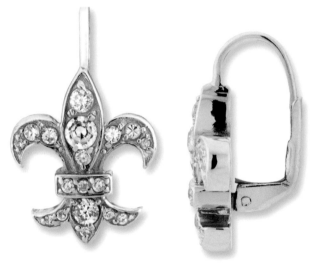

Fleur Drop Earrings

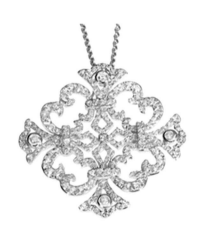

Miracles Pendant

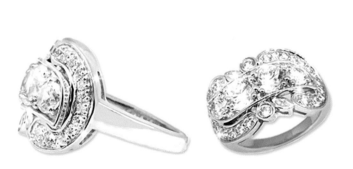

Lasting Love Ring (shown with side view)

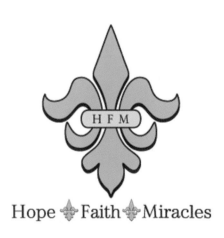

www.hopefaithmiracles.com

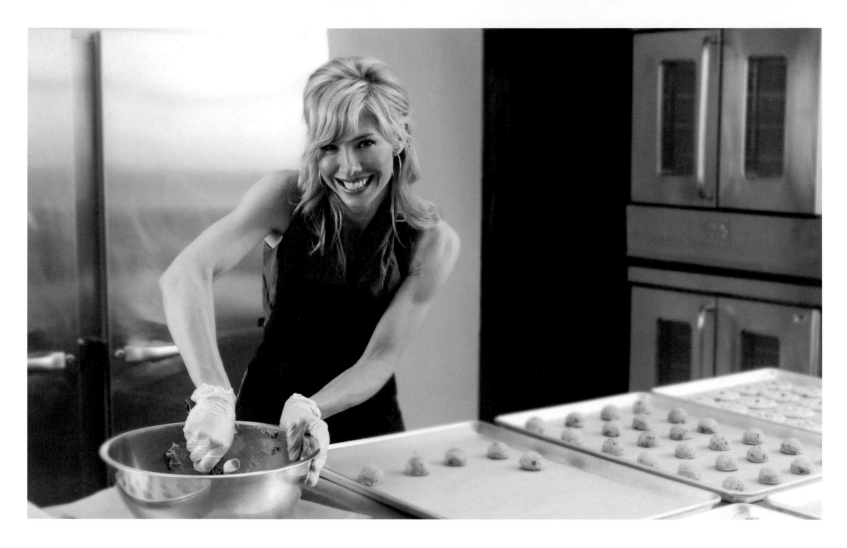

Celiac disease is a condition that damages the lining of the small intestine and prevents it from absorbing parts of food that are important for staying healthy. The damage is due to a reaction to eating gluten, which is found in wheat, barley, rye and possibly oats.—*U.S. National Library of Medicine*

I'm very passionate about educating people about celiac disease, which I have. You can have a gene test, which is 100 percent accurate as to whether or not you have one of the genes than can cause celiac. If you are feeling sick and ingesting gluten doesn't make you feel well (and you have the gene), it's probably a good idea to cut it out. I'm not a doctor, but that's my advice.

I say go to a doctor and seek out medical advice on how to get tested for celiac disease properly. Before I was diagnosed I thought I was going to die. I was being tested for everything. I'd never been so sick and this went on for years and years.

An actress with whom I worked on *As the World Turns* in New York looked at me one day and she said, "Oh, celiac disease." It was a miracle that I took a role on that show for seven months back in 2005 and met her.

Things are changing for the better in terms of awareness. It's been a great thing to have Miley Cyrus come out and say that she's gluten-free.

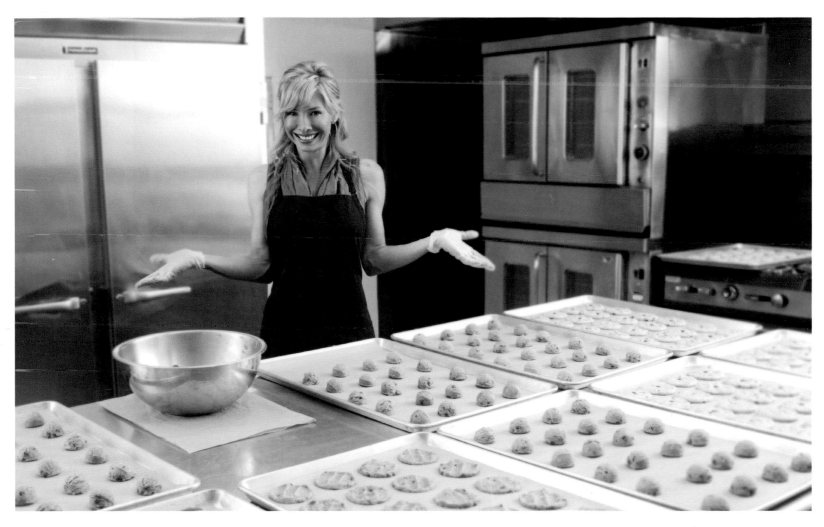

I shared what I learned about celiac disease when I went back onto *General Hospital*. I learned about (actress) Bergen Williams' story about surviving cancer and how she changed her diet. I asked her if she'd heard about gluten (which is related to celiac disease). She told me about her catering company, which makes gluten-free food. She developed this gluten-free, vegan, oil-free cookie and named it "The Sarah Brown." She called me one time and said, "Sarah, I'm here with Steven Hawking and he's a huge fan of 'The Sarah Brown' cookie that I made in your honor!"

You really are your own best health advocate. Nobody knows your body like you do. I've not knowingly ingested gluten since I was diagnosed. I'd rather jump off a building than cheat and have something that contained gluten.

www.eatmecookies.com.

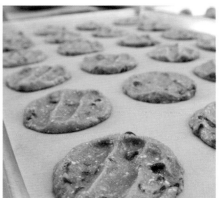

I love educating people about gluten!
—*Sarah Brown*

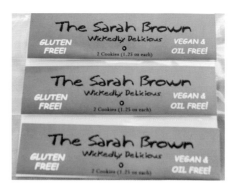

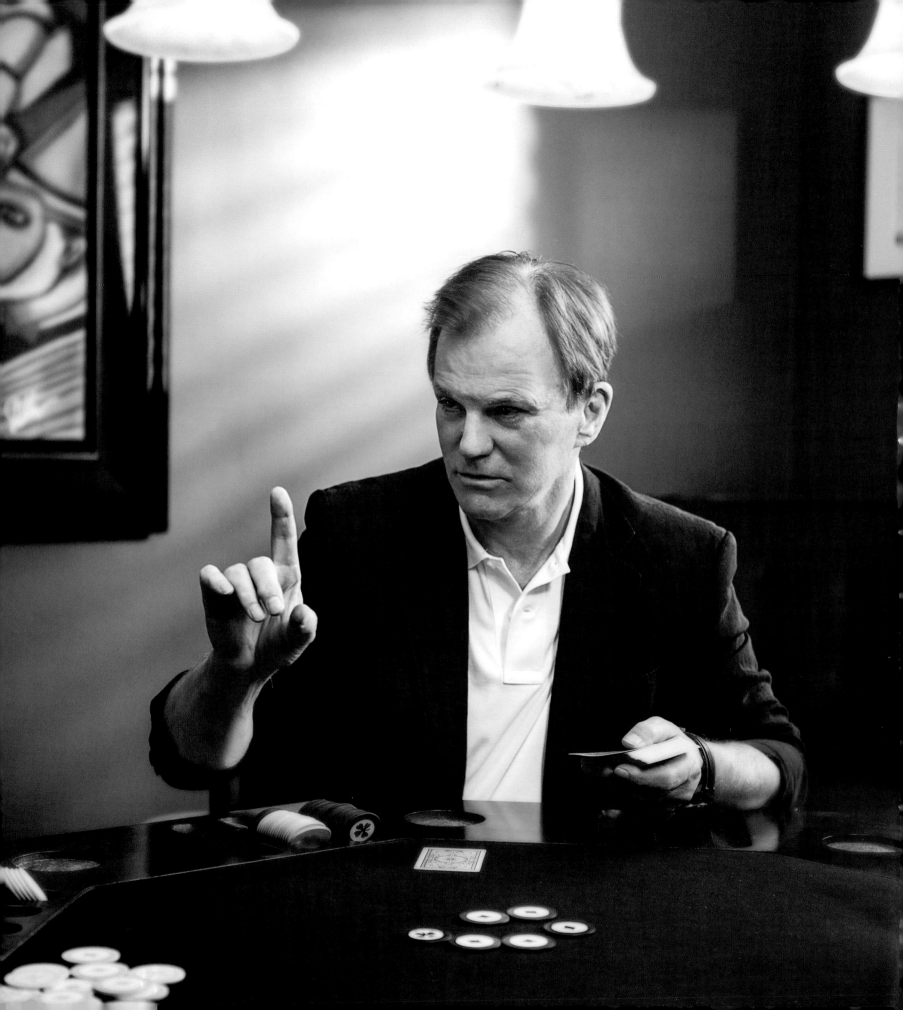

I've been playing poker with buddies for quite a while. The group's changed over the years because people will find work on game nights or they move away. When we started out we called ourselves "The Magnificent Seven" and we'd play every other weekend.

We've always gotten together at my house. I'm a good player, fortunately. It comes down to smarts, luck and having the right cards. It's like chess. You need to be aware of the cards and try to read your fellow players. A few guys over the years have talked more than they've paid attention. You could always count on them for the rent!

Playing poker with the guys isn't just about cards. When we get together we blow off steam and have a "boys' night." It's a good way to catch up, raise some hell and blow off some steam. We play for enough money that nobody's going to go broke, but enough so that you have to keep your mind on the game.

There's a tradition at the end of the night: everyone says how much they've won and how much they've lost. That keeps things in perspective.
—*Josh Taylor*

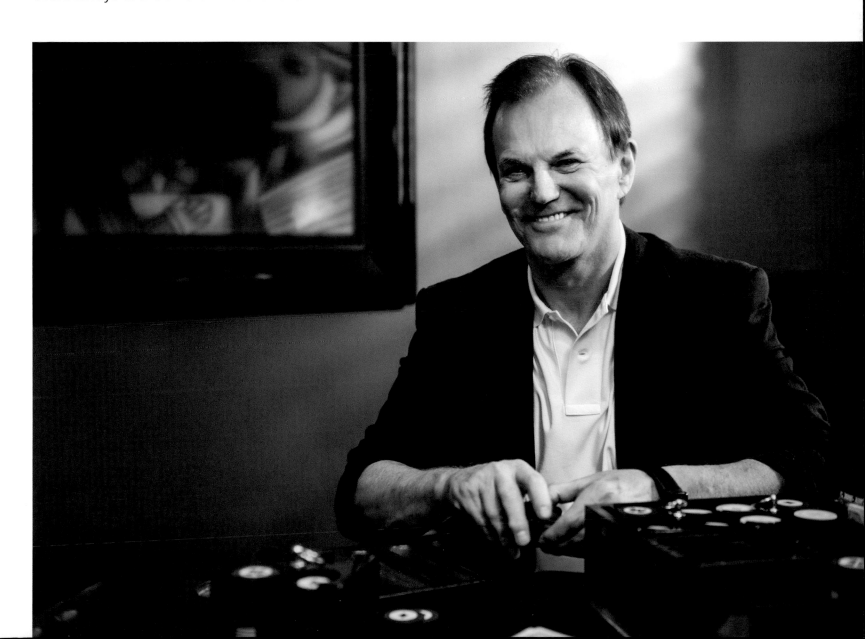

Bill and I recently completed our first novel, *Trumpet*. We found that the joy of writing is having some control and being able to give your characters the snappy lines that you've always wanted to have! Bill's said that writing is a wonderfully collaborative process and he's right. It has helped tie our marriage together more tightly. It really has. Together, we agreed on every word that went into the novel or else it didn't go in. We'd write separately from each other and then get together at the computer and read it out loud. We'd write together, too.

I've learned that waiting for inspiration and saying you're not inspired today is no way to get anything done. You must make your own deadlines and say "I'm going forward regardless." You have to do that.

(Writing has) given us a private world—it isn't about acting or our family life or our past life together. This gave us a world that we had created, in which only we knew what things happened to people we loved, our characters. Writing *Trumpet* together was a wonderful new experience.
—*Susan Seaforth Hayes*

Writing our memoir was a joining experience, but (the novel) was even more so—we had to end up with *one* voice. How did we know it was finished? One day you have to just say, "That's it! No more changes."
—*Bill Hayes*

I stay in college classes. I've been taking stand-up comedy classes, too. I've never liked a 'dirty' act. I've taken comedy classes [taught by] Jonathan Solomon. We had to figure out what our persona was going to be so that when we hit the stage we'd be ready. I'd been doing comedy about my kids. We got to the "persona" part of the class and I didn't know if anyone in the class knew I worked in television. One girl raised her hand and asked, "Why isn't she talking about being a soap star?" I wasn't going to make that part of what I did. The teacher said, "Yeah, that's a problem. We're going to have to change that because when you get up on stage, people will say, 'Oh, she's on Days of our Lives.'" You have to open up with who you are or else there's a disconnect between you and the audience. I love comedy. I've always wanted to do it. I ended up being on a soap opera for 35 years. So it's a great outlet for me. I love learning about the ins and outs and the dynamics of what makes things funny.
—*Deidre Hall*

Showing kindness to others has always been a big thing for me. When I was at Radio City Music Hall, I'd perform as one of the Rockettes in as many as five shows a day. I'd keep smiling throughout every performance and one day somebody asked me, "How can you keep doing that?" I said, "Because it's a different audience each time and they all deserve the best we have to give!"

I try to look at the good in everything. One of the things that makes me feel good is leaving a 20 percent tip for anyone who waits on me—always. They work very hard for their money. Many times I tip more than that if I like the person. That's important to me. It gives me a sense of "Wow, that's what we're here for." I really believe that's what we're here for—to help other people.

Not everyone learns that in life. I was given a test when I got sick with myasthenia gravis and I had to change. I had to reexamine myself and figure out what I had to do. One of the things it taught me was that it's not about you. It's about everyone else. It was truly a waking up experience for me. I think my positive outlook has played a role in my recovery.
—*Suzanne Rogers*

Whimsical, obscure events and occurrences make me laugh. Sometimes I laugh harder than I should. I'm tickled by things that are obscure and unusual. I love spontaneous things that you don't see coming that will completely jar you. It's a healthy thing to do. It's like our connection to outdoors. I would say my soul requires laughter.
—*Shawn Christian*

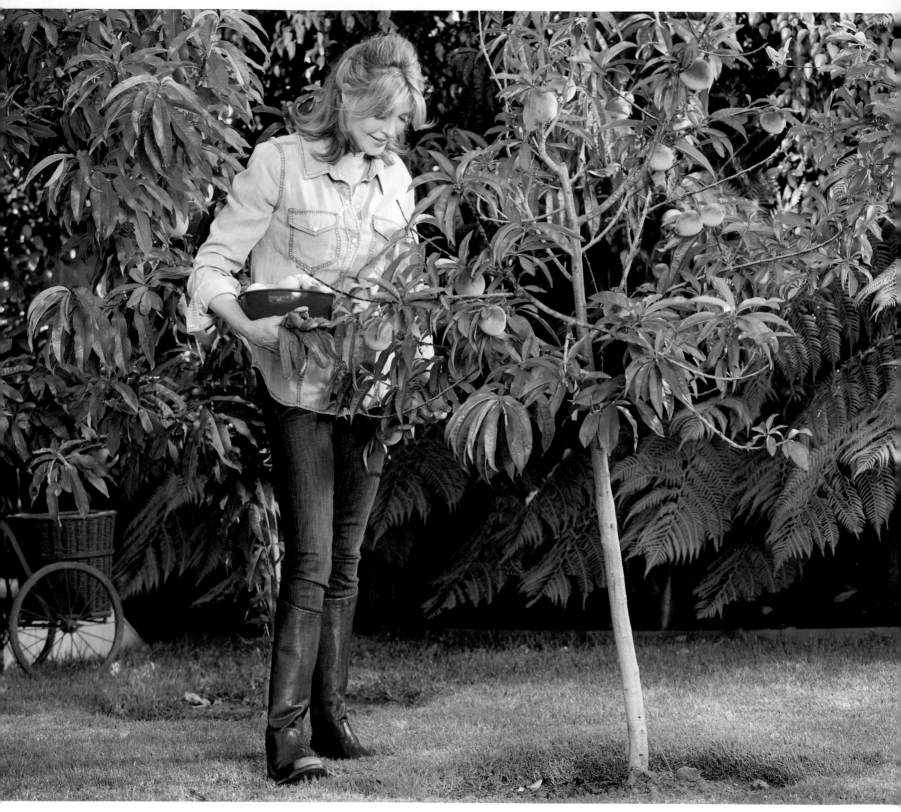

Every corner of my yard and
garden is dedicated to the foods
that enrich our bodies and lives.

—*Deidre Hall*

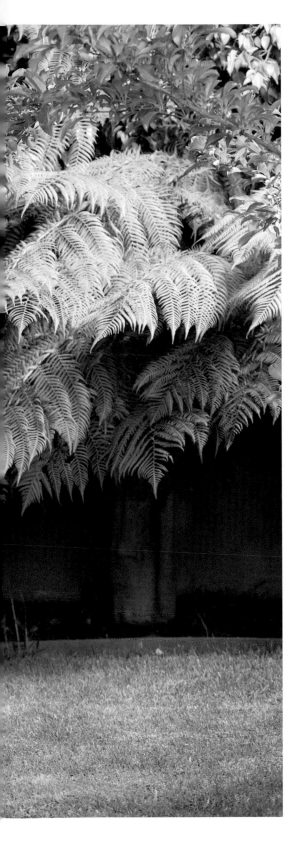

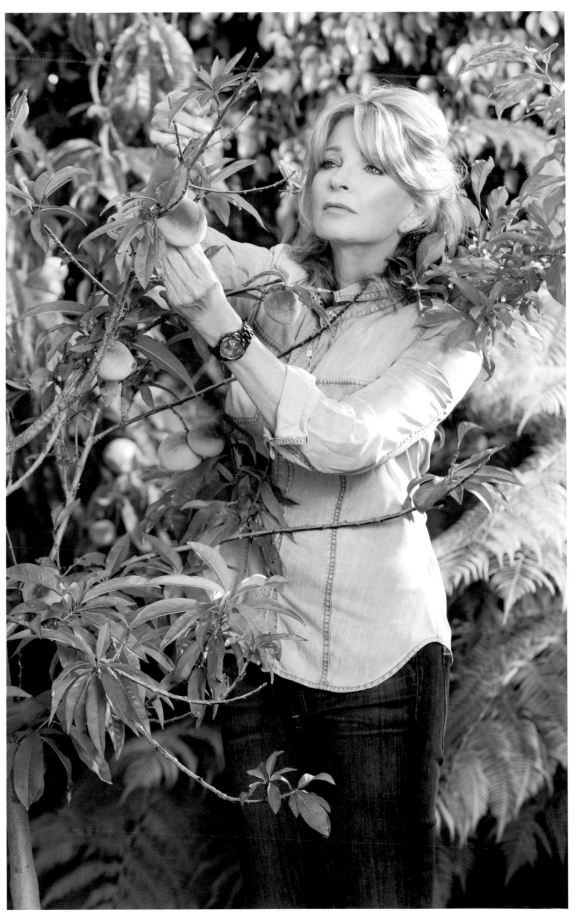

I shoot travel and landscape photography. I have a love of the outdoors. It's a relationship that goes together very well. I have shot quite a bit of landscape photography in North America and a fair amount in Southeast Asia and in Africa. I have portraits from all over the world.

What I enjoy about photography is that there are no limitations. In order to set up one photograph it's not unusual for me to go to a place to anticipate weather, light and time of day. I'll go to a place beforehand and look at the different atmospheric and structural conditions, shadows and balance of lighting. I spent a lot of time setting up different shots.

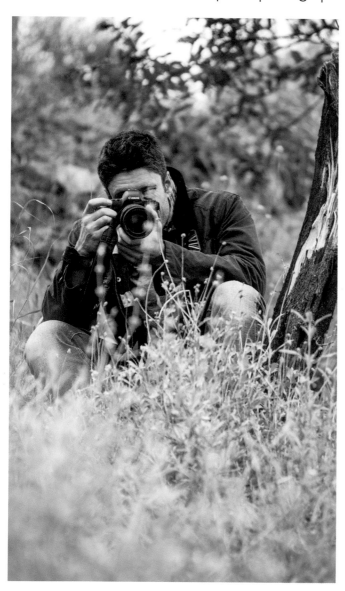

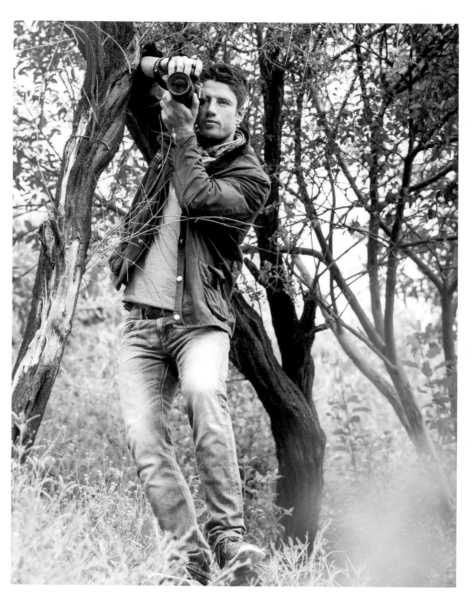

I feel that it's extremely important to have a number of different creative outlets.
—*James Scott*

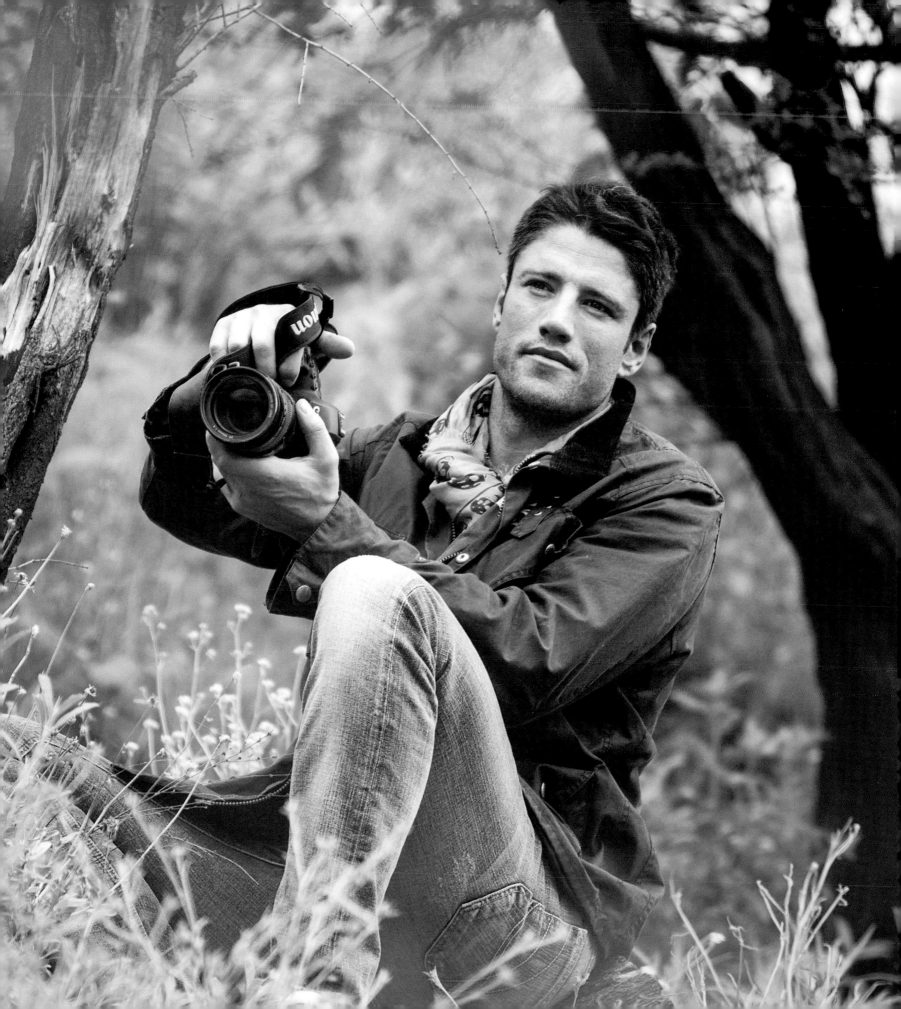

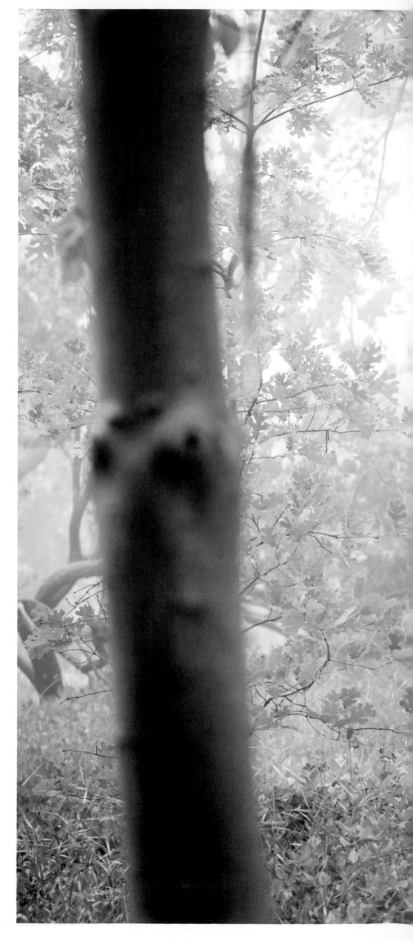

I look forward to the days
I spend at my lake house.
When I am here, I do the
things I love to do, such as
gardening. It's tough on the
back...but good for the soul.
—*Joseph Mascolo*

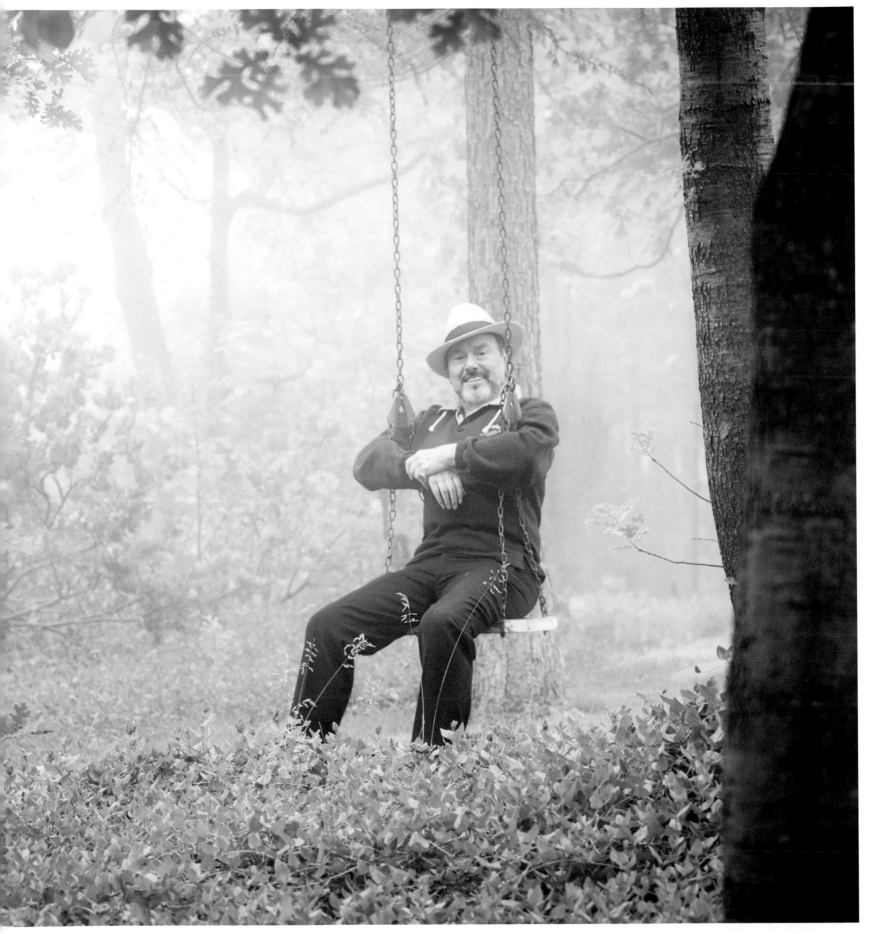

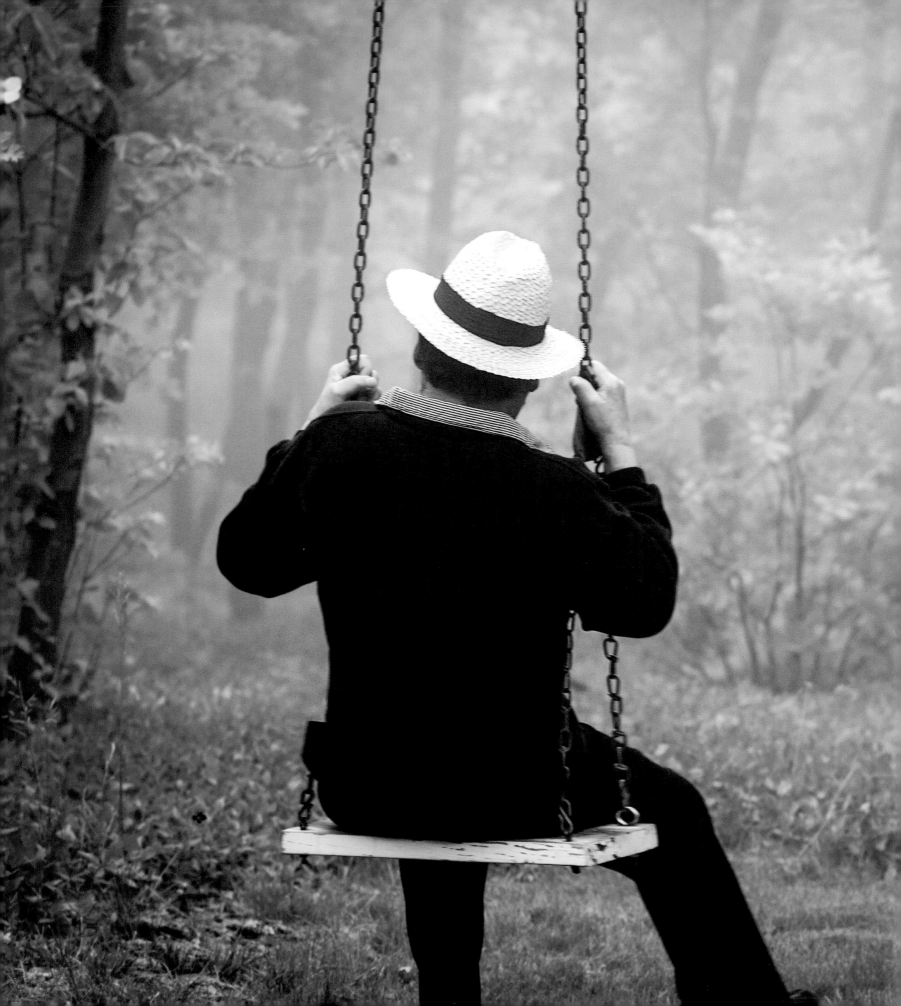

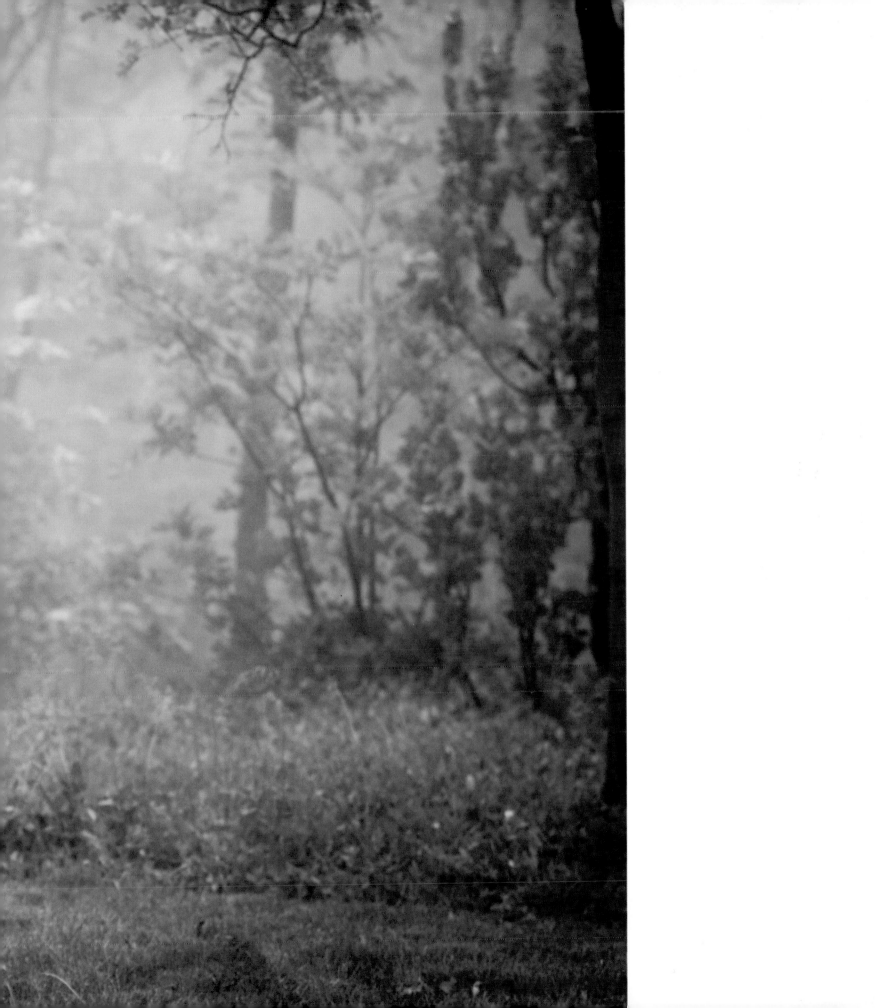

Photography by:

Tracey Morris Photography

www.traceymorris.com

Additional photography by:

John Russo Photography, Inc.

www.johnrussophoto.com

pages 58, 59, 106, 107, 109, 112, 113, 136, 137, 178, 179,

184, 186, 187, 198, 199, 219, 248, 249, 292, 296

The cast members of *Days of our Lives* have managed

to incorporate the following into their daily routines:

1. Eating regular diets of salmon (and other fish), greens and fruit
2. Drinking recommended daily amounts of water
3. Understanding the value of getting a good night's sleep
4. Stimulating their minds with outside hobbies, interests and passions
5. Finding fulfillment in giving back to others
6. Stretching routinely to stay flexible
7. Exercising regularly

which are all part of the key to Better Living!

SPECIAL THANKS TO: the cast of *Days of our Lives*, Elizabeth Gulick, Michael Maloney, Juliette Harris, Maya Frangie, Alexis Ellen, Joe Exclusive, Gianni CJ Valentino, Nick Schillace, Garry Allyn, Matthew Holman, Lee Harris, Bebe Booth, Deidre Decker, Alexis Phifer, Robert Morris, Irwin Miller, Amanda Tirador, Tom McIlwee, Staff at Corday Productions; Freddie Roach's Wild Card Boxing Club, Valencia Country Club, First Christian Church of North Hollywood, The Bistro Garden, Rose Hills Memorial Park, Chef's Kitchens, Paige Premium Denim, Eat Me Cookies; Meridian's Bodies in Motion, Northridge; The Great Greek Restaurant, Sherman Oaks; The Tipsy Pig, TheFremont Centre Theatre, Nazareth House Los Angeles, Habitat for Humanity, San Fernando; TPC Valencia Country Club, Neil Lane Jewelry, Lowe Show Horse Centre, Underwood Family Farms; It Girl Publicity; Sony Pictures Consumer Products.

INDEX